CELL BIOLOGY RESEARCH PROGRESS

TUMOR SUPPRESSORS

CELL BIOLOGY RESEARCH PROGRESS

Additional books in this series can be found on Nova's website under the Series tab.

Additional E-books in this series can be found on Nova's website under the E-books tab.

CANCER ETIOLOGY, DIAGNOSIS AND TREATMENTS

Additional books in this series can be found on Nova's website under the Series tab.

Additional E-books in this series can be found on Nova's website under the E-books tab.

CELL BIOLOGY RESEARCH PROGRESS

TUMOR SUPPRESSORS

SUSAN D. NGUYEN
EDITOR

Nova Science Publishers, Inc.
New York

For permission to use material from this book please contact us:
Telephone 631-231-7269; Fax 631-231-8175
Web Site: http://www.novapublishers.com

Library of Congress Cataloging-in-Publication Data

Tumor suppressors / editor, Susan D. Nguyen.
p. ; cm.
Includes bibliographical references and index.
ISBN 978-1-61761-986-1 (hardcover)
1. Antioncogenes. 2. Tumor suppressor proteins. I. Nguyen, Susan D.
[DNLM: 1. Genes, Tumor Suppressor. 2. Neoplasms--genetics. 3.
Neoplasms--prevention & control. 4. Tumor Suppressor Proteins. QZ 202]
RC268.43.T867 2011
612'.01575--dc22
2010036163

Published by Nova Science Publishers, Inc. † New York

Contents

Preface **vii**

Chapter 1 Aflatoxin B_1 and Acetaldehyde Mutational Patterns in the Tumour Suppressor Gene *TP53*: Experimental Fingerprints Using a Functional Assay and Relevance to Human Cancer Aetiology **1**
Vincent Paget, Mathilde Lechevrel and François Sichel

Chapter 2 Curative Therapy for Terminal Cancer? **25**
Doug Dix

Chapter 3 Breast Cancer Screening by Methylation Analysis of Tumor Suppressor Genes in Breast Fluid **43**
JS de Groot, KPM Suijkerbuijk, PJ van Diest and E van der Wall

Chapter 4 Rab GTPases as Potential Tumor Suppressors **71**
Christelle En Lin Chua, Yishan Lim, Ee Ling Ng and Bor Luen Tang

Chapter 5 Regulation of Neutrophil Function by Tumor Suppressor PTEN **89**
Subhanjan Mondal and Hongbo R. Luo

Chapter 6 Wnt Pathway-Independent Activities of the APC Tumor Suppressor **105**
Jenifer R. Prosperi and Kathleen H. Goss

Chapter 7 Emerging Roles of BRIT1/MCPH1 in Genome Maintenance and Tumor Suppression **133**
Guang Peng and Shiaw-Yih Lin

Chapter 8 The Role of Histone Deacetylase (HDAC) and EZH2 in Oncogenesis: Epigenetic Silencing of Tumor Suppressors **149**
Junpei Yamaguchi, Motoko Sasaki and Yasuni Nakanuma

Chapter 9 Functions of Kank1 and Carcinogenesis **161**
Naoto Kakinuma, Yun Zhu, Takunori Ogaeri, Jun-ichiro Suzuki and Ryoiti Kiyama

Chapter 10 The Relationship Between MicroRNA and Tumor Suppressors **175**
Douglus Wu and Mary Waye

Chapter 11 Biomarkers for Radiosensitivity and Radiosensitization Targets in Prostate Cancer **189**
WeiWei Xiao, Peter Graham, Carl Power and Yong Li

Chapter 12 Molecular Functions of the p53 Tumor Suppressor in the Apoptotic Response to DNA Damage **229**
Kiyotsugu Yoshida

Chapter 13 How does Tumor Suppressor FHIT Modulate Oxidative Stress and DNA Damage Checkpoints in Early Cancer? **243**
Hideshi Ishii and Toshiyuki Saito

Chapter 14 Role of the Tumor Suppressor PDCD4 in the Differentiation of the Skin **253**
Sachiko Matsuhashi, Takeshi Okawa and Yutaka Narisawa

Chapter Sources **263**

Index **265**

Preface

Chapter 1 - Mutations in the TP53 gene are the most common alterations in human tumours. TP53 mutational patterns have sometimes been linked to carcinogen exposure. In hepatocellular carcinoma (HCC), a specific G>T transversion in codon 249 is classically described as a fingerprint of aflatoxin B1 (AFB1) exposure. Likewise G>T transversions in codons 157 and 158 have been related to tobacco exposure in human lung cancers. However, controversies remain about the interpretation of TP53 mutational pattern in tumours as the fingerprint of genotoxin exposure. By using a functional assay, the Functional Analysis of Separated Alleles in Yeast (FASAY), the present study depicts the mutational pattern of TP53 in normal human fibroblasts after in vitro exposure to well-known carcinogens: AFB1 and acetaldehyde. These in vitro mutation patterns were then compared to those found in human tumours using the IARC database of TP53 mutations.

AFB1mutational pattern reveals that codon 245 is the main hot spot, whereas no mutations are found in codon 249. The locations of mutations within GG and GC/CG sequences are well in accordance with AFB1-adducts location data. In our assay, AFB1 mainly induces G>A transitions, followed by G>T and A>G mutations. This suggests that G>T transversion at codon 249 is likely the result of a selection bias in human HCC rather than a true fingerprint of AFB1 adducts. Indeed, a comparison of the mutation pattern with that found in human HCC excluding codon 249 reveals that the two spectra are quite similar. Furthermore, the similarity between our in vitro pattern with that identified in AFB1-induced mice lung tumours suggests that AFB1may be a potent lung carcinogen in humans.

Acetaldehyde mutational pattern is very different to the AFB1 one, showing mainly G>A transitions, many of them located in CpG sites in strong accordance with acetaldehyde interstrand adduct locations. One third of the mutations are located in TP53 hot-spots: codons 245, 248, 249 and 273. These results support the ability of acetaldehyde, the first metabolite of ethanol, to induce TP53 mutations during oesophageal and head and neck carcinogenesis. Indeed, ethanol may be considered as a true genotoxin in regard to these particular tumours.

Chapter 2 - Diets deficient in folic acid or thiamin or even one essential amino acid will stop tumor growth. The side effects can be tolerated when mild, or treated with small replacement doses of the missing nutrient. The difference in blood perfusion between tumors and normal tissue will carry replacement nutrients preferentially to normal tissue. Diets deficient in ascorbic acid, vitamin B12, niacin, pyridoxine, choline, or essential fatty acids may also be selectively toxic to tumors. Inositol, glucose, and selenium or cysteine in dietary excess or deficiency, and moderate doses of vitamin D, might also be beneficial.

Hyperthermia, exercise, herbal teas, resveratrol, and the visualization of tumor destruction may enhance the benefits of nutrient manipulation. Undernutrition may reverse tumor resistance to conventional chemotherapy, which should be revaluated following a duration of nutrient manipulation. Together, reasonable, convenient, inexpensive interventions against terminal cancer constitute the perfect placebo, empowering terminal patients with legitimate hope for remission or cure.

Chapter 3 - Breast cancer is the major cause of cancer death in the Western world. Despite the fact that women undergo imaging-based screening at regular intervals, many cancers are still discovered in between screening visits. This indicates an urgent need for novel screening and risk assessment modalities that could be of additive value to imaging-based screening.

Breast cancer is initiated and progresses by genetic and epigenetic events resulting in aberrant gene function. Epigenetic alterations occur through mechanisms other than changes in the primary nucleotide sequence of a gene. One of the most important epigenetic mechanisms is DNA methylation. The term DNA methylation describes the addition of a methyl group to a cytosine base in the DNA. In the normal situation DNA methylation is involved in the regulation of many cellular maintenance processes. However, during tumorigenesis, hypermethylation of promoters of tumor suppressor genes is associated with silencing of transcription. In this way methylation contributes to cancer initiation and progression. Methylation alterations frequently occur in early stages of tumor development and can also be detected in non-cancerous cells adjacent to the tumor, which indicates a methylation "field defect". Moreover, epigenetic changes are reversible and therefore potential therapeutic targets.

Analyzing DNA promoter methylation of tumor suppressor genes in nipple fluid could be a new screening modality. Nipple fluid is normally produced in small amounts in the ducts of non-lactating women and can be obtained by non-invasive vacuum aspiration. This fluid contains intact ductal epithelial cells together with free DNA derived from such cells, which can be analyzed for methylation aberrations. Using oxytocin nasal spray, nipple fluid can be aspirated from more than 90% of women, including high-risk women that previously underwent local or systemic treatment. We and others previously showed that methylation of a panel of tumor suppressor genes such as CCND2, SCGB3A1, APC, RASSF1 and RARB is associated with the presence of breast cancer. Using Quantitative Multiplex Methylation-Specific PCR, methylation alterations can reliably be assessed in the limited amounts of DNA present in nipple fluid.

In conclusion, analyzing patterns of promoter methylation of tumor suppressor genes in nipple fluid can potentially serve as a valuable breast cancer screening method. A large prospective study is currently ongoing in our institute to determine the added value of this modality to existing screening methods.

Chapter 4 - The Ras-associated binding (Rab) family of small GTPases serves as molecular switches in regulating vesicular membrane traffic in all eukaryotic cells. Although not conventionally categorized as oncogenes or tumor suppressors, aberrant expressions of several members of the Rab family in cancer tissues have nonetheless been noted. Recent findings have highlighted the potential of certain Rab family members acting both as oncogenic drivers, as well as tumor suppressors. Rab25's expression status, for example, could be an important determinant of progression and aggressiveness of breast and ovarian cancers. Paradoxically, its over-expression could also be tumor-suppressive. In general, deregulation of Rab expression could perturb proliferative or survival signaling pathways through spatial and temporal changes in growth factor receptor traffic and associated signaling. Furthermore, aberrant expression of Rabs may affect the modulation of the dynamics of cell adhesion components (such as integrins) and the cytoskeleton. This may in turn affect cancer cell migration, invasion and metastasis. Finally, deregulation of Rabs that are important in the differentiation of progenitor cells may impair differentiation and enhance tumorigenesis. We discuss in this chapter recent findings implicating Rabs in a variety of human cancers, and explore in particular, plausible mechanisms of how Rabs could be tumor-suppressive.

Chapter 5 - Identification of the first tumor supressor RB1, or the retinoblastoma gene laid the groundwork for identification of other tumor supressor genes. Over the years genetic evidences implied that at least one factor in chromosome 10 is an important tumor supressor. Partial or complete loss of chromosome 10 led to prostrate, bladder or brain cancer and when wild type chromosone 10 was reintroduced in glioblastoma cell lines it reduced the ability of these cells to form tumors in nude mice. Later through LOH analysis it was identified that the region 10q23 is the most common region of loss of chromosome 10 in prostrate cancer. Further analysis revealed that protein involved in these cancer is a protein tyrosine phosphatase with a large region homologus to chick tensin and was thus named PTEN standing for phosphatsase and tensin homolog deleted on chromosome 10. Following years unfolded that PTEN regulates the PI3K pathway by acting as a 3' phosphatase converting the product of PI3K, PtdIns(3,4,5)P3 to PtdIns(4,5,)P2.

Chapter 6 - The adenomatous polyposis coli (APC) tumor suppressor gene is commonly lost in both inherited and sporadic colorectal cancer and is frequently inactivated in many other human cancers. Moreover, Apc deficiency in animal models is sufficient for tumorigenesis in a diverse set of tissue types, demonstrating that APC loss not only correlates with cancer pathogenesis but drives tumor development. Over the last two decades since its identification, much attention has been devoted to deciphering the molecular mechanisms responsible for APC's tumor suppressor activity. The picture that is emerging is one of APC as a 'gatekeeper' of epithelial and tissue homeostasis by serving as a scaffold for multi-protein complexes, including the β-catenin destruction machinery. Although regulation of Wnt signaling by APC through β-catenin degradation has been well studied, separable Wnt-independent functions of APC have been identified. In this review, the authors will summarize the interaction of APC with junctional and polarity complexes, the cytoskeleton, nuclear proteins and apoptotic factors. Emerging evidence will be presented that supports the importance of these interactions in apical-basal and front-rear polarity, migration, differentiation, DNA replication, mitosis, DNA repair and apoptosis through Wnt pathway-independent mechanisms. The contribution of these processes to tumor development as a result of APC inactivation will be discussed. Lastly, we will address how the uncoupling of these activities from Wnt signaling may provide a therapeutic opportunity for treating APC-deficient cancers. Together, these generally under-appreciated, Wnt-independent aspects of APC function may significantly revise the accepted view of APC-mediated tumor suppression and, importantly, uncover novel strategies for cancer treatment.

Chapter 7 - BRIT1 (BRCT-Repeat Inhibitor of hTERT expression) was originally identified from the laboratory as an inhibitor of human telomere reverse transcriptase (hTERT) by a genome-wide genetic screen[1]. The amino acid sequence of BRIT1 was later matched to a putative disease gene called microcephalin (MCPH1). Dysfunction of BRIT1/MCPH1 causes an autosomal recessive genetic disease known as primary microcephaly, which is characterized by reduced brain size of patients[2]. In addition to neuronal development disorder, aberrations of BRIT1 have been identified in various human cancers including breast, ovarian and prostate cancer. In order to gain the mechanistic insights into how BRIT1 deficiency leads to the pathogenesis of the human diseases, the studies and studies from other groups indicate BRIT1 functions as an early DNA damage responsive protein to coordinate cellular responses to genotoxic stresses and maintain genomic stability. In this chapter, the authors only focus on the function of BRIT1 as a tumor suppressor gene in tumorigenesis. They will discuss the emerging roles of BRIT1 in orchestrating cellular responses to DNA damage including DNA damage signaling, checkpoint activation, and DNA repair. As genomic instability is a hallmark of cancer cells, we will further discuss in the context of cancer development, how BRIT1 functions as a novel tumor suppressor by providing cells with a fundamental genome maintenance mechanism against tumorigenesis and how BRIT1 deficiency may provide a unique opportunity for targeted therapeutics in cancer treatment.

Chapter 8 - Epigenetic mechanisms result in the silencing of genes without a change in their coding sequence. The most well-characterized alteration is DNA hypermethylation, and a modification of histones also contributes to tumor suppressor loss through epigenetic silencing.

Acetylation and deacetylation of histones play an important role in transcription regulation. The acetylation status of histones is determined by histone deacetylase (HDAC), and HDAC are strongly expressed in cancerous tissue. HDAC inhibitors are known to alter gene expression and to induce different phenotypes in various transformed cells, including growth arrest, apoptotic pathways and mitotic cell death. For example, the CDK inhibitor p21WAF1/CIP1 is one of most common genes induced by HDAC inhibitor.

Polycomb group proteins are epigenetic chromatin modifiers involved in cancer development. EZH2, one component of polycomb repressive complex, contain the signature domain providing the methylation active site, and its expression levels are abnormally elevated in malignant tissues. EZH2 mediates tumor suppressor genes such as p16INK4A and E-cadherin, affecting and controlling cell proliferation, differentiation and invasiveness in cancer cells. As a consequence, a down-regulation of EZH2 induces significant growth inhibitory effects and represses its invasiveness in carcinoma cells.

HDAC and EZH2 are strongly expressed in cancer cells and they seem to interact each other and contribute to oncogenesis. HDAC inhibitor (SAHA) decreases EZH2 expression itself in carcinoma cells, in addition to HDAC repression. This double-repression effect might be an important mechanism in the anticancer effect of SAHA. Furthermore, HDAC inhibitor and/or EZH2-repression using siRNA affect trimethylated and acetylated levels at p16INK4A and E-cadherin promoter, and the combined treatment increases the expression level of p16INK4A and E-cadherin synergistically. Consequently, functional links between EZH2 and HDAC contribute to an emerging view that all these types of epigenetic silencing machinery play an important role in abnormal control of gene expression in malignant cells. Therefore, EZH2 and HDAC may be promising targets for treatment strategy.

Chapter 9 - The Kank1 gene was found at 9p24 in a human chromosome showing loss of function through allelic loss/mutation/epigenetic modification in renal cell carcinoma cells. Loss or mutation of the gene has been found in cases of other diseases including cancers. The functions of the Kank1 protein, such as inhibition of cell migration, intracellular transport and cytokinesis, are discussed here in association with carcinogenesis/metastasis.

Chapter 10 - This review attempts to examine some of evidence that support the role of microRNA in tumor suppression, and to review those reports that shown promise of alteration of microRNAs as a strategy for cancer therapy. There are several ways that microRNA can affect tumor suppressors. Some reports have demonstrated that MicroRNA can act as tumor suppressors themselves (e.g. let-7, mir-125a), while others have shown that they act by affecting the up-stream regulators of tumor suppressors or downstream targets of oncogenes. The picture is also complicated by the fact that some microRNAs are regulated by other microRNAs (e.g. miR-16-1 precursor abolishes the expression of the mature miR-16), and some microRNAs can be regulated by oncogenes (e.g. miR-17-92 is regulated by c-Myc).

Chapter 11 - Prostate cancer (CaP) is the main cause of cancer death in men in Western countries. Radiation has been serving as an indispensable component of therapy for CaP patients. Local CaP recurrence after radiotherapy is a pattern of treatment failure attributable to radioresistance of cancer cells. Identification of predictive biomarkers for radioresistance offers the potential to select appropriate patients for multi-modality anti-cancer treatment or selection of an alternative modality.

Numerous membranous, cytoplasmic and intranuclear oncoproteins involved in prominent cell signaling pathways, such as PI3K/AKT, MAPK/ERK and apoptosis pathways, have been proven to contribute to the radioresistance of CaP. Assessing expression of these proteins will help to predict the radiation responsiveness of CaP patients.

The discovery of the existence of cancer stem cells (CSCs) provides another explanation of tumor recurrence after radiation. This is an interesting research area providing promise for overcoming cancer radioresistance. CSCs have been identified in CaP cells, which are more tumorigenic than the non-tumor initiating cells in vitro and in vivo studies. Understanding the mechanisms of radioresistance of the CSCs will help to overcome recurrence after radiotherapy in CaP patients.

In this chapter, we aim to discuss the biomarkers related to radioresistance in CaP from two aspects: the markers involved in major signaling pathways and those associated with CSCs. The potential beneficial effects associated with targeting these markers and overcoming the observed clinical radioresistance to current treatments and CaP recurrence are also discussed.

Chapter 12 - The tumor suppressor p53 has been implicated in many important cellular processes, including regulation of apoptotic cell death, in the cellular response to DNA damage. When cells encounter genotoxic stress, certain sensors for DNA lesions stabilize and activate p53. Eventually, p53 exerts its tumor suppressor function by transactivating numerous target genes. Active p53 is subjected to a complex and diverse array of covalent post-translational modifications, which selectively influence the expression of p53 target genes. In this context, the molecular basis for how p53 induces apoptosis has been substantially studied; however, the relative contribution of each downstream effecter is still to be explored. Moreover, little is known about precise mechanisms by which modified p53 is capable of apoptosis induction. A thorough understanding for the whole picture of p53 modification in apoptosis will be extremely valuable in the development of highly effective and specific therapies for caner patients. This review is focused on the current views regarding the regulation of cell fate by p53 in the apoptotic response to DNA damage.

Chapter 13 - Oxidative stress, a biochemical condition that is characterized by an imbalance between the presence of relatively high levels of toxic reactive species and antioxidative defense mechanisms, has been linked to various cellular philology and disorders characterized by cell death, such as stem cells of neural and hematopoietic systems. Recent studies indicate that common chromosome fragile sites, non-random targets of double stranded breaks under replication perturbation that are characteristic of tumors, paradoxically encode the tumor suppressor FHIT gene, which modulates response to oxidative stress and DNA damage. Since it is inactivated in precancer or early stages of carcinogenesis, we propose that the FHIT gene plays a role in the creation of cancer initiating cells. Mechanistic roles of FHIT in modulating oxidative stress and DNA damage checkpoints of cancer initiating cells are also discussed.

Chapter 14 - First isolated as an antigen gene involved in the cell cycle, the human programmed cell death 4 (PDCD4) gene mapped at 10q24. Mouse Pdcd4 was shown to suppress the transformation of JB6 mouse epidermal cells exposed to promoters such as TPA, inhibiting AP-1 transactivation. PDCD4 expression was down-regulated in many tumor tissues. PDCD4/Pdcd4 was classified as a protein synthesis regulator, because the protein associates with eIF4A, a component of the initiation complex of protein synthesis, thereby inhibiting cap-dependent translations. When cells are stimulated by mitogens, the PDCD4-protein is phosphorylated by S6K activated through Akt-mTOR signal transduction pathway and degraded in an ubiquitin-proteasome system, stimulating protein synthesis and carcinogenesis. Besides the regulation of translation, PDCD4/Pdcd4 also regulates transcriptions and induces apoptosis as it is over-expressed in tumor cells by plasmid transfection.

In the normal skin, PDCD4 expression was localized in differentiating cell layers of epidermis but was absent or less extent in PCNA-positive cell layers such as basal cell layers of epidermis or bulbar area of hair follicles. Apoptotic casepase systems were shown to be activated on the cornification of epidermis and on the induction of apoptosis by UVB irradiation which induced PDCD4 expression in HaCaT cells. These results indicates that PDCD4 may contribute for the differentiation of epidermal cells and hair follicles. In the transgenic mice specifically expressing Pdcd4 in epidermal cell lineages, the epidermis was resistant to carcinogenesis and the hair follicles underwent earlier catagen to show a shorter hair phenotype than the normal skin. This results support the idea that PDCD4 may contribute to the differentiation on the hair follicles. However, Pdcd4 nock-down mice showed normal development although the animals were more sensitive to carcinogenesis than normal siblings. PDCD4 might partly contribute to the differentiation of the skin.

In: Tumor Suppressors
Editor: Susan D. Nguyen

ISBN: 978-1-61761-986-1

Chapter 1

Aflatoxin B$_1$ and Acetaldehyde Mutational Patterns in the Tumour Suppressor Gene *TP53*: Experimental Fingerprints Using a Functional Assay and Relevance to Human Cancer Aetiology

Vincent Paget, Mathilde Lechevrel and François Sichel*

GRECAN EA1772-IFR 146 ICORE,
Université de Caen Basse-Normandie et Centre François Baclesse,
Av. du Général Harris, 14076 Caen-Cedex 05, France

Abstract

Mutations in the *TP53* gene are the most common alterations in human tumours. *TP53* mutational patterns have sometimes been linked to carcinogen exposure. In hepatocellular carcinoma (HCC), a specific G>T transversion in codon 249 is classically described as a fingerprint of aflatoxin B1 (AFB1) exposure. Likewise G>T transversions in codons 157 and 158 have been related to tobacco exposure in human lung cancers. However, controversies remain about the interpretation of *TP53* mutational pattern in tumours as the fingerprint of genotoxin exposure. By using a functional assay, the Functional Analysis of Separated Alleles in Yeast (FASAY), the present study depicts the mutational pattern of *TP53* in normal human fibroblasts after *in vitro* exposure to well-known carcinogens: AFB1 and acetaldehyde. These *in vitro* mutation patterns were then compared to those found in human tumours using the IARC database of *TP53* mutations.

* Corresponding author: François Sichel, GRECAN, Centre François Baclesse, 5 Av. du Général Harris, 14076 Caen-cedex 05, France. Tel +33.231.45.51.93, Fax +33.231.45.51.72, francois.sichel@unicaen.fr

AFB1mutational pattern reveals that codon 245 is the main hot spot, whereas no mutations are found in codon 249. The locations of mutations within GG and GC/CG sequences are well in accordance with AFB1-adducts location data. In our assay, AFB1 mainly induces G>A transitions, followed by G>T and A>G mutations. This suggests that G>T transversion at codon 249 is likely the result of a selection bias in human HCC rather than a true fingerprint of AFB1 adducts. Indeed, a comparison of the mutation pattern with that found in human HCC excluding codon 249 reveals that the two spectra are quite similar. Furthermore, the similarity between our *in vitro* pattern with that identified in AFB1-induced mice lung tumours suggests that AFB1may be a potent lung carcinogen in humans.

Acetaldehyde mutational pattern is very different to the AFB1 one, showing mainly G>A transitions, many of them located in CpG sites in strong accordance with acetaldehyde interstrand adduct locations. One third of the mutations are located in *TP53* hot-spots: codons 245, 248, 249 and 273. These results support the ability of acetaldehyde, the first metabolite of ethanol, to induce *TP53* mutations during oesophageal and head and neck carcinogenesis. Indeed, ethanol may be considered as a true genotoxin in regard to these particular tumours.

Keywords: acetaldehyde, aflatoxin B_1, *TP53*, mutation, hepatocarcinoma, lung carcinoma, head and neck carcinoma, esophagus carcinoma, FASAY.

Introduction

Mutations of the *TP53* tumour suppressor gene are the most frequent genetic alterations in human cancers [Soussi, 2007]. Characterisation of mutation spectra induced by carcinogens in appropriate target sequences provides information on the involvement of specific etiological factors in cancer development [Chang, 1993; Hussain, 1998; Hussain, 2000; Pfeifer, 2002]. Relationships between benzo(a)pyrene or UV irradiation and specific mutations commonly isolated in human lung or skin tumours have been respectively established by epidemiological and experimental studies. Hepatocarcinoma (HCC) is a striking example of geographical differences in the mutational *TP53* pattern linked to etiological factors. In high-risk areas, exposure to dietary aflatoxin B_1 (AFB_1) is described as a primary risk factor [Hussain, 2007], essentially associated with chronic infection by the HBV and HCV hepatitis viruses. AFB_1 is a hepatotoxin produced by the *Aspergillus flavus* and *A. parasiticus* fungi. This mycotoxin is primarily bioactivated in liver by cytochromes P450 1A2 (CYP1A2) and 3A4 (CYP3A4) to a genotoxic epoxide that forms N^7-guanine DNA adducts [Mace, 1997]. These adducts are acknowledged as being highly mutagenic [Smela, 2001]. In HCC from patients exposed to dietary AFB_1, AGG to AGT (G>T, arginine to serine) transversion at codon 249 is classically identified as the specific *TP53* mutation [Aguilar, 1993; Shen, 1996]. In addition, a link has been identified between a high frequency of this targeted mutation and strong AFB_1 exposure in high-risk areas [Hussain, 2007]. The concept of the genetic fingerprint of AFB_1 has also been endorsed by *in vitro* studies reporting the ability of AFB_1 to induce codon 249 transversion in normal hepatocytes or in liver epithelial cell lines expressing CYP [Aguilar, 1993; Mace, 1997]. Nevertheless a few studies failed to demonstrate the codon 249 as a hot spot [Chan, 2003; Sengstag, 1999].

Denissenko e*t al.* also demonstrated that AFB_1 adducts are not preferentially located on codon 249 of *TP53* [Denissenko, 1999]. These conflicting results raise the question of the true origin of this hot spot: as to whether it is the fingerprint of the AFB_1 adduct or the result of a selection process arising during HCC carcinogenesis.

Although AFB_1 is best known as a hepatocarcinogen following the ingestion of contaminated grains, nuts and oil seeds, this mycotoxin can also target the respiratory system. An experimental study has shown that AFB_1 is able to induce lung carcinoma in mice [Tam, 1999]. In order to study AFB_1 metabolic activation, the efficiency of lung cells was investigated in rabbits and mice [Massey, 2000]. The CYP2A13-catalysed metabolic activation *in situ* may play a critical role in human lung carcinogenesis related to inhalation exposure to AFB_1 [He, 2006]. In addition, Dvorackova [Dvorackova, 1976] reported a possible association between the occurrence of human lung cancer and inhalation exposure to AFB_1. Inhalation of AFB_1-contaminated grain dust may present a cancer hazard to exposed individuals in certain agricultural occupations [Hayes, 1984], e.g. handling of corn silage spoiled by AFB_1 could be a potential risk factor for human safety [Garon, 2006]. All of the above results support the hypothesis that the carcinogenic potential of AFB_1 may impact tissue other than the liver and may induce unusual and specific genetic alterations.

Long term exposure to alcohol is associated with a high incidence of several cancers, including cancers of the upper aero-digestive tract (oral cavity, oro-pharynx, hypopharynx and esophagus), liver, colo-rectum, breast, and, to a lesser extent, pancreas and lung [Boffetta, 2006a; Boffetta, 2006b; Poschl, 2004a]. Unlike tobacco, which is another known risk factor for esophageal cancer, the involvement of alcohol in carcinogenesis is unclear. Ethanol alone has generally not been found to induce cancer in experimental models [IARC, 1988]. There has not been any evidence that ethanol can be directly carcinogenic, but rather that it acts through indirect mechanisms [Poschl, 2004b]. Many functional alterations of cells may be attributed to ethanol itself. Indeed, previous studies demonstrated that ethanol exposure increased the metabolic activation of procarcinogens such as nitrosamines. Carcinogen bioactivation and detoxification depend on the target tissue studied, gender, and whether ethanol was administered acutely or chronically [Barnes, 2000; Seitz, 2007].

Alcohol is mainly metabolized into acetaldehyde, which is the primary metabolite obtained through the oxidation of ethanol by alcohol dehydrogenase (ADH) and *CYP2E1* in the liver but also in extra-hepatic tissues such as the esophagus [Lechevrel, 1999]. Acetaldehyde is then oxidized to acetate by aldehyde dehydrogenase (ALDH) [Quertemont, 2004; Yokoyama, 2003]. In addition, much higher levels of acetaldehyde can be produced through the microbial oxidation of ethanol by oral microflora [Homann, 2000]. So, exposure to acetaldehyde in the upper aero-digestive tract arises from both endogenous and bacterial production. These data have shown possible differences in microbial composition and relative concentrations among high and low acetaldehyde producers [Homann, 1997; Homann, 2000; Homann, 2001; Muto, 2000]. Poor oral hygiene is another important risk factor. An association with alcohol consumption greatly increases the risk of developing oral cavity cancers, this being even more pronounced for heavy drinkers [Homann, 2001; Rehm, 2003; Room, 2003]. Genotoxic effects of acetaldehyde in human cells include damage to DNA through multiple pathways, single and double strand breaks, oxygen reactive species (ROS) generation, DNA or protein/DNA cross-links, chromosomal aberrations, sister chromatin exchanges and gene mutations [Hecht, 2001; Noori, 2001; Singh, 1995]. Acetaldehyde reactions with DNA lead to various adducts, some of them proven to be mutagenic [Brooks, 2005; Hecht, 2001; Stein, 2006].

Indeed, AFB_1 and acetaldehyde are well-known human genotoxic carcinogens. These compounds were chosen owing to their large range of genotoxicity and pattern of DNA adducts, which makes them good candidates for a study about molecular fingerprint during carcinogenesis. In fact, controversies remain about the interpretation of *TP53* mutational pattern in tumours as the fingerprint of genotoxin exposure [Bitton, 2005]. As many *TP53* mutations found in tumours strongly affect p53 functional properties [Dearth, 2007], we used a functional assay, the Functional Analysis of Separated Alleles in Yeast (FASAY) [Ishioka, 1993], in order to describe mutational patterns of *TP53* after *in vitro* exposure of normal human cells to AFB_1 and acetaldehyde. In order to make a comparison with patterns related to human tumours, normal human cells were exposed to low and relevant concentrations of genotoxins (i.e. nM and mM ranges for AFB_1 and acetaldehyde, respectively). These *in vitro* patterns of mutations were then compared to those found in experimental and in human tumours using the IARC database of *TP53* mutations [Olivier, 2002].

Materials and Methods

Cell line and cell culture

Human diploid fibroblasts AG1521 (Coriell Institute, Camden, NJ) were grown at 37°C in a humidified atmosphere of 5% CO2 and 95% air, in Eagle's Minimal Essential Medium (MEM) supplemented with 10% inactivated foetal bovine serum (FBS). Before starting the study, we ensured that no *TP53* mutations were observed on AG1521 cells by sequencing genomic DNA using a Beckman Automated Sequencer (CEQ 8000). AFB_1 (Sigma, CAS number: 1162-65-8) and acetaldehyde (Acros Organics, CAS number: 75-07-0) were diluted in the MEM 10% FBS and left in medium culture for 2 hours at 37°C. During AFB_1 experiments, the medium was previously completed with 200µL (4%) of S9 liver microsomal fractions of phenobarbital and β-naphtoflavone treated rats (Biopredic, Rennes, France), NADPH 4µM and G6P 5mM. Culture plates were then washed three times with PBS 1X, before being re-incubated for 1 week with the new medium. As the doubling time of these cells is around 3 days, this post-incubation time has been chosen to allow 2 cell cycles for mutation fixation.

Cytotoxicity study

AG1521 fibroblasts were exposed to AFB_1 concentrations from 0.8 to 16µM in presence of S9-mix, and to acetaldehyde concentrations from 1 µM to 200 mM, for 2 hours at 37°C in 96-well microplates. The microplates were then washed three times with PBS 1X, and re-incubated for 3 days at 37°C. Cell cytotoxicity was evaluated in a XTT assay (Sigma) according to the Scuderio protocol [Scudiero, 1988].

RNA extraction and Reverse Transcription (RT)-PCR

Total RNA from cultured cells were extracted using an Rneasy Mini Kit (Qiagen) according to manufacturer instructions. Reverse-Transcription Polymerase Chain Reaction (RT-PCR) was performed using 1µg of RNA samples. The RT step was carried out with a reaction mixture containing 150ng of random primers (Invitrogen), 10U of *RNasin* (Promega) and 0.5mM dNTPs in a final volume of 20µl (Qiagen Omniscript kit). To amplify cDNA special primers were designed to contain a phosphorothioate linkage on 3' region: P3 [5'- ATT-TGA-TGC-TGT-CCC-CGG-ACG-ATA-TTG-AA(s)C -3'] and P4 [5'- ACC-CTT-TTT-GGA-CTT-CAG-GTG-GCT-GGA-GT(s)G -3']. Amplifications were performed under the following conditions: initial melting at 94°C for 3 min, 35 cycles of 94°C for 30 s, 62°C for 30 s and 72°C for 30s; followed by a final extension at 72°C for 7 min. Two microlitres of the cDNA reaction products were amplified in 25µl of *Pyrobest* buffer II (Takara) plus 1.25 units of *Pyrobest* DNA polymerase, 5% (v/v) dimethyl sulfoxide, and 2.5mM of each dNTP.

Preparation of vector pSS16

Twenty-five µg of pSS16 [Flaman, 1995; Ishioka, 1993], generously donated by J.M. Flaman (INSERM U614, Rouen, France), were digested for 2 hours at 37°C in 100µL of buffer REact® 2 (*Stu* I and *Hind* III buffer), plus 50 units of *Stu* I and 50 units of *Hind* III. The vector was rescued with GFX columns (Amersham Biosciences) and dephosphorylised by Calf Intestine Alkaline Phosphatase (CIP, QBiogene). After inactivation of CIP, the vector was extracted after gel purification using the GFX columns (Amersham Biosciences).

Yeast transformation

To test p53 status, yeast strain YIG397 [Flaman, 1995], generously donated by J. Cachot (LEMA, Université du Havre, France), was co-transformed with unpurified PCR products, linearised vector pSS16 and carrier DNA, using the lithium acetate procedure. It was then plated on synthetic minimal medium minus leucine and adenine for incubation over 3 days at 30°C followed by one or 2 days at 4°C. This second step was carried out to intensify the red coloration. This red coloration is induced by the accumulation of an intermediate product of adenine synthesis.

TP53 plasmid recovery from yeast and DNA sequencing

TP53-expressing plasmids were rescued from isolated red colonies. These red colonies were returned to culture and lysed with *Zymolyase* (MP-Biomedicals). QIAprep®Miniprep (Qiagen) was used to rescue plasmids. Before sequencing *TP53* cDNA was re-amplified with primers P5 [5'- TCT-GTC-ACT-TGC-ACG-TAC-TCC -3'] and P6 [5'- AGA-GGA-GCT-GGT-GTT-GTT-GG -3'], designed to cover exon 5 to exon 9. Two sets of primers were chosen to sequence the recombination sites on either side of the *TP53* cDNA: at 5' region primers PA [5'- CAG-TCA-GAT-CCT-AGC-GTC-GAG -3'] and PB [5'- CTC-CGT-CAT-

GTG-CTG-TGA-CT -3']; at 3' region primers PC [5'- AAG-GAA-ATT-TGC-GTG-TGG-AG -3'] and PD [5'- CAG-GCC-CTT-CTG-TCT-TGAAC -3'].

Sequence tools analysis

To analyse sequences of *TP53,* we used the Thierry Soussi database (http://p53.free.fr/) to obtain the *TP53* wild type sequence. We then used the Blast tool on NCBI (http://www.ncbi.nlm.nih.gov/) to perform sequence alignments. To compare different *TP53* mutational patterns, the IARC database (http://www-p53.iarc.fr/) was used.

Results

Cytotoxicity of AFB1 and acetaldehyde on AG1521 cells

Cell growth after exposure of AG1521 human fibroblasts to various concentrations of AFB_1 and acetaldehyde showed a concentration-dependent decrease (data not shown). This assay enabled us to establish an IC50 of 6.4µM for AFB_1 and of 25mM for acetaldehyde. These values are in agreement with other studies that have already used eukaryotic superior cells [He, 2006; Mace, 1997; Singh, 1995]. We decided to opt for exposure concentrations ranging from 16 to 800nM and from 0.1 to 7.5mM for AFB_1 and acetaldehyde, respectively. In both cases, the higher concentration corresponds to a growth inhibition of approximately 25%. Cytotoxicity was therefore low and resumption of culture was easier after exposure.

Rate of mutations

Tables 1 and 2 show the overall results for each compound. Every set of exposed and control cells was plated in triplicate. As reproducibility among triplicates was very high and was published elsewhere [Paget, 2008a; Paget, 2008b], it is only shown the total number of colonies for each triplicate.

Among the red colonies found in control cells, only a few ones bear mutations in the central part of *TP53*, i.e. exons 5 to 9. The other ones display non digested pSS16 or mutations located in the recombination sites, which were considered as artefacts. The two colonies bearing a mutation in the central part of *TP53* showed an AGT insertion in exon 7/8 which is likely a splicing defect rather than a true mutational event, as already described [Paget, 2008a, Paget 2008b, Billet 2010]. It is noteworthy that the rate of this splicing defect looks very close among the two experiments using AG1521 fibroblasts and also using another cell line, the A549 lung cells [Billet, 2010].

The rates of mutation were not concentration-dependant, which suggests a "plateau-effect" as described in other genotoxicity assays [Maron, 1983; Platel, 2009]. These rates were slightly decreasing at the top concentration with the two compounds, in relation with cytotoxicity. Overall, this suggests that lower concentrations would have been used with FASAY.

TP53 mutations in AFB_1 exposed normal human fibroblasts

Results of functional assays performed on normal human fibroblasts exposed to several AFB_1 concentrations are shown in table 1. 186 red colonies were screened and only 44 mutations were identified in *TP53* DNA binding domain for all tested AFB_1 concentrations. We can point out that among the latter mutations, the 3-base insertion is re-expressed at the same average in comparison with control samples: 3.8% (7/186) vs 3.6% (1/28), respectively (table 1). This mutation was not taken into account in the AFB_1 mutational spectrum.

Table 3 summarizes the mutations sequenced in AFB_1 exposed cells. Four mutations were one-base insertion or deletions, leading to frameshift. The remaining mutations were single nucleotide substitutions including 1 nonsense and 32 missense mutations. Many of these mutations occurred in well-known human tumour hot spots: codons 175, 245 and 282 (IARC database). The mutational pattern is depicted in Fig. 1B: G>A transitions were the most prevalent (13/37, 35%) among which 8 were located at CpG sites. They were followed by G>T transversions (8/37, 22%), A>G transitions (8/37, 22%), A>T (3/37, 8%) and A>C transversions (1/37, 3%).

In order to permit extensive comparison, we combined the AFB_1 mutational profile of our *in vitro* study with those found in AFB_1 induced lung tumours in mice [Tam, 1999] and in human HCC (IARC database) (Fig.1).

TP53 mutations in acetaldehyde exposed normal human fibroblasts

182 red colonies (44 to 47 colonies for each exposure concentration) were sequenced from acetaldehyde exposed cells (Table 2). Only 42 displayed mutations in exons 5-9. The remaining 140 red colonies were found to bear mutations at the recombination sites. Out of the 42 mutations found in exons 5-9 (Table 4.A.), 7 were the same 3-base insertion described in the control. Again, this mutation will not be taken into account in the acetaldehyde mutational spectra.

Three mutations were one-base insertion or deletion, leading to frameshift mutations. The remaining 32 mutations were single nucleotide substitutions, 2 of which were nonsense and 30 missense. Many of these mutations occurred in well-known human tumour hot-spots: codons 245, 248, 249, 273 (IARC database). The pattern of mutations is depicted in Fig. 2A: G>A transitions were the most prevalent (23/35, 66%); among them, 14 (40%) were located at CpG sites, followed by G>T transversions (4/35, 11%), A>G transitions (2/32, 6%) and A>T transition (2/32, 6%). To compare this mutational profile with those found in human tumours (IARC database), Fig. 2.B. and 2.C. illustrate respectively the pattern of mutations identified in esophageal SCC, excluding non-drinkers and in lung tumours, excluding non-smokers.

Table 1. Summary of yeast transformations for AFB_1 experiments. Results show pooled data of a relevant triplicate.

		Aflatoxin B_1 (nM)					
		Control cells	**16**	**32**	**160**	**320**	**800**
Yeast transformation							
Total number of colonies	A	1920	1839	1803	1893	1863	1962
Total number of red colonies	B	66	127	122	115	109	105
Recovering of red colonies and PCR step							
Analysed red colonies	C	28	45	38	34	29	40
Red colonies bearing *TP53* (PCR positive)	D	26	42	36	32	28	37
Red colonies bearing non digested pSS16 (C-D)	E	2	3	2	2	1	3
Sequencing step							
Colonies mutated on exons 5 to 9	F	1	12	10	8	7	7
AGT insertion in exon 7/8 (splicing defect)	G	1	1	1	2	1	2
"True" mutations (F-G)	H	0	11	9	6	6	5
Statistical analysis							
Total number of "true" mutations (HxB/C)		0	31.0	28.9	20.1	22.6	13.1
Rate of mutation (%) 100 x (HxB/C) / A		**0**	**1.69**	**1.60**	**1.07**	**1.21**	**0.67**

Table 2. Summary of yeast transformations for acetaldehyde experiments. Results show pooled data of a relevant triplicate.

		Acetaldehyde (mM)				
		Control cells	**0.1**	**1**	**3**	**7.5**
Yeast transformation						
Total number of colonies	A	4655	4598	4324	4271	4053
Total number of red colonies	B	155	284	273	319	305
Recovering of red colonies and PCR step						
Analysed red colonies	C	36	45	47	44	46
Red colonies bearing *TP53* (PCR positive)	D	31	43	44	40	43
Red colonies bearing non digested pSS16 (C-D)	E	5	2	3	4	3

Sequencing step						
Colonies mutated on exons 5 to 9	F	1	14	11	10	7
AGT insertion in exon 7/8 (splicing defect)	G	1	2	2	2	1
"True" mutations (F-G)	H	0	12	9	8	6
Statistical analysis						
Total number of "true" mutations (HxB/C)		0	75.7	52.3	58.0	39.8
Rate of mutation (%) 100 x (HxB/C) / A		**0**	**1.65**	**1.21**	**1.36**	**0.98**

Table 3. Summary of *TP53* mutations observed in red colonies from AFB_1-exposed human fibroblasts

(Mutated bases are given in bold, GG or CC sequences are highlighted in strong grey, CG or GC sequences are highlighted in light grey)

(A) Summary of *TP53* mutations in exon 5 to 9 already found in control cells

Number	Exon	Codon	Base change	Amino acid insertion
1 → 7	7-8	261	AGT→AGT **AGT**	Pro→Pro Pro

(B) Summary of *TP53* mutations in exon 5 to 9 found only in exposed cells

Number	Exon	Codon	Base change	Amino acid substitution	Nature of mutation
8	5	129	CCT G**C**C CTC→G**A**C	Ala→Asp	Missense
9	5	141	ACC TGC CCT>TG**T** CC		Frameshift
10	5	144	GTG C**A**G CTG>C**G**G	Leu→Pro	Missense
11	5	145	CAG C**T**G TGG>C**C**G	Leu→Pro	Missense
12	5	151	ACA **C**CC CCG>**T**CC	Pro→Ser	Missense
13	5	155	GGC A**C**C CGC>A**A**C	Thr→Asn	Missense
14 → 15	5	170	ATG **A**CG GAG>**G**CG	Thr→Ala	Missense
16	7	174	GTG **A**GG C>GGC		Frameshift
17	7	175	AGG C**G**C TGC**>**C**A**C	Arg→His	Missense
18 → 20	7	179	CAC **C**AT GAG>**A**AT	His→Asn	Missense
21	7	194	CAT C**T**T ATC>C**C**T	Leu→Pro	Missense
22	7	216	AGT **G**TG GTG>**A**TG	Val→Met	Missense
23 → 25	8	220	CCC **T**AT GAG>**C**AT	Tyr→His	Missense

Table 3 (Continued)

Number	Exon	Codon	Base change	Amino acid substitution	Nature of mutation
26	8	234	CAC TA**C** AAC>TA**A**	Tyr→Stop	Nonsense
27 → 28	8	244	ATG G**G**C GGC>G**A**C	Gly→Asp	Missense
29	8	245	GGC GGC ATG>G**A**G C		Frameshift
30	8	245	GGC **G**GC ATG>**T**GC	Gly→Cys	Missense
31 → 35	8	245	GGC **G**GC ATG>**A**GC	Gly→Ser	Missense
36	8	265	CTA C**T**G GGA>C**G**G	Leu→Arg	Missense
37	8	265	CTA C**T**G GGA>C**A**G	Leu→Gln	Missense
38	8	282	GAC C**G**G CGC>C**A**G	Arg→Gln	Missense
39	8	283	CGG C**G**C ACA>C**A**C	Arg→His	Missense
40	8	288	GAG A**A**T CTC>A**T**T	Asn→Ile	Missense
41	8	293	AAA **G**GG GAG>GGG AG		Frameshift
42	8	295	GAG C**C**T CAC>C**A**T	Pro→His	Missense
43	8	296	CCT **C**AC CAC>**T**AC	His→Tyr	Missense
44	9	305	ACT A**A**G CGA**>**A**T**G	Lys→Met	Missense

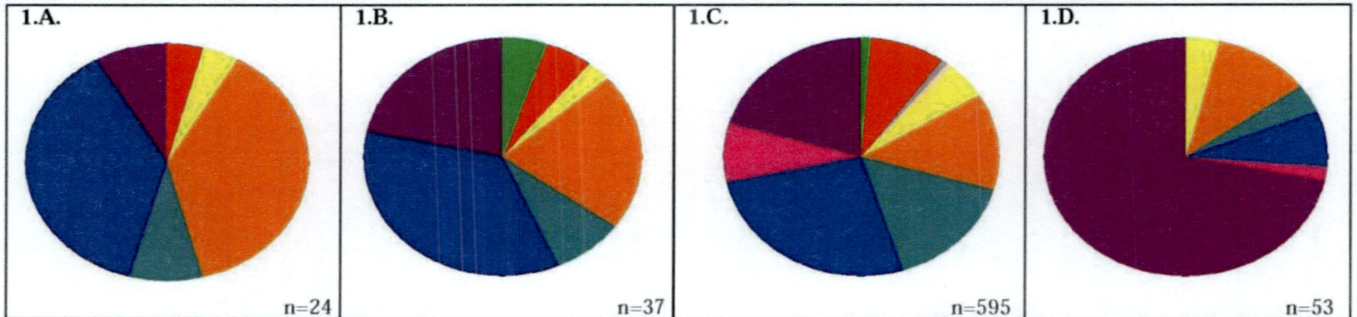

Type of mutation	(**1.A.**) AFB_1 *in vivo* lung (mouse)		(**1.B.**) AFB_1 *in vitro* (FASAY)		(**1.C.**) HCC / 249-		(**1.D.**) HCC/AFB_1+	
Insertions	0	(0%)	2	(5.4%)	6	(1.0%)	0	(0%)
Deletions	1	(4.2%)	2	(5.4%)	54	(9.1%)	0	(0%)
Tandem	0	(0%)	0	(0%)	5	(0.8%)	0	(0%)
Complex	0	(0%)	0	(0%)	3	(0.5%)	0	(0%)
A:T>C:G	1	(4.2%)	1	(2.7%)	29	(4.9%)	2	(3.8%)
A:T>G:C	9	(37.5%)	8	(21.6%)	79	(13.3%)	6	(11.3%)
A:T>T:A	2	(8.3%)	3	(8.1%)	91	(15.3%)	2	(3.8%)
G:C>A:T	9	(37.5%)	13	(35.1%)	157	(26.4%)	4	(7.5%)
G:C>C:G	0	(0%)	0	(0%)	49	(8.2%)	1	(1,9%)
G:C>T:A	2	(8.3%)	8	(21.6%)	122	(20.5%)	38	(71.7%)
Total (n)	24	(100%)	37	(100%)	595	(100%)	53	(100%)

Figure 1. A-D. Mutation patterns of human *TP53*. (n)= number of mutations. (A) *In vivo* AFB_1-induced mutations in mouse lung tumours [Tam, 1999]. (B) *In vitro* AFB_1-induced mutations (FASAY). (C) HCC, codon 249 excluded (noted HCC/249-) (IARC database). (D) HCC, documented AFB_1exposure (noted AFB_1+) (IARC database).

Discussion

The tumour suppressor p53 plays a crucial role in the cellular response to various stresses, such as oncogene activation or DNA damage, regulating many target genes that induce cell-cycle arrest, DNA repair, apoptosis, senescence and metabolism [Green, 2006; May, 1999; Menendez, 2007]. Most mutations in the *TP53* gene compromise p53 functions and *TP53* mutations are found in most human cancers.

By using functional assay (FASAY), we showed that AFB_1 and acetaldehyde impair the functionality of p53 and we were able to describe mutational patterns. It should be emphasised that mutagenic response was obtained at low and biologically relevant concentrations. With AFB_1, our three lowest concentrations (16, 32 and 120 nM) are close to seric concentrations found in healthy subjects living in high AFB_1-exposure areas: e.g., from 16 to 290 nM in Nigeria [Onyemelukwe, 1981] and from 16 to 42 nM in Egypt [Hassan, 2006]. With acetaldehyde, mutations occurred at concentrations as low as 100 μM, which is lower than concentration of acetaldehyde found in saliva which has been measured at up to 140 μM after a 0.5 g/kg dose of ethanol in volunteers [Homann, 1997] and up to 400 μM after a concomitant exposure to alcohol and tobacco [Salaspuro, 2004].

AFB_1 Mutational Pattern

AFB_1 is the most widely known chemical hepatocarcinogen in humans and animals. Through its numerous features, this mycotoxin is an attractive and useful experimental tool for investigating the relationship between genetic fingerprint and environmental carcinogen exposure. Involvement of AFB_1-induced p53 mutant in human HCC has been established in geographical regions associated with high dietary exposure [Hussain, 2007]. The mutations, classically described in these liver tumours exhibit a specific hot spot mutation at *TP53* codon 249, resulting in an arginine to serine amino-acid substitution [Bressac, 1991; Hsu, 1991].

In this work we have validated a new approach to study the functional status of p53 in normal human cells exposed to AFB_1 by using the FASAY functional assay. We have therefore described a differential mutational pattern of AFB_1 which is in support of the hypothesis that codon 249 of the human *TP53* is not a hot spot for AFB_1 outside a hepatic carcinogenesis context.

AFB_1 requires metabolic activation to damage DNA. The epoxidation is the major bioactivation pathway which results in DNA alkylating species. AFB_1-8, 9-epoxide targets the N^7 position of guanine leading to several DNA adducts whose principal is 8,9-dihydro-8-(N^7-guanyl)-9-hydroxyaflatoxine B_1 (AFB_1-N^7-Gua) [Essigmann, 1977]. The positively charged imidazole ring of this adduct promotes depurination, resulting in apurinic site (AP) formation. Alternatively, after the imidazole ring-opening, stable species of AFB_1 formamidopyridine (AFB_1-FAPY) occur only under slightly basic conditions. These three types of DNA damage were proven to be mutagenic, leading mainly to G>T transversions and G>A transitions [Smela, 2001], as observed in our experimental pattern.

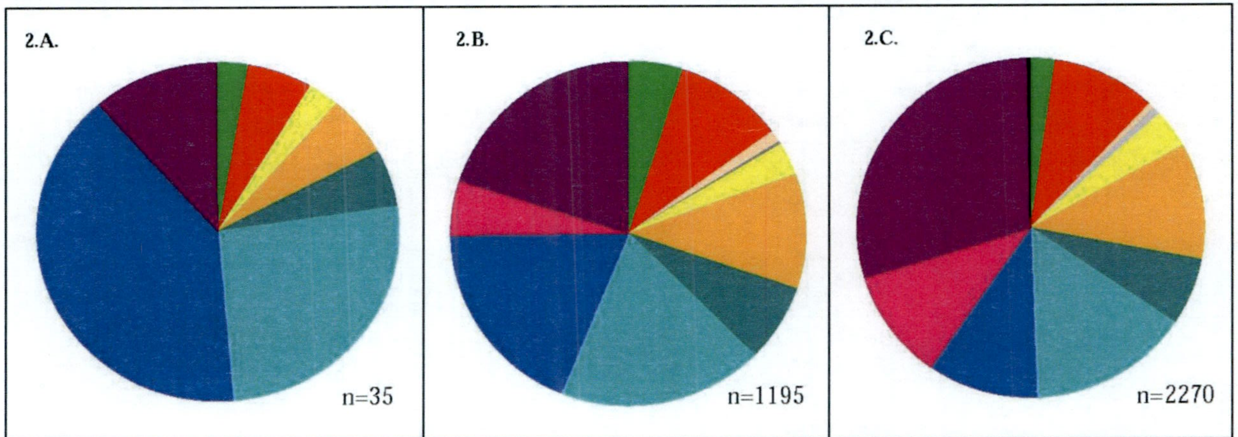

Type of mutation	(2.A.) Acetaldehyde *in vitro*	(2.B.) Esophagus SCC excluding non-drinkers	(2.C.) Lung tumours excluding non-smokers
Insertions	1 (2.9%)	60 (5.0%)	52 (2.3%)
Deletions	2 (5.7%)	118 (9.9%)	216 (9.5%)
Tandem	0 (0%)	16 (1.3%)	17 (0.7%)
CC Tandem	0 (0%)	1 (0.1%)	1 (0.1%)
Complex	0 (0%)	0 (0%)	17 (0.7%)
A:T>C:G	1 (2.9%)	38 (3.2%)	83 (3.7%)
A:T>G:C	2 (5.7%)	128 (10.7%)	253 11.1%)
A:T>T:A	2 (5.7%)	87 (7.3%)	140 (6.2%)
G:C>A:T	9 (25.7%)	221 (18.4%)	341 15.0%)
G:C>A:T at CpG	14 (40.0%)	225 (18.8%)	237 (10.4%)
G:C>C:G	0 (0%)	62 (5.2%)	237 (10.4%)
G:C>T:A	4 (11.4%)	238 (19.9%)	671 (29.5%)
Not available	0 (0%)	1 (0.1%)	5 (0.2%)
Total (n)	35 (100%)	1195 (100%)	2270 (100%)

Figure 2. A-C. Mutation pattern of human *TP53*. (n) = number of mutations. (2.A.) *In vitro* acetaldehyde-induced mutations. (2.B.) Esophageal SCC tumours excluding non-drinkers (IARC database). (2.C.) Lung tumours excluding non-smokers (IARC database).

Table 4. Summary of *TP53* mutations observed in red colonies from human fibroblasts exposed to acetaldehyde

(A) Summary of *TP53* mutations in exon 5 to 9 already found in control cells

Number	Exon	Codon	Base change	Amino acid insertion
1 → 6	7-8	262-263	AGT→AGT **AGT**	Pro→Pro Pro

(B) Summary of *TP53* mutations in exon 5 to 9 found only in exposed cells

Number	Exon	Codon	Base change	Amino acid substitution	Nature of mutation
7	5	128	C**C**T→C**T**T	Pro→Leu	Missense
8	5	141	TGC CCT →TG**T** CCC T		Frameshift
9	5	151	C**C**C→C**T**C	Pro→Leu	Missense
10	5	171	GA**G**→GA**T**	Glu→Asp	Missense
11	5	178	C**A**C→C**G**C	His→Arg	Missense
12	5	178	**C**AC→**A**AC	His→Asn	Missense
13	5	178	**C**AC C→ACC		Frameshift
14 → 16	7	245	**G**GC→**A**GC (CpG)	Gly→Ser	Missense
17	7	247	**A**AC→**G**AC	Asn→Asp	Missense
18 → 21	7	248	C**G**G→C**A**G (CpG)	Arg→Gln	Missense
22	7	249	A**G**G→A**A**G	Arg→Lys	Missense
23	7	249	A**G**G→A**A**G	Arg→Lys	Missense
24	8	262	C**C**T→C**T**T	Pro→Leu	Missense
25 → 26	8	267	**C**GG→**T**GG (CpG)	Arg→Trp	Missense
27 → 28	8	273	**C**GT→**T**GT (CpG)	Arg→Cys	Missense
29 → 30	8	278	C**C**T→C**T**T	Pro→Leu	Missense
31 → 33	8	283	C**G**C→C**A**C (CpG)	Arg→His	Missense
34	8	286	**G**AA→**A**AA	Glu→Lys	Missense
35 → 36	8	288	A**A**T→A**T**T	Asn→Ile	Missense
37 → 38	8	298	**G**AG→**T**AG	Glu→Stop	Nonsense
39	8	299	**C**CC CCA G→CCC CAG		Frameshift
40	8	299	C**T**G→C**G**G	Leu→Arg	Missense
41	9	309	**C**CC→**T**CC	Arg→Ser	Missense

AFB_1 epoxide binds preferentially double stranded DNA on guanine within sequences containing G or C rather than A or T [Benasutti, 1988; Misra, 1983; Muench, 1983, Yu, 1990]. This guanine-alkylating is enhanced in highly transcribed areas [Irvin, 1985]. Indeed, Denissenko *et al.* examined adducts localisation in *TP53* exon 7 in HepG2 cells [Denissenko, 1999]. They demonstrated that adducts were located only on guanine residues, mainly within GG sequences and, to a lesser extent, CG or GC sequences. The most targeted codons were 244, 245 and 248, followed by 247, 249 and 250. Moreover, cytosine methylation has been found to greatly enhance guanine alkylation at CpG sites [Chen, 1998]. It should be emphasised that this clearly demonstrates that the high frequency of mutations in codon 249 in HCC was not attributable to a particular reactivity of AFB_1 towards this codon. In our model of normal fibroblasts, we also observed that the codon 249 of *TP53* is not a mutational hotspot for AFB_1. Indeed the codons 244 and 245 were preferred targets for mutations. Moreover, 24 mutations out of 37 (65%) arose from G:C base pairs (21 substitutions, 3 deletions/insertions). Among these 24 mutations, in accordance with adduct studies [Denissenko, 1999], 19 were located within GG sequences and 2 within CG or GC sequences (21 out of 24; 88%). Furthermore, two out of the 3 remaining mutations concerned a guanine within GT sequences, another putative reactive guanine-residue according to Benasutti rules [Benasutti, 1988].

One surprising feature of our spectrum is the high frequency of mutations located on A:T base pairs: 12 substitutions and one deletion out of 37 mutations (35%). This suggests that non- targeted mutations may occur through a translesion synthesis mechanism, as previously described with benzo[a]pyrene-*N2*-dG adducts. Indeed, the Pol eta enzyme is able to misincorporate an erroneous base in front of the adduct or in the 3' position in an acellular system [Rechkoblit, 2002]. To our knowledge, the ability of human translesional polymerases to bypass AFB_1 adducts has never been studied. However, in *E. coli* cells, studies using modified plasmids bearing AFB_1-N7-Gua adducts have shown that a significant proportion of induced mutations were non-targeted mutations located at the 5' side of the adduct [Bailey, 1996]. Another study has shown that the AFB_1-FAPY adduct may also be responsible for non- targeted mutations in *E. coli* [Smela, 2002], some of which relating to A:T base pairs. It is noteworthy that among the 13 mutations we found on A:T base pairs, 11 (85 %) were contiguous to GG or GC sequences. This percentage is very close to that of G:C base pair mutations located in GG or GC sequences: 88%. This strongly suggests that, in accordance with all available literature data on reactivity of AFB_1 epoxide towards different DNA sequences, the vast majority of *TP53* mutations found in our experimental model should be induced by adducts located in GG and GC/CG sequences, A:T base pair mutations being generated by a non-targeted translesion synthesis process.

With our functional assay using normal human cells, we observed an unusually high frequency of G>A transitions. Indeed, Smela *et al.* reported that the G>T transversion was the most frequently observed mutation induced by AFB_1 *in vitro* and *in vivo* [Smela, 2001]. However, two *in vivo* studies have reported that G>A were predominant in *c-Ki-ras* oncogene in rat HCC [Soman, 1993] and in *TP53* lung carcinoma in mice [Tam, 1999]. Two biological processes have been found to affect the G>T / G>A ratio in *TP53* after AFB_1 exposure *in vitro*. Firstly, the methylation of cytosine in CpG sequences enhances G>A transitions [Chan, 2003]. Secondly, the bioactivation of AFB_1 by human CYP1A2 favours G>A transitions on codon 250 in comparison to CYP3A4 [Mace, 1997]. Despite the fact that firstly, the methylation status of *TP53* in our model was unknown and, secondly, we used a double induced rat microsomal fraction allowing the expression of both CYP1A2 and CYP3A, we are unable to conclude on the possible involvement of such processes in our model.

The pattern of mutations of *TP53* in human HCC in high AFB_1 exposure areas is well documented. This pattern shows a high prevalence of G>T transversions (approximately 70% in the IARC database, see fig 1.D), especially on codon 249 which represent around 50% of the total mutations (IARC database). All of the mutations described on codon 249 were G>T transversions. It should be noted, as previously discussed, that codon 249 is not a major site of adduct formation [Denissenko, 1999]. Furthermore, epidemiological studies have suggested that this particular mutation is enhanced by co-infection with hepatotropic viruses such as HBV [Ming, 2002; Shen, 1996]. An *in vitro* study has shown that expression of the HBx viral oncogen in human liver cell lines dramatically increases the prevalence of mutation on codon 249 [Sohn, 2000]. When currently considered, these results are in support of a clonal selection of cells bearing this mutation during HCC carcinogenesis. Consequently, this hot spot appears as the result of a selection bias, which may explain the discrepancy between experimental *in vitro* data using FASAY [Chan, 2003; Sengstag, 1999; this study] and human HCC pattern. Indeed, when the mutations in codon 249 are excluded from the HCC pattern (Fig.1C.), the average of G>T transversions reaches 21%, which is close to our own experimental data (22%). These two spectra are rather similar (Fig.1B. and 1C.), with the exception of the prevalence of the G>C transversion which represents 8% in the HCC pattern and is absent in our experimental pattern.

Acetaldehyde Mutational Pattern

In contrast to AFB_1, mutagenicity of acetaldehyde is poorly documented. Only one previous study described the mutagenic effects of acetaldehyde in human cells, using *HPRT* as reporter gene [Noori, 2001]. That study agreed with our own in showing that the most frequent mutation was G:C>A:T transition (47% for *HPRT* and 66% for *TP53*). However, the location on CpG-sites was more prevalent in *TP53*. This discrepancy could be partly explained by the different percentage of CpG sites between *HPRT* and *TP53*. In fact, they represent 1.1% in *HPRT* and 3.7% in *TP53*. The second most frequently found mutations in our work are G:C>T:A (11%), the other mutations being present on A:T bases pairs or corresponding to deletions or insertions. We found more than 75% of our mutations on G:C base pairs, suggesting a preferential location of acetaldehyde-induced damage on guanine. The formation of DNA adducts produced by acetaldehyde has been widely studied. The major adduct produced is *N2*-ethylidene-dG; however, condensation of acetaldehyde could lead to more complex adducts such as *N2*-propano-dG, exocyclic dG adducts or interstrand cross links (ICL) between two opposite dG in CpG sequences [Hecht, 2001; Stein, 2006]. Furthermore, it has been demonstrated that ICL are formed only in the 5'- CpG -3', not in the 5'- GpC -3' sequence [Lao, 2005]. Although acetaldehyde could react with dA and dC at the nucleoside level [Vaca, 1995], the vast majority of DNA adducts target dG. This fact could explain why these genetic alterations occur mainly on G:C base pairs, as shown on different human genes such as *TP53* (this study) and *HPRT* [Noori, 2001].

The mutagenicity of various acetaldehyde adducts has been studied using chemically modified plasmids. Whether the major *N2*-ethylidene-dG adduct is mutagenic is questionable, many studies showing efficient repair in mammalian cells [Brooks, 2005]. However, exocyclic adducts have been proved to be mutagenic in human cells, leading to G>T, G>A and, to a lesser extent, G>C mutations [Stein, 2006]. We did not observe G>C transversion in the *TP53* gene, but G>T and G>A mutations together accounted for 75% of the mutations found. Interestingly, these kinds of mutations have been linked to the polymerases involved in translesion synthesis, Pol iota inducing G>A transition and Pol eta G>T transversion [Yang, 2003]. Studies with the chemically stable ICL of acetaldehyde occurring in CpG sequences showed that both G>T and G>A mutations are induced [Liu, 2006]. It should be emphasized that 16 out of the 35 mutations we found (46 %) are G>A or G>T mutations located in CpG sequences. Furthermore, in accordance with the sequence specificity of ICL on CpG, and not in GpC sequences as previously stated [Lao, 2005], we did not observe any G>A transition in GpC sequences. Taken together, these results strongly suggest that acetaldehyde exerts a mutagenic effect in human cells mainly through ICL. In summary, our results are in accordance with predicted mutations using chemically modified plasmids. Indeed, G>A transitions found in CpG sequences of *TP53,* which are classically linked to the spontaneous deamination of 5-methylcytosine, could also be ascribed to acetaldehyde ICL in alcohol-related tumours.

As previously stated, the main interest of the FASAY is to allow comparison of mutational patterns with those found in human tumours. So, we have compared mutations induced by acetaldehyde to those observed on squamous cell carcinoma of the esophagus, excluding non-drinkers (IARC database: 1195 referenced mutations) (Fig. 2.B.). However, as the mutational spectrum described in esophageal SCC results from multiple exposure to tobacco and alcohol [Launoy, 1997; Tuyns, 1977], we have also displayed the mutational spectrum of *TP53* in lung cancers, excluding non-smokers (2270 referenced mutations) in order to delineate mutations induced by these two etiological factors (Fig. 2.C.). In all three mutational spectra G:C>A:T and G:C>T:A are the two most observed mutations (Fig. 2.). Even if there are some similarities between these spectra, some major differences can be highlighted and explained. Firstly, we found a much greater percentage of G:C>A:T (66%) than in esophageal SCC in drinkers (37%) and also than in smokers lung cancers (25%). At the same time, we found less G:C>T:A transitions (11%), a mutation classically ascribed to B[a]P in tobacco smoke, than in esophageal SCC in drinkers (20%) and also than in smokers lung cancers (30%). These differences suggest that the G>A and G>T mutations found in esophageal SCC in drinkers are linked to both alcohol and tobacco exposure. These results suggest also that the excess of G:C>A:T in esophageal compared to lung cancers may be explained by alcohol exposure leading to acetaldehyde production. Another main difference can be noted on G:C>C:G. We did not find this kind of mutation at all, whereas it accounts for 5% of mutations in esophageal SCC, and 10% in lung cancers in smokers. Furthermore, a comparison of these mutations has shown a higher prevalence in smokers than in non-smokers [Hernandez-Boussard, 1998]. Together, these observations strongly suggest that G:C>C:G mutations are linked to tobacco exposure rather than to alcohol.

We have also compared the position of acetaldehyde-induced mutations (35 mutations distributed on 19 codons) with the IARC database. In order to be close to alcohol exposure only, we have selected mutations from oesophageal SCC by including non-smokers and excluding non-drinkers (54 referenced mutations distributed on 40 codons). In our study, about half of the mutations in the acetaldehyde pattern (16/35) are localized on codons already mutated in such tumours. Furthermore, codons 245, 248, 273 and 286, which are hyper-mutated in esophageal SCC in drinkers and non-smokers, represent nearly 29% (10/35) of all acetaldehyde-induced mutations. These data show the ability of FASAY to recover tumour hot-spots, although no selection of mutated cells occurs during the assay.

It should also be emphasised that the mutational patterns found after acetaldehyde and AFB_1 exposure are quite different, acetaldehyde inducing twice as many G>A transitions and 3 times less G>A transitions than AFB_1. The location of mutations is also different: main mutated codons being 178, 245, 248 and 283 after acetaldehyde exposure and 179, 220 and 245 after AFB_1 exposure. Codon 245, a major hot spot in human tumours, was found to be the only shared codon in the two spectra. This highlights the ability of FASAY to qualitatively discriminate mutagens.

Conclusion

In conclusion, the mutational pattern of human fibroblasts exposed to AFB_1 is in well accordance with adducts location data. Although it appears different from the mutational pattern of human HCC, the discrepancy is highly reduced if mutations located on the 249 codon are excluded. When considered concurrently, these results reinforce other studies which have suggested that G>T transversions on codon 249 were likely the result of a selection bias in human HCC rather than a true fingerprint of AFB_1 adducts. Furthermore, our *in vitro* spectrum is quite similar to that identified in AFB_1-induced lung tumours in mice. Indeed, AFB_1 is a pulmonary carcinogen among animals [Donnely, 1996a], a pneumotoxic among humans [Donnely, 1996b], and it has also been suggested that AFB_1 could be a human lung carcinogen among occupationally exposed workers [Hayes, 1984]. Our results on human fibroblasts suggest that it may be interesting to study the mutagenicity of AFB_1 in human pulmonary cells by using FASAY.

Results obtained with acetaldehyde are in accordance with predicted mutations found in the literature. Indeed, we have found a high frequency of G:C>A:T and G:C>T:A, in CpG sequences of *TP53*. These mutations, which are classically linked to the spontaneous deamination of 5-methylcytosine, could also be ascribed to acetaldehyde-induced ICL in alcohol-related tumours. Furthermore, we showed that the *in vitro* mutational pattern of acetaldehyde looks like those found in human alcohol-related tumours such as esophageal SCC. Taken together, these results strongly suggest that that alcohol acts as a true genotoxin in head and neck and oesophageal tumours through acetaldehyde production [Paget, 2008a]. This present study gives a strong biological plausibility to epidemiological studies which have definitively shown that alcohol acts as a non threshold carcinogen in such cancers [Baan, 2007].

Finally, the ability of FASAY to study different biological materials including either normal and cancerous differentiated cells, or cancer stem cells, offers the exciting perspectives to study mutational patterns in order to improve our knowledge of human chemical carcinogenesis.

Acknowledgments

The authors thank J.M. Flaman (INSERM U614, Université de Rouen, France) and J. Cachot (LEMA, Université du Havre, France) for their assistance and advice in FASAY and for the gift of yeast strain and vectors, G. Abéguillé and M. Duval for their technical assistance in DNA sequencing and Pr K. Meflah, director of the Centre de Lutte Contre le Cancer François Baclesse, for his support. V. Paget is a recipient of a fellowship from the Ligue Nationale Contre le Cancer, Comité de l'Orne. Research was supported by grants from the Ligue Nationale Contre le Cancer, Comité de l'Orne.

References

Aguilar F., Hussain S.P., Cerutti P. (1993) Aflatoxin B_1 induces the transversion of G-->T in codon 249 of the p53 tumor suppressor gene in human hepatocytes, *Proc. Natl. Acad. Sci. U.S.A.*, 90, 8586-8590.

Baan R., Straif K., Grosse Y., Secretan B., El Ghissassi F., Bouvard V. *et al.* (2007) *Lancet Oncol.*, 8, 292-293.

Bailey E.A., Iyer R.S., Stone M.P., Harris T.M., Essigmann J.M. (1996) Mutational properties of the primary aflatoxin B_1-DNA adduct, *Proc. Natl. Acad. Sci. U.S.A.*, 93, 1535-1539.

Barnes S.L., Singletary K.W., Frey R. (2000) Ethanol and acetaldehyde enhance benzo[a]pyrene-DNA adduct formation in human mammary epithelial cells, *Carcinogenesis*, 21, 2123-2128.

Benasutti M., Ejadi S., Whitlow M.D., Loechler E.L. (1988) Mapping the binding site of aflatoxin B_1 in DNA: systematic analysis of the reactivity of aflatoxin B_1 with guanines in different DNA sequences, *Biochemistry*, 27, 472-481.

Billet S., Paget V., Garçon G., Heutte N., André V., Shirali P., Sichel F. (2010) Benzene-induced mutational pattern in the tumour suppressor gene TP53 analysed by use of a functional assay, the functional analysis of separated alleles in yeast, in human lung cells. *Arch. Toxicol.*, 84, 99-107.

Bitton A., Neuman M.D., Barnoya J, Glantz S.A. (2005) The p53 tumour suppressor gene and the tobacco industry: research, debate, and conflict of interest. *Lancet*, 365, 531-540.

Boffetta P., Hashibe M. (2006a) Alcohol and cancer, *Lancet Oncol.*, 7, 149-156.

Boffetta P., Hashibe M., La Vecchia C., Zatonski W., Rehm J. (2006b) The burden of cancer attributable to alcohol drinking, *Int. J. Cancer*, 119, 884-887.

Bressac B., Kew M., Wands J., Ozturk M. (1991) Selective G to T mutations of p53 gene in hepatocellular carcinoma from southern Africa, *Nature*, 350, 429-431.

Brooks P.J., Theruvathu J.A. (2005) DNA adducts from acetaldehyde: implications for alcohol-related carcinogenesis, *Alcohol*, 35, 187-193.

Chan K.T., Hsieh D.P., Lung M.L. (2003) In vitro aflatoxin B_1-induced p53 mutations, *Cancer Lett.*, 199, 1-7.

Chang F., Syrjanen S., Tervahauta A., Syrjanen K. (1993) Tumourigenesis associated with the p53 tumour suppressor gene, *Br. J. Cancer*, 68, 653-661.

Chen J.X., Zheng Y., West M., Tang M. (1998) Carcinogens preferentially bind at methylated CpG in the p53 mutational hot spots, *Cancer Res.*, 58, 2070-2075.

Dearth L.R., Qian H., Wang T., Baroni T.E., Zeng J., Chen S.W. *et al.* (2007) Inactive full-length p53 mutants lacking dominant wild-type p53 inhibition highlight loss of heterozygosity as an important aspect of p53 status in human cancers. *Carcinogenesis*, 28, 289-298.

Denissenko M.F., Cahill J., Koudriakova T.B., Gerber N., Pfeifer G.P. (1999) Quantitation and mapping of aflatoxin B_1-induced DNA damage in genomic DNA using aflatoxin B1-8,9-epoxide and microsomal activation systems, *Mutat. Res.*, 425, 205-211.

Donnelly P.J., Devereux T.R., Foley J.F., Maronpot R.R., Anderson M.W., Massey T.E. (1996a) Activation of K-ras in aflatoxin B_1-induced lung tumors from AC3F1 (A/J x C3H/HeJ) mice, *Carcinogenesis*, 17, 1735-1740.

Donnelly P.J., Stewart R.K., Ali S.L., Conlan A.A., Reid K.R., Petsikas D., Massey T.E. (1996b) Biotransformation of aflatoxin B_1 in human lung, *Carcinogenesis*, 17, 2487-2494.

Dvorackova I. (1976) Aflatoxin inhalation and alveolar cell carcinoma, *Br. Med. J.*, 1, 691.

Essigmann J.M., Croy R.G., Nadzan A.M., Busby Jr. W.F., Reinhold V.N., Buchi G., Wogan G.N. (1977) Structural identification of the major DNA adduct formed by aflatoxin B_1 in vitro, *Proc Natl. Acad. Sci. U.S.A.*, 74, 1870-1874.

Flaman J.M., Frebourg T., Moreau V., Charbonnier F., Martin C., Chappuis P., Sappino A.P., Limacher I.M., Bron L., Benhattar J. (1995) A simple p53 functional assay for screening cell lines, blood, and tumors, *Proc. Natl. Acad. Sci. U.S.A.*, 92, 3963-3967.

Garon D., Richard E., Sage L., Bouchart V., Pottier D., Lebailly P. (2006) Mycoflora and multimycotoxin detection in corn silage: experimental study, *J. Agric. Food Chem.*, 54, 3479-3484.

Green D.R., Chipuk J.E. (2006) p53 and metabolism: Inside the TIGAR, *Cell*, 126, 30-32.

Hassan A.M., Sheashaa H.A., Abdel Fatah M.F., Ibrahim A.Z., Gaber O.A. (2006) Does aflatoxin as an environmental mycotoxin adversely affect the renal and hepatic functions of Egyptian lactating mothers and their infants? A preliminary report, *Int. Urol. Nephrol.*, 38, 339-342.

Hayes R.B., van Nieuwenhuize J.P., Raatgever J.W., ten Kate F.J. (1984) Aflatoxin exposures in the industrial setting: an epidemiological study of mortality, Food Chem. *Toxicol.*, 22, 39-43.

He X.Y., Tang L., Wang S.L., Cai Q.S., Wang J.S., Hong J.Y. (2006) Efficient activation of aflatoxin B_1 by cytochrome P450 2A13, an enzyme predominantly expressed in human respiratory tract, *Int. J. Cancer*, 118, 2665-2671.

Hecht S.S., McIntee E.J., Wang M. (2001) New DNA adducts of crotonaldehyde and acetaldehyde, Toxicology, 166, 31-36.

Hernandez-Boussard T.M., Hainaut P. (1998) A specific spectrum of p53 mutations in lung cancer from smokers: review of mutations compiled in the IARC p53 database, *Environ. Health Perspect.*, 106, 385-391.

Homann N., Jousimies-Somer H., Jokelainen K., Heine R., Salaspuro M. (1997) High acetaldehyde levels in saliva after ethanol consumption: methodological aspects and pathogenetic implications, *Carcinogenesis*, 18, 1739-1743.

Homann N., Tillonen J., Meurman J.H., Rintamaki H., Lindqvist C., Rautio M., Jousimies-Somer H., Salaspuro M. (2000) Increased salivary acetaldehyde levels in heavy drinkers and smokers: a microbiological approach to oral cavity cancer, *Carcinogenesis*, 21, 663-668.

Homann N., Tillonen J., Rintamaki H., Salaspuro M., Lindqvist C., Meurman J.H. (2001) Poor dental status increases acetaldehyde production from ethanol in saliva: a possible link to increased oral cancer risk among heavy drinkers, *Oral Oncol.*, 37, 153-158.

Hsu I.C., Metcalf R.A., Sun T., Welsh J.A., Wang N.J., Harris C.C. (1991) Mutational hotspot in the p53 gene in human hepatocellular carcinomas, *Nature*, 350, 427-428.

Hussain S.P., Harris C.C. (1998) Molecular epidemiology of human cancer: contribution of mutation spectra studies of tumor suppressor genes, *Cancer Res.*, 58, 4023-4037.

Hussain S.P., Harris C.C. (2000) Molecular epidemiology and carcinogenesis: endogenous and exogenous carcinogens, *Mutat. Res.*, 462, 311-322.

Hussain S.P., Schwank J., Staib F., Wang X.W., Harris C.C. (2007) TP53 mutations and hepatocellular carcinoma: insights into the etiology and pathogenesis of liver cancer, *Oncogene*, 26, 2166-2176.

IARC (1988) Alcohol drinking. IARC Working Group, Lyon, 13-20 October 1987, IARC Monogr. *Eval. Carcinog. Risks Hum.*, 44, 1-378.

Irvin T.R., Wogan G.N. (1985) Quantitative and qualitative characterization of aflatoxin B_1 adducts formed in vivo within the ribosomal RNA genes of rat liver DNA, *Cancer Res.*, 45, 3497-3502.

Ishioka C., Frebourg T., Yan Y.X., Vidal M., Friend S.H., Schmidt S., Iggo R. (1993) Screening patients for heterozygous p53 mutations using a functional assay in yeast, *Nat. Genet.*, 5, 124-129.

Lao Y., Hecht S.S. (2005) Synthesis and properties of an acetaldehyde-derived oligonucleotide interstrand cross-link, *Chem. Res. Toxicol.*, 18, 711-721.

Launoy G., Milan C.H., Faivre J., Pienkowski P., Milan C.I., Gignoux M. (1997) Alcohol, tobacco and oesophageal cancer: effects of the duration of consumption, mean intake and current and former consumption. *Br. J. Cancer*, 75, 1389-1396.

Lechevrel M., Casson A.G., Wolf C.R., Hardie L.J., Flinterman M.B., Montesano R., Wild C.P. (1999) Characterization of cytochrome P450 expression in human oesophageal mucosa. *Carcinogenesis* 20, 243-248.

Liu X., Lao Y., Yang I.Y., Hecht S.S., Moriya M. (2006) Replication-coupled repair of crotonaldehyde/acetaldehyde-induced guanine-guanine interstrand cross-links and their mutagenicity, *Biochemistry*, 45, 12898-12905.

Mace K., Aguilar F., Wang J.S., Vautravers P., Gomez-Lechon M., Gonzalez F.J., Groopman J., Harris C.C., Pfeifer A.M. (1997) Aflatoxin B_1-induced DNA adduct formation and p53 mutations in CYP450-expressing human liver cell lines, *Carcinogenesis*, 18, 1291-1297.

Maron D.M., Ames B.N. (1983) Revised methods for the Salmonella mutagenicity test, *Mutat. Res.*, 113, 173-215.

Massey T.E., Smith G.B., Tam A.S. (2000) Mechanisms of aflatoxin B_1 lung tumorigenesis, *Exp. Lung Res.*, 26, 673-683.

May P., May E. (1999) Twenty years of p53 research: structural and functional aspects of the p53 protein, *Oncogene*, 18, 7621-7636.

Menendez D., Inga A., Jordan J.J., Resnick M.A. (2007) Changing the p53 master regulatory network: Elementary, my dear Mr Watson, *Oncogene*, 26, 2191-2201.

Ming L., Thorgeirsson S.S., Gail M.H., Lu P., Harris C.C., Wang N., Shao Y., Wu Z., Liu G., Wang X., Sun Z. (2002) Dominant role of hepatitis B virus and cofactor role of aflatoxin in hepatocarcinogenesis in Qidong, China, *Hepatology*, 36, 1214-1220.

Misra R.P., Muench K.F., Humayun M.Z. (1983) Covalent and noncovalent interactions of aflatoxin with defined deoxyribonucleic acid sequences, *Biochemistry*, 22, 3351-3359.

Muench K.F., Misra R.P., Humayun M.Z. (1983) Sequence specificity in aflatoxin B_1--DNA interactions, *Proc. Natl. Acad. Sci. U.S.A.*, 80, 6-10.

Muto M., Hitomi Y., Ohtsu A., Shimada H., Kashiwase Y., Sasaki H., Yoshida S., Esumi H. (2000) Acetaldehyde production by non-pathogenic Neisseria in human oral microflora: implications for carcinogenesis in upper aerodigestive tract, *Int. J. Cancer*, 88, 342-350.

Noori P., Hou S.M. (2001) Mutational spectrum induced by acetaldehyde in the HPRT gene of human T lymphocytes resembles that in the p53 gene of esophageal cancers, *Carcinogenesis*, 22, 1825-1830.

Olivier M., Eeles R., Hollstein M., Khan M.A., Harris C.C., Hainaut P. (2002) The IARC TP53 database: new online mutation analysis and recommendations to users. *Hum. Mutat.*, 19, 607-614.

Onyemelukwe G.C., Ogbadu G. (1981) Aflatoxin levels in sera of health first time rural blood Hassan A.M., Sheashaa H.A., Abdel Fatah M.F., Ibrahim A.Z., Gaber O.A. (2006) Does aflatoxin as an environmental mycotoxin adversely affect the renal and hepatic functions of Egyptian lactating mothers and their infants? A preliminary report, *Int. Urol. Nephrol.*, 38, 339-342.

Paget V., Lechevrel M., Sichel F. (2008a) Acetaldehyde-induced mutational pattern in the tumour suppressor gene TP53 analysed by use of a functional assay, the FASAY (functional analysis of separated alleles in yeast), *Mutat. Res.*, 652, 12-19.

Paget V., Sichel F., Garon D., Lechevrel M. (2008b) Aflatoxin B1-induced TP53 mutational pattern in normal human cells using the FASAY (Functional Analysis of Separated Alleles in Yeast). *Mutat. Res.*, 656, 55-61.

Pfeifer G.P., Denissenko M.F., Olivier M., Tretyakova N., Hecht S.S., Hainaut P. (2002) Tobacco smoke carcinogens, DNA damage and p53 mutations in smoking-associated cancers, *Oncogene*, 21, 7435-7451.

Platel A., Nesslany F., Gervais V., Marzin D. (2009) Study of oxidative DNA damage in TK6 human lymphoblastoid cells by use of the in vitro micronucleus test: Determination of No-Observed-Effect Levels. *Mutat Res.*, 678, 30-37.

Poschl G., Stickel F., Wang X.D., Seitz H.K. (2004a) Alcohol and cancer: genetic and nutritional aspects, *Proc. Nutr. Soc.*, 63, 65-71.

Poschl G., Seitz H.K. (2004b) Alcohol and cancer, Alcohol Alcohol. 39 155-165.

Quertemont E. (2004) Genetic polymorphism in ethanol metabolism: acetaldehyde contribution to alcohol abuse and alcoholism, Mol. *Psychiatry*, 9, 570-581.

Rechkoblit O., Zhang Y., Guo D., Wang Z., Amin S., Krzeminsky J., Louneva N., Geacintov N.E. (2002) trans-Lesion synthesis past bulky benzo[a]pyrene diol epoxide N2-dG and N6-dA lesions catalyzed by DNA bypass polymerases, *J. Biol. Chem.*, 277, 30488-30494.

Rehm J., Room R., Monteiro M., Gmel G., Graham K., Rehn N., Sempos C.T., Jernigan D. (2003) Alcohol as a risk factor for global burden of disease, *Eur. Addict. Res.*, 9, 157-164.

Room R., Graham K., Rehm J., Jernigan D., Monteiro M. (2003) Drinking and its burden in a global perspective: policy considerations and options, *Eur. Addict. Res.*, 9, 165-175.

Salaspuro V., Salaspuro M. (2004) Synergistic effect of alcohol drinking and smoking on in vivo acetaldehyde concentration in saliva, *Int. J. Cancer*, 111, 480-483.

Scudiero D.A., Shoemaker R.H., Paull K.D., Monks A., Tierney S., Nofziger T.H., Currens M.J., Seniff D., Boyd M.R. (1988) Evaluation of a soluble tetrazolium/formazan assay for cell growth and drug sensitivity in culture using human and other tumor cell lines, *Cancer Res.*, 48, 4827-4833.

Seitz H.K., Stickel F. (2007) Molecular mechanisms of alcohol-mediated carcinogenesis, *Nat. Rev. Cancer*, 7, 599-612.

Sengstag C., Morbe J.L., Weibel B. (1999) Codon 249 of the human TP53 tumor suppressor gene is no hot spot for aflatoxin B_1 in a heterologous background, *Mutat. Res.*, 430, 131-144.

Shen H.M., Ong C.N. (1996) Mutations of the p53 tumor suppressor gene and ras oncogenes in aflatoxin hepatocarcinogenesis, *Mutat. Res.*, 366, 23-44.

Singh N.P., Khan A. (1995) Acetaldehyde: genotoxicity and cytotoxicity in human lymphocytes, *Mutat. Res.*, 337, 9-17.

Smela M.E., Currier S.S., Bailey E.A., Essigmann J.M. (2001) The chemistry and biology of aflatoxin B(1): from mutational spectrometry to carcinogenesis, *Carcinogenesis*, 22, 535-545.

Smela M.E., Hamm M.L., Henderson P.T., Harris C.M., Harris T.M., Essigmann J.M. (2002) The aflatoxin B(1) formamidopyrimidine adduct plays a major role in causing the types of mutations observed in human hepatocellular carcinoma, *Proc. Natl. Acad. Sci. U.S.A.*, 99, 6655-6660.

Sohn S., Jaitovitch-Groisman I., Benlimame N., Galipeau J., Batist G., Alaoui-Jamali M.A. (2000) Retroviral expression of the hepatitis B virus x gene promotes liver cell susceptibility to carcinogen-induced site specific mutagenesis, *Mutat. Res.,* 460, 17-28.

Soman N.R., Wogan G.N. (1993) Activation of the c-Ki-ras oncogene in aflatoxin B_1-induced hepatocellular carcinoma and adenoma in the rat: detection by denaturing gradient gel electrophoresis, *Proc. Natl. Acad. Sci. U.S.A.*, 90, 2045-2049.

Soussi T. (2007) p53 alterations in human cancer: more questions than answers, *Oncogene*, 26, 2145-2156.

Stein S., Lao Y., Yang I.Y., Hecht S.S., Moriya M. (2006) Genotoxicity of acetaldehyde- and crotonaldehyde-induced 1,N(2)-propanodeoxyguanosine DNA adducts in human cells, *Mutat. Res.*, 608, 1-7.

Tam A.S., Foley J.F., Devereux T.R., Maronpot R.R., Massey T.E. (1999) High frequency and heterogeneous distribution of p53 mutations in aflatoxin B_1-induced mouse lung tumors, *Cancer Res.*, 59, 3634-3640.

Tuyns A.J., Pequignot G., Jensen O.M. (1977) [Esophageal cancer in Ille-et-Vilaine in relation to levels of alcohol and tobacco consumption. Risks are multiplying], *Bull. Cancer*, 64, 45-60.

Vaca C.E., Fang J.L., Schweda E.K. (1995) Studies of the reaction of acetaldehyde with deoxynucleosides, *Chem. Biol. Interact.*, 98, 51-67.

Yang I.Y., Miller H., Wang Z., Frank E.G., Ohmori H., Hanaoka F., Moriya M. (2003) Mammalian translesion DNA synthesis across an acrolein-derived deoxyguanosine adduct. Participation of DNA polymerase eta in error-prone synthesis in human cells, *J. Biol. Chem.*, 278, 13989-13994.

Yokoyama A., Omori T. (2003) Genetic polymorphisms of alcohol and aldehyde dehydrogenases and risk for esophageal and head and neck cancers, *Jpn. J. Clin. Oncol.*, 33, 111-121.

Yu F.L., Bender W., Geronimo I.H. (1990) Base and sequence specificities of aflatoxin B_1 binding to single- and double-stranded DNAs, *Carcinogenesis*, 11, 475-478.

In: Tumor Suppressors
Editor: Susan D. Nguyen

ISBN: 978-1-61761-986-1

Chapter 2

Curative Therapy for Terminal Cancer?

Doug Dix
Department of Health Science
University of Hartford
West Hartford, CT 06117, USA

Summary

Diets deficient in folic acid or thiamin or even one essential amino acid will stop tumor growth. The side effects can be tolerated when mild, or treated with small replacement doses of the missing nutrient. The difference in blood perfusion between tumors and normal tissue will carry replacement nutrients preferentially to normal tissue. Diets deficient in ascorbic acid, vitamin B12, niacin, pyridoxine, choline, or essential fatty acids may also be selectively toxic to tumors. Inositol, glucose, and selenium or cysteine in dietary excess or deficiency, and moderate doses of vitamin D, might also be beneficial. Hyperthermia, exercise, herbal teas, resveratrol, and the visualization of tumor destruction may enhance the benefits of nutrient manipulation. Undernutrition may reverse tumor resistance to conventional chemotherapy, which should be revaluated following a duration of nutrient manipulation. Together, reasonable, convenient, inexpensive interventions against terminal cancer constitute the perfect placebo, empowering terminal patients with legitimate hope for remission or cure.

Problem

When curative therapy has run its course and failed, patients are left with two options: palliative care or unconventional medicine. The former can extinguish hope, and, in that way, aggravate anxiety, pain, nausea, and depression [1]. The latter can be burdensome, expensive, and futile or harmful [2]. There's a clear need for a third option, one that supports legitimate hope for remission while being convenient, inexpensive, and safe. Manipulation of critical nutrients can fill this need.

Approach to a Solution

Tumors are poorly vascularized [3]. This is one reason chemotherapy fails. Cytotoxic drugs only trickle into tumors while pouring into normal tissue [4]. Dietary deprivation of essential nutrients, e.g., vitamins and amino acids, turns this table to therapeutic advantage, as replacement doses will only trickle into tumors while rescuing normal tissue [5-6].

It's natural to want to test this theory in animals before recommending it to patients, but animals differ from humans in nutrient requirements and metabolism [7]. And animals aren't capable of a placebo effect. What's needed as the third option is the perfect placebo. Nutrient manipulation is that because it makes sense but hasn't been tested. Physicians can be honest [8]. And most patients want honesty [9]. Nutrient manipulation might work. There's reason to hope. And because this approach hasn't been tested, there are no thorny issues of inefficacy. Because nutrient manipulation is convenient, inexpensive, and relatively safe, it will do little harm. And terminal patients have little to lose.

Curative therapy begins with education. Terminal patients must be taught that tumors are dangerous because they grow, and that growth depends on cell division, which requires DNA replication, and protein and lipid synthesis. Cells must double their biomass in order to divide. Most normal cells are not engaged in cell division. They're not replicating DNA, and are less dependent on protein and lipid synthesis than dividing cells. Normal cells that are engaged in division, e.g., bone marrow and gastrointestinal epithelium, can be halted for a time without threatening the host. It's reasonable, therefore, to expect inhibition of cell division to be selectively toxic to tumors. This is the rationale for conventional cytotoxic chemotherapy. The fact that such therapy can cure advanced leukemia and testicular cancer validates the rationale.

Advanced cancer is labeled "terminal" when it becomes resistant to chemotherapy. It does this by evolving mechanisms to hide from or destroy cytotoxic drugs. Nutrient manipulation is unlike cytoxic chemotherapy because it cannot be resisted. Without key nutrients, cells cannot make DNA, protein, or lipid, and cell division is impossible. This is how nutrient manipulation can cure terminal cancer.

Water-Soluble Vitamins

Vitamins are organic chemicals, which in trace amounts are essential to survival but cannot be made by the body. They must be ingested. Some are water-soluble, i.e., they're not stored in the body and can be washed out of food before ingestion. And some of these are essential to cell division.

Without folic acid, cells can't make purines or thymidylic acid. Without thiamin they can't make ribose or deoxyribose. Without these precursors, cells can't make DNA or RNA. Without RNA, cells can't make protein. Without DNA and protein, cells can't divide. And tumor cells that can't divide aren't dangerous.

Diets devoid of these vitamins will stop tumors in their tracks. It's textbook biochemistry, as are the side effects of anemia and beriberi. These side effects can be tolerated when mild. But the beauty of the approach comes from the theoretical ability to selectively rescue normal cells with small replacement doses of the missing vitamins.

The poor perfusion that protects tumors from cytotoxic drugs will thwart access to small replacement doses of vitamins. The success of high dose methotrexate therapy with leukovorin rescue can be explained in part by analogy [10-11]. More methotrexate gets into the tumor because of the high dose, but less leukovorin gets into the tumor than into normal tissue because of the perfusion difference between tumors and normal tissue.

A palatable diet for achieving folic acid deficiency has been published [12]. Diets based on polished rice are famous for inducing thiamin deficiency [13]. Almost any food can be rendered free of all water-soluble vitamins by shredding and boiling it repeatedly in large volumes of water. The resulting mash is unappetizing. It can be improved by baking, broiling, frying, or toasting, and flavored with sugar, starch, salt, vinegar, alcohol, water-soluble-vitamin-free oils and fats, as well as artificial ingredients. Non-targeted water-soluble vitamins and minerals must be replaced as supplements.

Other water-soluble vitamins that are essential to proliferating cells include ascorbic acid, vitamin B12, niacin, pyridoxine, biotin, choline, and inositol. These vitamins can be removed by the method described above, i.e., shredding all food and boiling it repeatedly in large volumes of water. Vitamin B12 is naturally absent from plant foods. Removal of ascorbic acid will lead to scurvy, of vitamin B12 to pernicious anemia and subtle nerve damage, of niacin to pellagra, of pyridoxine to lymphopenia, seborrheic dermatitis, and peripheral neuropathy, of choline to fatty liver and changes in blood lipids, and of inositol to alopecia and eczema.

Ascorbic acid protects folate reductase, which catalyzes the generation of tetrahydrofolic acid, which, in its methenyl and formyl forms, is necessary for purine and thymidylic acid synthesis. Vitamin B12 recycles tetrahydrofolic acid. In the absence of vitamin B12, tetrahydrofolic acid is trapped in a methyl form that prevents purine and thymidylic acid synthesis. Proliferating cells require biomass and need NADH and NADPH to make it [14]. Without NADPH, cells can't make ribose, deoxyribose, or free fatty acids. This deficiency precludes synthesis of nucleic acids and membranes. Because proliferating cells make more proteins than normal cells, they're more dependent on amino acid transamination, transulfuration, and decarboxylation, and the vitamin necessary for those reactions, pyridoxine. Diets deficient in pyridoxine might be selectively toxic to tumors [15]. Pyridoxine deficiency might be particularly effective against lymphocytic leukemia, as lymphopenia is a symptom of pyridoxine deficiency.

Dividing cells must double their lipid content, and require biotin and NADPH to make the necessary free fatty acids. Biotin deficiency precludes lipid synthesis, and might be selectively toxic to tumors. Biotin is also required for purine synthesis. But biotin deficiency cannot easily be achieved by removing biotin from food because normal intestinal flora produce biotin. Consumption of the raw egg-white protein, avidin, can cause biotin deficiency, but raw eggs are a source of Salmonella, which is particularly dangerous to terminal cancer patients. Heating eggs to kill Salmonella destroys avidin. Perhaps a method can be developed for killing Salmonella in eggs, e.g., by ionizing radiation, while sparing avidin. Or perhaps eggs can be screened for Salmonella to identify those that could be safely consumed raw. Or perhaps avidin can be obtained from some other safe source. Without safe avidin, however, biotin deficiency is an impractical, although tantalizing, weapon.

Pyridoxine deficiency might mimic some of the effects of biotin deficiency, as pyridoxine is required in the first step of sphingosine synthesis. Without pyridoxine, ceramides cannot be made. These N-acyl sphingosine derivatives function as membrane components and powerful signaling molecules. Some ceramides enhance hypoxic injury, while others inhibit it [16]. Cancer cells are resistant to hypoxic injury [17]. Disturbing their ability to make ceremides might make them less so.

Two other water-soluble vitamins have less clearly defined roles and toxicities, but may be worthy of exploration. Choline is a component of phospholipids [lecithins] that function in membranes and mediate mitogenic signals. It is an essential nutrient for humans [18]. Metabolites of choline are found in higher concentration in breast cancer than in benign breast lesions or normal breast tissue [19]. Choline will be removed from food by repeated shredding and boiling, as described above, but diets deficient in choline have been described [20-21]. Choline deficiency might be particularly effective against lymphocytic leukemia because it has been linked to increased lymphocyte apoptosis [22].

Inositol is an essential nutrient that has the potential to be selectively toxic to tumors in excess [23] or deficiency [24]. Inositol is a component of a large variety of important signaling lipids [25-26]. Alternating pulses of inositol excess and deficiency might be worthy of exploration. The consequence of inositol deficiency is alopecia and eczema.

Essential Amino Acids

Dietary proteins deficient in one or more essential amino acids [leucine, isoleucine, valine, phenylalanine, tryptophan, threonine, lysine, and methionine] are well known [27]. Rice, wheat, and corn are deficient in lysine. Corn is also deficient in tryptophan. Legumes [beans, soybeans, peas, lentils, and peanuts] are deficient in methionine, but rich in lysine. Prepared diets for treating phenylketoneuria [PKU] are deficient in phenylalanine. Prepared diets for treating maple syrup urine disease are deficient in leucine, isoleucine, and valine. Essential amino acid deficiency will cause protein malnutrition, which can be tolerated for a time, and then relieved by addition of the missing essential amino acid.

Essential Fatty Acids

Water-insoluble vitamins are not directly linked to cell proliferation, but essential fatty acids are worthy of consideration as anti-tumor agents. Linoleic, linolenic, and aracidonic acids are polyunsaturated fatty acids that are required in trace amounts in the diet. They function as membrane components and precursors of prostaglandins and can be deficient in popular low-fat diets. The popular trend to replace polyunsaturated with monounsaturated fats and to use commercial fat substitutes aggravates the risk of essential fatty acid deficiency [28]. Depleting arachidonic acid from the diet is a means of reducing prostaglandins and thromboxanes. Asprin is another means to this end as it inhibits conversion of arachidonic acid to prostaglandins. Anecdotal evidence [but not controlled clinical trial] suggests that asprin can prevent some cancers [29]. The conspicuous consequence of essential fatty acid deficiency is dermatitis, which can be tolerated for a time, and then relieved by addition of polyunsaturated oil to the diet.

Activation of the blood coagulation pathway is essential to metastasis, and thromboxanes are components of that pathway. Anticoagulants prolong survival in cancer patients [30]. Perhaps essential fatty acid deficeincy, will do the same.

Synergy

Inhibition of two sequential steps in a biochemical pathway can, on occasion, yield synergy, as when trimethoprim is used in combination with sulfamethoxazole against sensitive microbes. Such synergy against terminal cancer might be found in combination deficiencies of methyl-donors, i.e., folic acid, vitamin B12, ascorbic acid, choline, and methionine. Tryptophan deficiency enhances the impact of niacin deficiency, and *vice versa,* and deficiency of the two nutrients might be synergistically toxic to tumors. Combination deficiencies of thiamin, niacin, tryptophan, and, if safe avidin is available, biotin should be explored for synergistic toxicity to tumors. Low-protein diets might enhance the impact of essential amino acid depletion as some nonessential amino acids have a sparing effect on essential amino acids. Nonessential cysteine reduces the need for methionine, as does nonessential tyrosine for phenylalanine. Perhaps asprin in combination with essential fatty acid deficiency would be synergistically toxic to tumors.

Minerals and Trace Elements

Diets deficient in water-soluble vitamins will tend to be deficient also in minerals and trace elements. These nutrients can be replaced as supplements, but physicians must insure that consumption of minerals and trace elements is neither deficient nor excessive. This may require regular monitoring of serum concentrations.

Disruption of critical sulfhydryl-disulfide equilibria causes rapid lysis of mouse leukemia cells in culture [31]. If this phenomenon applies to human cancer cells *in vivo,* cysteine supplements might be beneficial. Selenium maintains glutathione homeostasis and might be beneficial in excess or deficiency [32]. Using cysteine and/or selenium in excess or deficiency against terminal cancer is purely speculative, however. No data suggests that manipulating either nutrient will kill cancer cells. This is in contrast to the previously mentioned nutrient manipulations, each of which has a biochemical basis for efficacy.

Tumor Lysis Syndrome

Nutrient depletion has the potential to kill advanced cancer cells quickly, and, in that way, cause tumor lysis syndrome [33]. This is a potentially life-threatening complication of rapid tumor destruction. The safe route is to gently taper off toward nutrient deficiency rather than suddenly eliminating nutrients from the diet. But terminal patients may not have time for this safe route. They should be full partners in deciding how fast to deplete nutrients. Those who choose to suddenly eliminate critical nutrients should be aware of the risks, and their physicians should be ready to support them with hydration, allopurinol, electrolytes, etc., in the event of tumor lysis syndrome.

Diet Optimization

Should nutrient deficiencies be used together in combination, or individually in sequence, or as small combinations in sequence? Which combinations or sequences are optimal?

Much research can be devoted to finding the optimal diet. Should essential nutrients be deprived simultaneously or sequentially? Should the nutrients be depleted or eliminated? Would a diet deficient, but tolerable, in folic acid, thiamin, ascorbic acid, vitamin B12, niacin, and pyridoxine as well as one or more essential amino acids, as well as choline, inositol, and essential fatty acids provide the best anti-tumor effect? Or, would better control come from severe sequential depletion, e.g., a folic acid – free diet that was maintained until anemia became intolerable, followed by a thiamin-free diet until beriberi became intolerable, followed by an ascorbic acid-free diet until scurvy became intolerable, followed by a vitamin B12-free diet until pernicious anemia became intolerable, followed by a niacin-free diet until pellagra became intolerable, followed by a diet depleted in one or more essential amino acids until protein-malnutrition became intolerable, followed by a pyridoxine-free diet until leucopenia and dermatitis became intolerable, followed by a choline-free diet until liver and blood lipid changes became intolerable, followed by an inositol-free diet until eczema became intolerable, followed by a diet free of essential fatty acids until dermatitis became intolerable, and then beginning again with a folic-acid free diet? What sequence of depletions at what levels of severity would be optimal? It is likely that the correct answer will vary among patients and tumors. Presently, the correct answer is not as important as engaging the patient in pursuit of a reasonable answer.

In sequence, nutrient depletion would maintain a block on tumor growth while permitting some, or all, normal cells to recover.

It is possible that every tumor is unique, and probable that this is the case for every advanced tumor [34-35]. Tumor individuality is the rationale for personalizing cancer therapy. It is reasonable, therefore, to encourage patients to take the lead in designing the protocol to attack their cancer. In this way, each patient can optimize his/her preferences for food taste and texture and his/her ability to tolerate side effects. Personal preference will enhance compliance and maximize the placebo effect. From the outset, physicians must emphasize that patients are breaking new ground. No nutrition depletion protocol has been tested against terminal cancer. Every protocol will probably require some modification, and some protocols will likely be ineffective.

Research

Because no prescription medicines are utilized in the nutrient manipulation protocols, physician-permission is not required. Patients can prepare the modified diets in their own kitchens. But physician-oversight is essential for patient-safety and scientific credibility. To collect data, physicians will need to elicit informed-consent from their patients and pass institutional human-investigations review.

If the anecdotal research is to lead to objective conclusions, physicians will need to record methods, materials, and results. Each patient's prognosis should be quantified according to objective criteria [36]. This will permit the search for correlations between prognosis and response to nutrient manipulation.

Measurements on tumor burden and serum nutrient levels are essential before beginning any protocol and at regular intervals during intervention. Physicians should watch for side effects and be ready to begin rescue efforts when side effects become serious. From the beginning, patients should be full partners in this effort. Any lessening in tumor burden should be communicated to patients to enhance compliance and embellish the placebo effect. Failure to observe a decrease in tumor burden after achieving serum nutrient depletion is reason to consider modifying the protocol. Patients should be fully prepared for this possibility from the beginning so as not lose hope or diminish the placebo effect.

Selective Toxicity

Nutrient manipulation does not end with dietary depletion of water-soluble vitamins, and essential amino- and fatty acids. Tumors, unlike most normal tissues, are locked into glycolysis [37]. This is the consequence of the cancer cell's metabolic commitment to continuous proliferation and not hypoxia, as it applies even to well-oxygenated tumors, e.g., leukemias [38] and airway tumors [39]. Metastatic tumor cells are locked into proliferative metabolism [40]. Metabolic commitment to continuous proliferation is the biochemical trait that is common to all cancer cells and missing from most, if not all, normal cells. It is the appropriate target for selective toxicity. Deprivation of nutrients needed for proliferation should be selectively toxic to leukemia cells and solid tumor cells and metastatic cells irrespective of their states of oxygenation.

Tumors are heterogeneous collections of cells. At any given time, some are hypoxic or anoxic and dormant or necrotic, while others are well-oxygenated and actively dividing [41-42] . It may not be possible to kill all cells in a given tumor at one time, and it probably isn't necessary. Some tumor cells seem to have stem cell-like properties. They're responsible for sustaining and spreading tumors [43-44]. Because they're in active proliferation metabolism, they'll be killed by nutrient manipulation. Dormant cells may be invulnerable to nutrient manipulation. But dormant cells aren't dangerous unless they begin dividing, in which case, they'll be killed by nutrient manipulation.

Nutrient Excess

Because tumor cells are locked into glycolysis, hyperglycemia increases lactic acid synthesis in tumors. Poor perfusion retards dissipation from tumors, and, as a result, lactic acid accumulates to the detriment of tumors [45-46]. Hyperglycemia, therefore, may be beneficial in combination or sequence with nutrient depletion. Patients may achieve hyperglycemia by frequent consumption of candy or sugary beverages.

Hyperglycemia will release insulin, which may precipitate hypoglycemia, which can also be toxic to tumors [47]. Terminal cancer patients might try some repetitive glucose tolerance testing, i.e., quick consumption of large quantities of sugar followed by fasting for 2-3 hours, followed by quick consumption of large quantities of sugar, etc.

There are hints that moderate doses of vitamin D can be beneficial against some cancers [48-49].

Embellishments

Hyperthermia [hot baths, electric blanket treatments, or sauna sessions] might be effective in its own right and might enhance the selective toxicity of hyperglycemia [50-52]. Hyperthermia can be comforting to terminal patients. Exercise might be beneficial psychologically as well as physiologically [53-55]. And there is rarely any harm in herbal teas [56] or visualizing tumor cell destruction [57]. These therapeutic embellishments give terminal patients opportunities to stay active in fighting their cancer. This can bolster legitimate hope for remission or cure. For patients who need to fight for survival, such hope is the means to quality life-time. Such hope can translate into effective cancer control.

Resistance Reversal

Whenever cancer cells are treated with cytotoxic drugs, resistance is a risk, and, unless the drugs are used in short-term combination, inevitable. This is the primary reason for the failure of chemotherapy to cure cancer. But resistance to the nutrient manipulations described above is inconceivable. Tumor cells cannot acquire the ability to make DNA, RNA, protein, and lipid without the vitamins and essential amino- and fatty acids. Without new DNA, RNA, protein, and lipid, tumor cells cannot divide. And tumor cells that can't divide aren't dangerous. Physicians should convince patients of these facts.

Nutrient deprivation as described above, blocks *de novo* synthesis of nucleotides, protein, and lipid. Tumor cells can circumvent drugs that block *de novo* synthesis by enhancing pathways to salvage pre-formed metabolites. With nutrient deprivation, however, this mechanism of resistance is impossible because the body isn't making the needed metabolites.

Physicians should carefully explain the biochemical basis for nutrient depletions, helping patients trace the pathways to cell division and nucleic acid and protein and lipid synthesis to see precisely how depletions of the above nutrients will stop tumor growth. Patients must be convinced that tumor growth is impossible without DNA replication and new protein and membrane synthesis and that these syntheses are impossible without the above nutrients.

Chemotherapy triggers an arms race. Tumors survive by evolving resistance mechanisms [58]. Membrane transporter proteins rank among the most important means to multidrug resistance. They are induced by oxidation-reduction signals made in response to chemotherapeutics. Glutathione is the single most important redox signaling metabolite [59]. This is a reason to consider manipulating glutathione concentration with cysteine and/or selenium in dietary excess or deficiency.

Hypoxia induces HIF-1 alpha, which then activates genes that permit cancer cells to flourish in hypoxic environments [60]. As nutrient deprivation kills hypoxic cells and terminal patients take a vacation from chemotherapy, natural selection may favor tumor cells with more drug-sensitive phenotypes. After a period of nutrient manipulation, standard curative chemotherapy should be reconsidered, particularly if terminal patients are in the mood for a new go-around.

Cancer cells increase SIRT1 in response to hypoglycemia [61]. Pulses of hyperglycemia might be beneficial not only for the localized lactic acid in generates, but also for suppressing SIRT1. Resistance to chemotherapy is enhanced by SIRT1 and by DNA methylation [62]. Deficiencies in methyl-donors, e.g., methionine, choline, folic acid, and vitamin B12 may reverse resistance by preventing methylation [63-64]. In normal cells, hypomethylation can cause cancer [63-64]. Terminal cancer patients deficient in methionine, choline, folic acid, or vitamin B12, should be monitored closely and rescued quickly.

Analogy and Precedent

Nutrient deprivation is the protocol of choice against obesity, non-insulin dependent diabetes mellitus, and atherosclerosis. It shrinks atherosclerotic plaque [65]. This is interesting because plaque resembles a benign tumor, with growth due in part to the proliferation of smooth muscle cells, which normally are non-proliferative [66]. Amino acid diets that have been used against Crohn's disease may, with depletion of one or more essential amino acids, be useful in the above protocol against cancer [67]. Conversely, provision of nutrients in abundance has not been found effective against terminal cancer [68]. Supplementation with folic acid, vitamin B6, and vitamin B12 did not reduce the risk of developing cancer [69]. Nutrient deprivation is a natural and reasonable intervention for terminal patients who want to fight for remission or cure.

Nutrient deprivation is the natural response to cancer. The vast majority of terminal cancer patients exhibit anorexia and cachexia [70]. This is often assumed to be harmful. In fact, anorexia and cachexia may be no more harmful against terminal cancer than fever is against infection. But to the extent that anorexia and cachexia is caused by fear or depression, it can be alleviated by the above nutritional manipulations.

The fetus fulfills the definition of a benign tumor, and undernutrition has a profound effect on the fetus, precisely when it is growing in cell number or size [71-72]. It is not unreasonable to imagine that anorexia- cachexia is the body's last, best defense against cancer. Calorie restriction is the most effective non-pharmacological intervention against aging and metabolic disease [73-74]. Patients on nutrient deprivation protocols should consume large quantities of water to wash out the targeted nutrients, protect against kidney stones and tumor lysis syndrome, and create a condition of caloric restriction [75]. In response to this condition, patients' basal metabolic rate will decline. They'll need less nutrition as a result. Tumors, on the other hand, continually select for faster- dividing, more nutrient-demanding, cells. Patients on undernutrition therapy will take the metabolic advantage from their tumors [76]. When they do that, resveratrol [found in red grapes, red grape juice, and red wine] may be beneficial [77].

Placebo

Among the various definitions of "suppress", two pertain to cancer: 1) "to inhibit the growth or development of", and 2) "to exclude from consciousness." Surgery, radiation, and chemotherapy, target the former. When they succeed, the latter follows as a corollary. When they fail, the latter becomes impossible.

Too-often, terminal cancer patients are obsessed with cancer, and that obsession can ruin their remaining time. Pain, nausea, anxiety, panic, depression, and loneliness are corollaries of cancer obsession. Palliative care can alleviate some corollaries, while aggravating others. Not all terminal patients are ready, willing, or able to surrender hope of remission or cure. And young cancer patients and their families are never ready to surrender [78]. For terminal patients who need to fight after conventional medicine has run it's course and failed, nutrient manipulation is ideal, first because it will "inhibit the growth or development of" cancer, and second because it gives terminal patients permission to "exclude from consciousness" the cancer obsession, and doing that can unleash the placebo effect, which may "inhibit the growth or development of" cancer.

The placebo effect is an ancient and revered fact of medical research. Anecdotal evidence suggests it works against cancer [79]. Controlled clinical trials show it can suppress benign epidermal tumors, i.e. warts [80]. When a physician pronounces a hex on warts, they tend to disappear. Warts are caused by members of the same group of viruses [papiloma] that cause cervical and genital cancers, and possibly laryngeal and oral cancers, and lung cancer. We should not quickly dismiss the potential utility of placebos against terminal cancer. But the placebo effect is currently out of vogue against terminal cancer because patient's emotional functioning did not predict survival [81]. The absence of objective evidence for a placebo effect against terminal cancer, together with the inherently deceptive nature of placebo therapy makes physicians reluctant to employ it. Nutrient manipulation as described above gives physicians cause to revaluate. The protocol should work. There's no need for deception, and no advantage in denying patients the benefits of a placebo effect.

Take a closer look at what Coyne et al have accomplished [81]. It's interesting and important but not a refutation of the placebo effect. Perhaps the placebo effect works by altering emotions, but there is no proof of that, and even if there were, there's no reason to assume that the emotions measured by Coyne et al. are identical to those created by a placebo. To have a chance at a placebo effect, treatment must be recommended in the identical manner that an effective drug is recommended. It may well be that the placebo effect is mediated by faith in the physician, or reason, instead of emotion [82]. Nutrient manipulation as described above can be recommended by physicians in the same manner as they recommend effective medicine. And physicians can give patients reason to believe nutrient manipulation will kill tumors.

Aging as Tumor Suppression

The aging process is the greatest carcinogen [83]. But it is also the greatest tumor suppressor. Cancers that exhibit peak incidence rates in childhood, e.g., retinoblastoma, neuroblastoma, rhabdomyosarcoma, Wilms' tumor, osteogenic and Ewing's sarcomas, and acute lymphoblastic leukemia are rare in older subjects. Testicular cancer, which peaks in middle-age, is rare in younger and older subjects. Clearly, no accumulative process, e.g., environmental exposure, DNA damage, telomere shortening, can account for this age-specificity.

It is tempting to ignore cancers that exhibit peak risks in childhood or middle age as special cases because they are rare. All common cancers, at first glance, exhibit "approximately exponential increases" in risk with advancing age. Close inspection, however, shows those patterns not to be even approximately exponential. Risk for the common cancers increases at a continuously decreasing rate, i.e., risk approaches a plateau. For some cancers, the plateau and subsequent decline in risk at very old age is conspicuous [84].

What causes the suppression of cancer at advancing age? Senescence. At least, that's currently the best bet. Beyond a certain age, cells lose the ability to divide, and are, therefore, no longer vulnerable to cancer [85]. Senescence may explain the exponential increase with age in risk of death from all causes. As dying cells are no longer replaced, cancer becomes less likely, but death from tissue failure more so.

A Theory of Carcinogenesis

What causes cancer? Oncogenes and tumor suppressor genes get the spotlight. But aging genes are more important, giving, and taking away, permission for the cancer genes to act.

Two copies of the retinoblastoma gene seem necessary to cause retinoblastoma [86]. Inheriting one of these genes shortens the time to cancer, but only until age 7 or so. After that, retinoblastoma is rare. The aging process, e.g., senescence, prevents it.

Inheriting genes for breast cancer or adenomatous polyposis or nonpolyposis colorectal cancer makes cancer almost inevitable. These inherited cancers occur at earlier ages than the spontaneous variety, but not much earlier, never before age 20, or so [87-88]. Something about the aging process prevents carcinogenesis before some tissue-specific, critical age. I suggest it is, once again, senescence. Cancer occurs when cells with cancer-causing mutations are free to divide. Perhaps in breast and colon and most epithelial tissues, the stem cells are committed to terminal differentiation until some critical age.

Survivors of the atomic bomb were at increased risk from a variety of cancers, but only at the ages those cancers normally appeared [89]. The blast of mutagens did not substantially shorten the time to cancer. Mutations can be inherited and they can accumulate over all ages, but they only exert carcinogenic influence over a rather short, tissue-specific, age-interval. The distribution of risk over this interval is unimodal for cancers that peak in childhood or middle-age. By extrapolation, that distribution is unimodal for cancers that peak in old age. The unimodal or approximately Gaussian distribution of risk suggests a stochastic process.

A theory of carcinogenesis must explain what happens at the critical age and over the critical interval to enable carcinogenesis. It is reasonable to focus this explanation on cells with the capacity for repeated cell division, i.e., stem cells.

There is evidence that many tissues contain two populations of stem cells, one active, the other quiescent [90]. In some tissues, the quiescent population may consist of differentiated cells which harbor the potential to dedifferentiate [91-93]. Over time, the quiescent population accumulates mutations, some of which are carcinogenic. But those mutations remain dormant unless or until quiescent cells are recruited into active division, which only begins when the active population is depleted. Perhaps this does not occur until after some critical tissue-specific age. Stochastic recruitment from the quiescent pool would explain the unimodal, approximately Gaussian shape of the variation of risk with age. Tissues with limited ability to regenerate, tend not to spawn cancer [94-98].

Inflammation is the response to injury. It predisposes to cancer because injury depletes the active stem cell pool and hastens recruitment from the quiescent pool. By this theory, tobacco and sunlight are carcinogenic not only because they cause mutations, but because they injure cells hastening the replacement of active stem cells from the quiescent pool. High metabolic rate and hyperthermia may do the same.

Childhood cancers are rare because young cells have little time to acquire mutations. Adult cancers are common because the quiescent cells have much time to acquire mutations.

Undernutrition reduces metabolic rate and may delay recruitment from the quiescent pool [99]. It may pressure tumors to favor cells that divide slowly, or not at all. Tumor cells may respond to undernutrition by reverting to normal. It's an optimistic thought with placebo value.

Beyond Placebo

Curative therapy for terminal cancer is an open book. As new, reasonable, convenient, inexpensive, and relatively safe interventions are discovered, they can be added to the list. In this way, patients who want to fight on after conventional medicine has failed can be supported in their efforts without compromising the integrity of conventional medicine. But in the end, and there is always an end, all efforts are futile, for death is inevitable, and before death, suffering, if only from fear of death, is routine.

Suffering can seem impossible to endure. In some forms, it is impossible. In some forms, it is more than that. But despite our best efforts, suffering isn't likely to become extinct. And while it exists, it is our incentive to change perspective on what we think. Who are we, really, and where are we headed, and what matters and what doesn't?

In the final analysis, death can't matter. In truth, it is an illusion. True self, like true love, true gravity, true anything, can never change. The bodies we inhabit change because they aren't true, and can't be us if we are true. Despite the pain, sorrow, fear, agony, and more that our bodies endure, there is reason to celebrate, for nothing true is lost or gained. Only boundaries seem rearranged, and boundaries never matter. In all that does matter, we are the same, now and forever. [100].

Acknowledgment

Dr. Patricia Cohen gave valuable criticism and advice.

References

[1] M. Fisch,, P. J. Loehrer, J. Kristeller, et al. *J. Clinical Oncology*, 21, 1937-43, 2003.

[2] A. Vickers, Alternative cancer cures: "unproven" or "disproven"?, *CA Cancer J. Clinicians*, 54, 110-18, 2004.

[3] A. A. Manzoor, T. Schroeder, M. W. Dewhirst, One-stop-shop tumor imaging: Buy hypoxia, get lactate free. *J. Clinical Investigation*, 118, 1616-19, 2008.

[4] P. Olson, D. Hanahan, Breaking the cancer fortress. *Science*, 324, 1400-01, 2009.

[5] P. Cohen, D. Dix, On the role of folate deficiency in cancer therapy, *Clinical Chemistry*, 34, 1945-46, 1988.

[6] D. Dix, "Legacy" in *Natural Literacy: How to Learn What We Yearn to Know*, Hamilton, Lanham MD. 2008, p. 141-45.

[7] H. A. Harper, V. W. Rodwell, P. A. Mayes, *Review of Physiological Chemistry*, Lang, Los Altos, CA, 1979,

[8] J. C. Tilburt, E. J. Emanuel, T. J. Kaptchuk, F. A. Curlin, F. G. Miller, Prescribing "placebo treatments": results of a national survey of U. S. internists and rheumatologists. *BMJ* 337, a1938, 2008.

[9] A. A. Wright, B. Zhang, A. Ray, et al., Associations between end-of-life discussions, patient mental health, medical care near death, and caregiver bereavement, *JAMA*, 300, 1665-73, 2008.

[10] J. Sterba, L. Dusek, R. Demlova, D. Valik, Pretreatment plasma folate modulates the parmacodynamic effect of high-dose methotrexate in children with acute lymphoblastic leukemia and non-Hodgkin lymphoma: "Folate overrescue" concept revisited. *Clinical Chemistry*, 52, 692-700, 2006.

[11] B. J. Spieger, K. Kennedy, R. Maze et al., Comparison of long-term neurocognitive outcomes in young children with acute lymphoblastic leukemia treated with cranial radiation or high-dose or very high dose intravenous methotrexate. *J. Clinical Oncology*, 24, 3858-84, 2006.

[12] V. Herbert, A palatable diet for producing experimental folate deficiency in man. *American J. Clinical Nutrition*, 12, 17-20, 1963.

[13] S. Davidson, R. Passmore, *Human Nutrition and Dietetics*, Williams and Wilkins, Baltimore, 1970.

[14] M. G. Vander Heiden, L. C/ Cantley, C. B. Thompson, Understanding the Warburg effect: The metabolic requirements of cell proliferation. *Science*, 324, 1029-33, 2009.

[15] G. P. Tryfiates, R. E. Bishop, A. J. Murgo, Vitamin B6 and cancer: A novel pyridoxal-5-phosphate conjugate in tumor cells and blood of cancer patients. *Anticancer Research*. 11, 1281-84, 1991.

[16] C. M. Crowder, Ceramides – friend or foe in hypoxia? *Science*, 324, 343-44, 2009.

[17] M. C. Brahimi-Horn, J. Chiche, J. Pouyssegur, Hypoxia and cancer. *J. Molecular Medicine*, 85, 1301-07, 2007.

[18] S. H. Zeisel, K. A. DaCosta, P. D. Franklin, E. A. Alexander, J. T. Lamont, N. F. Sheary, A. Beiser, Choline; an essential nutrient for humans. *FASEB Journal*, 5, 2093-98, 1991.

[19] R. Katz-Brull, D. Seger, D. Rivenson-Segal, E. Rushkin, H. Degani, Metabolic markers of breast cancer. Enhanced choline metabolism and reduced choline-ether-phospholipid synthesis. *Cancer Research*, 62, 1966-70, 2002.

[20] R. A. Jacobs, D. J. Jewden, M. A. Allman-Farinelli, M. E. Swendseid. Folate nutriture alters choline status of women and men fed low choline diets. *J. Nutrition*, 129, 712-17, 1999.

[21] K. A. DaCosta, C. G. Gaffney, L. M. Fischer, S. H. Zeisel, Choline deficiency in mice and humans is associated with increased plasma homocysteine concentration after a methionine load. *American J. Clinical Nutrition*, 81, 440-44, 2005.

[22] K A. Da Costa, M. D. Niculescu, C. N. Craciunescu, L. M. Fischer, S. H. Zeisel, Choline deficiency increases lymphocyte apoptosis and DNA damage in humans. *American J. Clinical Nutrition*, 84, 88-94, 2006.

[23] I. Uucenik, A. M. Shamsuddin, Cancer inhibition of inositol hexaphosphate [IP5] and inositol, From laboratory to clinic. *J. Nutrition*, 133, 37785-845, 2003.

[24] Y. Sun, Y. Mochizuki, P. W. Materuj, Inositol 1,2,4, Trisphosphate 5/6 kinase inhibits tumor necrosis factor-induced apoptosis. *J. Biological Chemistry* 278, 43645-53, 2003.

[25] T. Balla, Z. Szentpetery, Y. J. Kim, Phosphoinositide signaling: New tools and insights. *Physiology* 24, 231-44, 2009.

[26] J. C. Otto, P. Kelly, S. T. Chiou, J. D. York, Alterations in an inositol phosphate code through synergistic activation of a G protein and inositol phosphate kinases, *Proceedings National Academy Science*, 104, 15653-58, 2007.

[27] E. S. West, W. R. Todd, H. S. Mason, J. T. Van Bruggen, *Textbook of Biochemistry*, Macmillian, N. Y., 1966.

[28] E. Siguel, Diagnosing essential fatty acid deficiency. *Circulation*, 97, 2580-83, 1998.

[29] N. Cook, U. M. Lee, J. M. Gaziano, D. Gordon, P. M. Ridker, J. E. Manson, C. H. Hennekens, J. E. Buring, *JAMA*, Low-dose asprin in the primary prevention of cancer: The women's health study: a randomized controlled trial, 294, 47-55, 2005.

[30] G. L. Van Sluis, T. M. H. Niers, C. T. Esmon, W. Tigchelaar, D. J. Richel, H. R. Buller, C. J. F. Van Noorden, C. A. Spek, Endogenous activated protein C limits cancer cell extravasation through sphingosine-1-phosphate receptor 1-mediated vascular endothelial barrier enhancement, *Blood*, 114, 1968-73, 2009.

[31] D. E. Dix, Leukemia cell lysis by sulfhydryl reagents and thiols, *Life Sciences,* 19, 973-78, 1976.

[32] A. J. Duffield-Lillico, M. E. Reid, B. W. Turnbull, G. F. Combs, E. N. Slate, L. A. Fischbach, J. R. Marshall, L. C. Clark, Baseline characteristics and the effect of selenium supplementation on cancer incidence in a randomized clinical trial, A summary report of the national cancer prevention clinical trial. *Cancer Epidemiology, Biomarkers, and Prevention*, 11, 630-39, 2002.

[33] J. Held-Warmkessel, How to prevent and manage tumor lysis syndrome, *Nursing* 2010, 40, 26-31 2010.

[34] J. Couzin, Probing the roots of race and cancer, *Science*, 315, 592-94, 2007.

[35] J. Kaiser, Looking for a target on every tumor, *Science*, 326, 218-220, 2009.

[36] M. H. Ebell, Determining prognosis for patients with terminal cancer. *American Family Physician*, 72, 668-69, 2005.

[37] V. S. Shapot, Some biochemical aspects of the relationship between the tumor and the host. *Advanced Cancer Research*, 15, 253-56, 1972.

[38] R. G. Jones, C. B. Thompson, Tumor suppressors and cell metabolism: A recipe for cancer growth. *Genes & Development*, 23, 537-48, 2009.

[39] Y. Fan, K. G. Dickman, W-X Zong, Akt and c-Myc differentially activate cellular metabolic programs and prime cells to bioenergetic inhibition. *J. Biological Chemistry*, 285, 7324-33, 2010.

[40] M. C. Brahimi-Horn, J. Chiche, J. Pouyssegur, Hypoxia signaling controls metabolic demand. *Current Opinion Cell Biology*, 19, 223-29, 2007.

[41] L. H. Dang, C. Bettegowda, D. L. Huso, K. W. Kinzler, B. Vogelstein, Combination bacteriolytictherapy for the treatment of experimental tumors, *Proceedings National Academy Science*, 98, 15155-60, 2001.

[42] R. K. Jain, N. S. Forbes, Can engineered bacteria help control cancer? *Proceedings National Academy Science*, 98, 14748-50, 2001.

[43] J. M. Rosen, C. T. Jordan, The increasing complexity of the cancer stem cell paradigm, *Science*, 324, 1670-73, 2009.

[44] J. Kaiser, Cancer's circulation problem, *Science*, 327, 1072-74, 2010.

[45] S. Kohnoe, Y. Cmi., I. Takahashi, M. Yoshida, Y. Maehara, K. Sugimachi, Hypoxia and acidity increase the cytotoxicity of mitomycin C and caraboquone to human tumor cells in vitro. *Anticancer Research*, 11, 1401-04, 1991.

[46] S. Osinsky, L. Bubnouskala, T. Sergienko, Tumor pH under induced hyperglycemia and efficacy of chemotherapy. *Anticancer Research*, 7, 199-202, 1987.

[47] R. L. Aft, F. W. Zhang, D. Gius, Evaluation of 2-deoxy-D-glucose as a chemotherapeutic agent: mechanism of cell death. *British J. Cancer*, 87, 805-12, 2002.

[48] Pamela Goodwin, Breast Cancer Research Foundation and Mt. Sinai Hospital, Toronto.

[49] W. B. Grant, Vitamin D may reduce prostate cancer metastasis by several mechanisms. *American J. Pathology*, 173, 1589-90, 2008.

[50] R. Twombly, International study of hyperthermia spurs hopes in U.S. advocates. *J. National Cancer Institute* 102, 79-81, 2010.

[51] A. Bakshandeh-Bath, A. S. Stolitz, N. Homann, Preclinical and clinical aspects of Carboplatin and Gemcitabine combined with whole-body hyperthermia for pancreatic adenocarcinoma. *Anticancer Research*, 29, 3069-77, 2009.

[52] C. Krause, K. Klottermann, C. Mauz-Korholz, Molecular mechanisms and gene regulation of Melphalan- and hyperthermia- induced apoptosis in Ewing sarcoma cells. *Anticancer Research*, 28, 2585-93, 2008.

[53] M. A. Fiatarone, E. F. O'Neill, N. D. Ryan, K. M. Clements, G. R. Solares, M. E. Nelson, S. B. Roberts, J. J. Dehayias, L. A. Lipsitz, W. J. Evans, Exercise training and nutritional supplementation for physical frailty in very elderly people. *New England J. Medicine* 330, 1769-75, 1994.

[54] M. D. Holmes, W. Y. Chen, C. H. Kroenke, G. A. Coldnitz. Physical activity and survival after breast cancer diagnosis. *JAMA*, 293, 2470, 2005.

[55] K. S. Courneya, R. J. Segal, J. R. Mackey, et al. Effects of aerobic and resistance exercise in breast cancer patients receiving ajuvant chemotherapy: A multicenter randomized controlled trial. *J. Clinical Oncology*, 25, 4396-4404, 2007.

[56] B. R. Cassileth. "Questionable Therapies" in *Cancer Medicine*, eds. R. C. Bast, D. w. Kufe, R. Pollock, R. R. Weichseelbaum, J. F. Holland, E. Frei., B. C. Decker, Hamilton, 2000, p. 50-54.

[57] Associated Press, CIGNA offers free video game [RE-MISSION] for young cancer patients, *USA Today*, 5/30/07 [available on CIGNA website].

[58] S. Raguz, E. Yague, Resistance to chemotherapy: new treatments and novel insights into an old problem. *British J. Cancer* 99, 387-91, 2008.

[59] M. T. Kuo, Redox regulation of multidrug resistance in cancer chemotherapy. *Antioxidant Redox Signaling*, 11, 99-132, 2009.

[60] G. Powis, L. Kirkpatrick, Hypoxia inducible factor-1 alpha as a cancer drug target. *Molecular Cancer Therapy*, 3, 647-54, 2004.

[61] X Liang, T. Finkel, D. Shen, J. Yin, A. Azalos, M. M. Gottesman, SIRT1 contributes in part to cisplatin resistance in cancer cells by altering mitochondria metabolism, *Molecular Cancer Research*, 6, 1499-1506, 2008.

[62] B. Segura-Pacheco, E. Perez-Cardenas, L. Taja-Chayeb, A. Chavez-Blanco, A. Revilla-Vazquez, L. Benitez-Bribiesca, A. Duenas-Gonzalez, Global DNA hypermethylation-associated cancer chemotherapy resistance and its reversion with the demethylating agent hydralazine. *J. Translational Medicine*. 4, 32, 2006.

[63] M. Pufulete, R. Al-Ghnaniem, A. Khushai, P. Appleby, N. Harris, S. Gout, P. W. Emery, T. A. B. Sanders, Effect of folic acid supplementation on genomic DNA methylations in patients with colorectal adenoma. *Gut*, 54, 648-53, 2005.

[64] L. Brunaud, J. M. Alberto, A. Ayav,P. Gerard, F. Namour, L. Antunes, M. Braun, J. P. Bronowicki, L. Bresler, J. L. Gueant. Effects of vitamin B12 and folate deficiencies on DNA methylation and carcinogenesis in rat liver. *Clinical Chemistry Laboratory Medicine* 41, 1012-19, 2003.

[65] I. Shai, J. D. Spence, D. Schwarzfuchs, Y. Henkin, Dietary intervention to reverse carotid atherosclerosis, *Circulation*, 121, 1200-08, 2010.

[66] J. L. Johnson, A. H. Baker, K. Oka, L. Chan, A. C. Newby, Cl L. Jackson, S. J. George, Suppression of atherosclerotic plaque progressional instability by tissue inhibitor of metalloproteinase-2. *Circulation*, 113, 2435-44, 2006.

[67] J. C. Mansfield, M. H. Giaffer, C. D. Holdsworth, Controlled trial of oligopeptide versus amino acid diet in treatment of Crohn's disease. *Gut*, 36, 60-66, 1995.

[68] D. Y. Kim, S. M. Lee, K. E. Lee, H. R. Lee, J. H. Kim, K-W Lee, J. S. Lee, S. N. Lee, An evaluation of nutrition support for terminal cancer patients at teaching hospitals in Korea. *Cancer Research Treatment*, 38, 214-17, 2006.

[69] S. Zhang, Effect of continued folic acid, vitamin B6, Vitamin B12 on cancer risk in women, *JAMA*, 300, 2012-21, 2008.

[70] S. Perboni, A. Inui, Anorexia in cancer: role of feeding-regulatory peptides. Philosphical Transactions of the Royal Society London B *Biological Science*, 361, 1281-89, 2006.

[71] S. J. Atwoood, K. Codling, R. Shrimpton, *Strategy to Reduce Maternal and Child Undernutrition*, UNICEF, East Asia and Pacific Regional Office, 2003., p. 9

[72] Department for International Development, UK, *The Neglected Crisis of Undernutrition: Evidence for Action,* PRD 139, 2009.

[73] C. Canto, J. Auwerx, Caloric restriction. *Trends in Endocrinology and Metabolism*, 20, 325-31, 2009.

[74] R. J. Colman, R. M. Anderson, S. C. Johnson, E. K. Castman, J. Kosmatka, et. al. Caloric restriction delays disease onset and mortality in Rhesus monkeys. *Science*, 325, 201-04, 2009.

[75] S. Imai, SIRT1 and caloric restriction: an insight into possible trade-offs between robustness and frailty. *Current Opinion Clinical Nutrition Metabolic Care,* 12, 350-56, 2009.
[76] L. Raffaghello, C. Lee, F. M. Safdie, et al., Starvation-dependent differential stress resistance protects normal but not cancer cells against high-dose chemotherapy. *Proceedings of the National Academy of Science,* 105, 8215-20, 2008.
[77] K. J. Pearson, J. A. Baur, K. N. Lewis, et al. Resveratrol delays age-related deterioration and mimics transcriptional aspects of dietary restriction without extending life span. *Cell Metabolism*, 8, 157-68, 2008.
[78] J. Couzin, In their prime, and dying of cancer. *Science* 317, 1160-62, 2007.
[79] J. Lenzer, The body can beat terminal cancer – sometimes. *Discover*, September 2007.
[80] L. Thomas, "On Warts" in *The Medusa and the Snail*, Bantam Books, N.Y. 1979, p. 61-65.
[81] J. C. Coyne, T. F. Pajak, J. Harris, A. Konski, B. Movsas, K. Ang, D. Brunner Watkins, Emotional well-being does not predict survival in head and neck cancer patients: A Radiation Therapy Oncology Group study. *Cancer*, 112, 2326-28, 2008.
[82] L. Wang, In clinical trials and in the clinic, What is the placebo's effect? *JNCI*, 95, 6-7, 2003.
[83] D. Dix, On the role of genes relative to the environment in carcinogenesis. *Mechanisms of Ageing and Development*, 124, 323-32, 2003.
[84] A. Nejako, B. Aranton, D. Dix, Carcinogenesis: A cellular model for the age-dependance, *Anticancer Research*. 25, 1385-90, 2005.
[85] J. Campisi, Suppressing cancer: The importance of being senescent. *Science*, 309, 886-87, 2005.
[86] A. Knudson, Mutation and cancer: Statistical study of retinoblastoma, *Proceedings of the National Academy of Science*, 68, 820-23, 1971.
[87] J. Litton, G. Hortobagyi, B. Arun, et al., Breast cancer patients with high risk gene diagnosed 6 years earlier than generation before. Poster Session, M. D. Anderson Cancer Center, 2009.
[88] J. Amos-Landgraf, L. N. Kwong, W. F. Dove, a target-selected APC-mutant rat kindred enhances the modeling of familial human colon cancer, *Proceedings of the National Academy of Science*, 104, 4036-41, 2007.
[89] Y. Simizu, H. Kato, W. Scull, Studies of the mortality of A-bomb survivors. *Radiation Research*, 121, 120-41, 1990.
[90] L. Li, H. Clevers, Coexistence of quiescent and active adult stem cells in mammals. *Science*, 327, 542-45, 2010.
[91] K. S. Zaret, M. Grompe, Generation and regeneration of cells of the liver and pancreas. *Science*, 322, 1490-94, 2008.
[92] N. Toshinori, S. Manju, N. Yo-ichi, R. E. Braun, S. Yoshida, Functional hierarchy and reversibility within the murine spermatogenic stem cell compartment. *Science*, 328, 62-67, 2010.
[93] J. b. Gurdon, D. A. Melton, Nuclear reprogramming in cells, *Science*, 322, 1811-15, 2008.
[94] O. Bergmann, R. D. Bhardwaj, S. Bernard, et al. Evidence for cardiomyocyte renewal in humans, *Science*, 324, 98-101, 2009.
[95] C. E. Murry, R. T. Lee, Turnover after the fallout, *Science*, 324, 47-48, 2009.

[96] M. C. Subang, P. M. Richardson, Nuclear power for axonal growth, *Science*, 326, 238-240, 2009.

[97] D. L. Moore, M. G. Blackmore, Y. Hu et al., KLF family members regulate intrinsic axon regeneration ability, *Science*, 326, 298-301, 2009.

[98] D. L. Stocum, Acceptable nagging, *Science*, 318, 754-55, 2007.

[99] L. Fontana, L. Partridge, V. D. Longo, Extending healthy life span – from yeast to humans. *Science*, 328, 321-26, 2010.

[100] D. Dix, Natural Literacy: How to Learn What We Yearn to Know, Hamilton, *Lanham*, MD, 2008, p. 144-146.

In: Tumor Suppressors
Editor: Susan D. Nguyen

ISBN: 978-1-61761-986-1

Chapter 3

Breast Cancer Screening by Methylation Analysis of Tumor Suppressor Genes in Breast Fluid

JS de Groot, KPM Suijkerbuijk, PJ van Diest and E van der Wall
Harvard Medical School, Boston, Massachusetts, USA

Abstract

Breast cancer is the major cause of cancer death in the Western world. Despite the fact that women undergo imaging-based screening at regular intervals, many cancers are still discovered in between screening visits. This indicates an urgent need for novel screening and risk assessment modalities that could be of additive value to imaging-based screening.

Breast cancer is initiated and progresses by genetic and epigenetic events resulting in aberrant gene function. Epigenetic alterations occur through mechanisms other than changes in the primary nucleotide sequence of a gene. One of the most important epigenetic mechanisms is DNA methylation. The term DNA methylation describes the addition of a methyl group to a cytosine base in the DNA. In the normal situation DNA methylation is involved in the regulation of many cellular maintenance processes. However, during tumorigenesis, hypermethylation of promoters of tumor suppressor genes is associated with silencing of transcription. In this way methylation contributes to cancer initiation and progression. Methylation alterations frequently occur in early stages of tumor development and can also be detected in non-cancerous cells adjacent to the tumor, which indicates a methylation "field defect". Moreover, epigenetic changes are reversible and therefore potential therapeutic targets.

Analyzing DNA promoter methylation of tumor suppressor genes in nipple fluid could be a new screening modality. Nipple fluid is normally produced in small amounts in the ducts of non-lactating women and can be obtained by non-invasive vacuum aspiration. This fluid contains intact ductal epithelial cells together with free DNA derived from such cells, which can be analyzed for methylation aberrations. Using oxytocin nasal spray, nipple fluid can be aspirated from more than 90% of women, including high-risk women that previously underwent local or systemic treatment. We and others previously showed that methylation of a panel of tumor suppressor genes such as *CCND2, SCGB3A1, APC, RASSF1* and *RARB* is associated with the presence of breast cancer. Using Quantitative Multiplex Methylation-Specific PCR, methylation alterations can reliably be assessed in the limited amounts of DNA present in nipple fluid.

In conclusion, analyzing patterns of promoter methylation of tumor suppressor genes in nipple fluid can potentially serve as a valuable breast cancer screening method. A large prospective study is currently ongoing in our institute to determine the added value of this modality to existing screening methods.

Introduction

Breast cancer is the leading cause of cancer death in women worldwide and the incidence of breast cancer is expected to rise further. Therefore, breast cancer is a global burden of disease, indicating an urgent need for improvement in diagnosis and treatment. [1] Several hormonal and lifestyle factors have been identified as risk factors for the development of breast cancer, but the most well-established risk factor is the presence of a germ line mutation in the *BRCA1* or *BRCA2* genes. The cumulative breast cancer risk at the age of 70 years is 57% in *BRCA1* and 49% in *BRCA2* mutation carriers. [2] Regular screening by clinical breast examination, mammography or MRI is offered to these high-risk women, but not all carcinomas are detected by these exams. Brekelmans et al. found that the sensitivity of physical examination every 6 months and mammography every year is 74% in women with breast cancer risk over 15%. Sensitivity was even less (56%) in *BRCA1/2* mutation carriers and in women under the age of 40 years [3], which is partly accounted for by the higher breast density at younger age. Moreover, there is evidence that *BRCA1* and *BRCA2* germline mutation carriers have an increased radiosensitivity [4], which possibly results in an expected very limited net benefit from annual mammographic screening for *BRCA1/2* mutation carriers. [5] The overall sensitivity of MRI is significantly better than that of mammography at the cost of specificity. However, difficulties can be caused by an atypical manifestation of hereditary breast cancers at both mammography and MR imaging. [6;7]

Currently, the most effective ways of primary prevention of breast cancer in high-risk women are prophylactic bilateral mastectomy and prophylactic oophorectomy. In women with a *BRCA1* or *BRCA2* mutation, prophylactic bilateral total mastectomy seems to be associated with considerable reduction of the breast cancer risk, albeit incomplete. In a follow-up study of Meijers et al. no cases of breast cancer were observed after prophylactic mastectomy after a mean follow-up of 2.9 years, although eight breast cancers developed in women under regular surveillance after a mean follow-up of 3.0 years (p=0.003). [8] Hartmann et al. conducted a retrospective study of women with a family history of breast cancer undergoing bilateral prophylactic mastectomy and used the sisters of the high-risk probands as a control group. Prophylactic mastectomy resulted in a 90% reduction in breast cancer incidence and breast cancer mortality. [9] The surgical morbidity of prophylactic mastectomy is low, but few studies have yet addressed quality-of-life issues in women who have opted for prophylactic mastectomy. [10]

This all indicates the need for novel screening modalities that could be of additive value to imaging-based screening. Opportunities for the detection of breast cancer exist at three biological levels: systemically via the blood, at the whole organ level, and within the individual ducto-lobular structures of the breast. By targeting the ducto-lobular units, the site where breast cancer originates can be assessed. The different techniques for accessing and scrutinizing the ducto-lobular systems offer the potential to sample the microenvironment of the breast. [11] One way of accessing this microenvironment is the collection of nipple fluid. Nipple fluid, that contains breast epithelial cells, their free DNA and proteins secreted by them, is produced in small amounts in the breast ducts of non-lactating women (Figure 1) and can be collected by non-invasive vacuum-aspiration. Breast cancer develops by stepwise accumulation of interacting epigenetic and genetic events over time [12], with DNA promoter hypermethylation as the most frequently occurring event in cancer cells. [13] Methylation plays an important role in normal cells as well as in tumor development. Therefore, methylation patterns in nipple fluid may potentially serve as an additive and valuable screening method for breast carcinogenesis. [14]

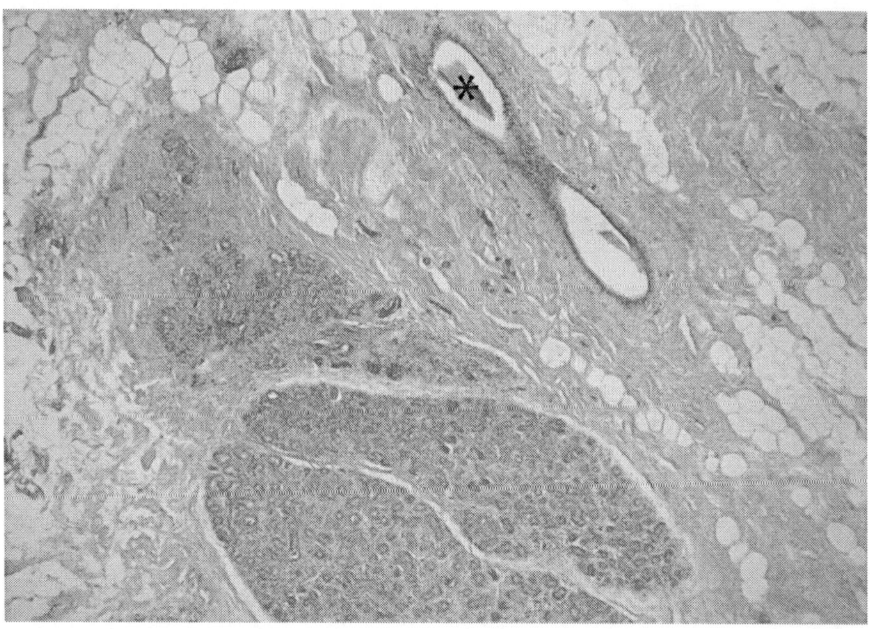

Figure 1. Nipple fluid (marked with *) in a mammary duct of normal breast tissue (H&E staining).

DNA Promoter Hypermetylation and Cancer

Cancer initiation and progression is driven by the accumulation of inherited and/or acquired DNA aberrations. These alterations may be genetic or epigenetic in nature. [15;16] Epigenetic modifications are changes in DNA structure that do not involve base sequence changes. [17] Compared with genetic events, epigentic alterations occur more often. [18] Epigenetic

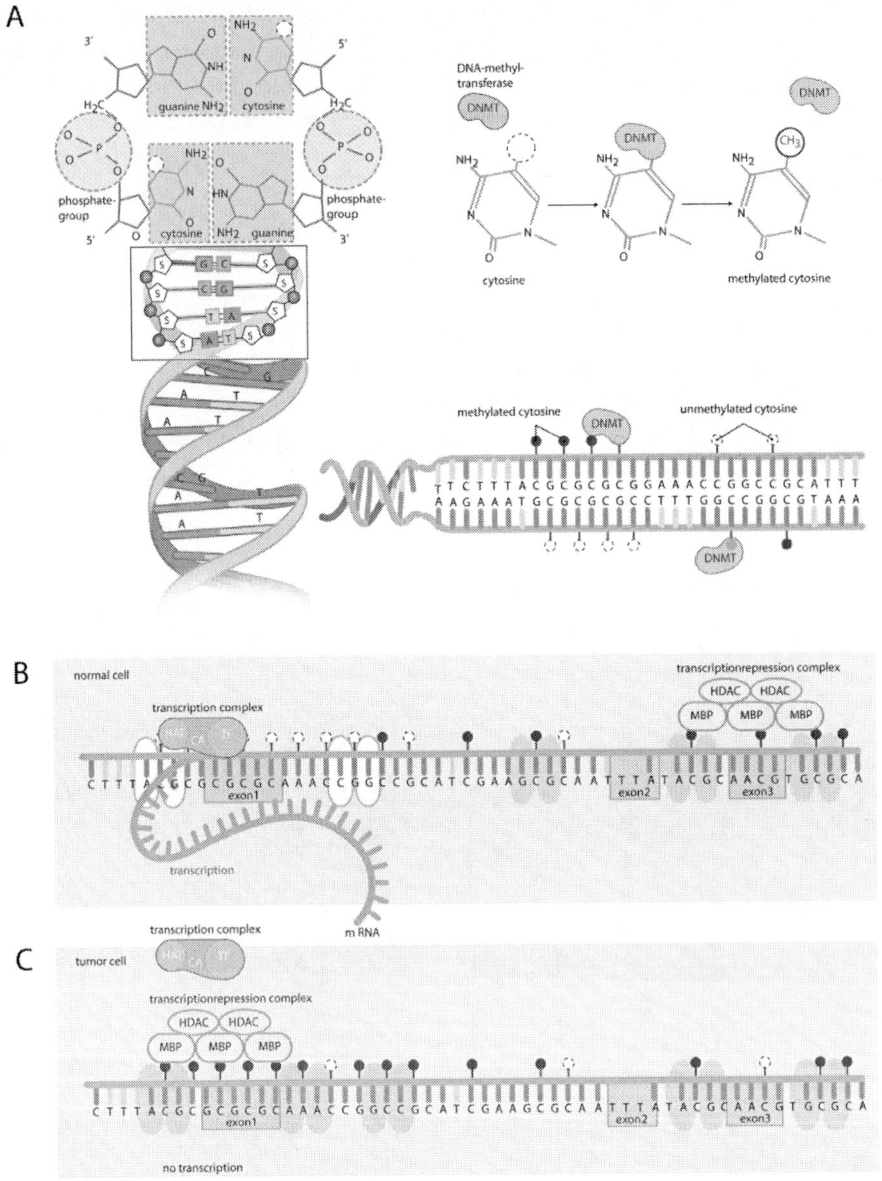

Figure 2. DNA promoter hypermethylation. This figure is reprinted with the permission of and adjusted from the original figure in *Nederlands Tijdschrift voor Geneeskunde*. [141] A. Methylation of the 5' carbon of a cytosine nucleotide by DNA methyltranferase (DNMT). DNMTs are enzymes catalyzing methylation of cytosine with S-adenosylmethionine as the donor of the methylgroup (CH_3). B. In a healthy cell the CpG island in the promoter region of a tumor suppressor gene is not methylated (exon 1) and the gene can be transcribed. The transcription complex consisting of histoneacetyltranferases (HATs), transcription factors (TF) and coactivators (CA) can bind the DNA where transcription starts. In this way unmethylated DNA is protected against DNMTs and transcription repression complexes consisting of methylcytosine binding proteins (MBPs) and histonedeacetylases (HDACs). In the rest of the genome (exon 2 and exon 3), outside the promoter region, CpG dinucleotides are methylated and bound to repressive MBP-HDAC complexes. C. In a cancer cell this situation is reversed. CpG islands are methylated, which blocks transcription of tumor suppressor genes and thereby inactivate these genes. DNMTs methylate CpG dinucleotides in the promoter region and MBP-HDAC complexes bind the DNA where normally the transcription starts.

regulation has been known to involve three interacting events: DNA methylation, histone modifications and nucleosomal remodelling. These processes modulate chromatin structure leading to activation or silencing of gene expression. Alterations in gene expression through aberrant epigenetic regulation in cells can lead to initiation, promotion and maintenance of carcinogenesis. [19] This chapter will further focus on DNA promoter hypermethylation as epigenetic event.

The process of methylation comprises the addition of a methyl group to the DNA. In mammals methylation is only possible on a CpG dinucleotide, where a cytosine is methylated that precedes 5' a guanosine in the DNA sequence. [16] These CpG dinucleotides are not evenly distributed over the genome. In the body of the genome there is a relative paucity of CpG dinucleotides. In the normal situation 80% of these CpG dinucleotides present in the body of the genome are methylated. [16] This helps to suppress unwanted transcription and is needed in X-chromosome inactivation and genetic imprinting. [13;16;20] However, in almost half of the human genome DNA clusters of CpG dinucleotides can be found in promoter regions, where transcription of DNA into RNA starts. [16] In normal cells, most CpG islands are unmethylated and transcription of the gene can take place (Figure 2B). In cancer cells, the patterns of DNA methylation are shifted and transcription is repressed. [16] When this occurs in tumor suppressor genes, carcinogenesis is initiated or enhanced (Figure 2C).

The process of DNA methylation (Figure 2A) is mediated by the DNA methyltransferase enzymes, DNMT1, DNMT3a, and DNMT3b. These enzymes transfer a methyl group to the cytosine in a CpG dinucleotide and catalyze methylation. [16;21] When a methyl group has bound to a cytosine, it is possible for methyl-CpG binding domains (MBD) proteins MeCP2, MBD1, MBD2, MBD3, MDB4, and Kaio, a methyl cytosine binding protein, to bind to the methyl-cytosines. MBDs cause the methylated DNA to be in a compacted chromatin environment through interactions with histone deacetylases (HDACs), histone methyltransferases (HMTs), and ATP-dependent chromatin remodelling enzymes. The compacted state of the DNA suppresses transcription of the gene. [21;22]

As described earlier, DNA methylation is one of the epigenetic changes that interacts with other epigenetic processes such as histone modifications, and nucleosomal remodelling of the DNA. DNA is wrapped around histone proteins to form the nucleosome. [21;23] The amino terminal tails of the histones protrude and can be modified by acetylation, methylation, phosphorylation, ubiquitination, and sumoylation. Modifications of the histones influence the transcription state of the DNA and can either suppress or promote DNA transcription. In a permissive state, the DNA can be transcribed. A permissive state of the DNA is characterised by hyperacetylation of histones H3 and H4 and di- and trimethylation of histone H3 at lysine 4 (H3K4). A compact chromatin structure suppresses DNA transcription and is marked by di- and tri-methylation of H3K9, tri-methyation of H3K27, and tri-methylation of H4K20. [15;21;24] Histone acetylation is regulated by histone acetyltransferases (HATs) and HDACs. HATs add acetyl groups that stabilize an open structure, in contrast to HDACs which deacetylate histones. [25] Other proteins involved in epigenetic regulation are Polycomb group (PcG) proteins [26;27], which are epigenetic chromatin modifiers. [19;22] Until now the exact mechanisms are unknown, but it is clear that the processes of DNA methylation, histone modification and nucleosomal remodelling interact with each other. [21]

Its reversible nature makes methylation an attractive therapeutic target. [26;27] This certainly is the case for haematological malignancies, but also in solid cancer beneficial effects have been demonstrated. Moreover, methylation has shown to have prognostic value and predicts response to treatment. [26;27] Above all, significant clinical benefit is to be expected of methylation as a biomarker for early detection of cancer. [28]

Promoter Methylation Assays

There is a panoply of different assays for determining promoter hypermethylation. Globally, the majority of assays are either restriction-enzyme based or bisulphite-conversion based techniques.

Restriction-enzyme methylation assays rely on the action of methylation-sensitive and/or methylation-dependent enzymes that cleave the unmethylated or the methylated DNA respectively. Methylation-Specific Multiplex Ligation-dependent Probe Amplification (MS-MLPA) is an example of a restriction-enzyme based assay. In MS-MPLA methylation-sensitive endonucleases are used to analyze the amount of methylated and unmethylated DNA. [29] Restriction-enzyme based methods are said to have several technical limitations, such as the limitation of enzyme-recognition sites and incomplete restriction-enzyme digestion in DNA originating from formaldehyde fixed material leading to false positive results. [19;30] In contrast to this, in a recent study, there was a strong correlation between a restriction enzyme based and a sodium bisulphite based methylation assay on DNA from paraffin embedded tissue. [31]

The technique of sodium bisulphite (NaBi) conversion of genomic DNA has been developed by Frommer et al. NaBi treatment results in a conversion of cytosine to uracil, but 5-methylcytosine is not affected. The DNA can be sequenced and amplified by PCR with two sets of strand-specific primers. [32] Genomic sequencing of NaBi treated DNA is a direct way to assess methylation status which is often referred to as the gold standard. Disadvantages are its laborious nature and limited potential for analyzing heterogenous DNA samples. [31] A more simple way to detect hypermethylation is a methylation-specific PCR (MSP).

Table 1. Tumor suppressor genes known to be involved in DNA promoter hypermethylation in breast cancer.

Gene	Aliases	Chromosomal location	Description	Reference
APC	*Adenomatous polyposis coli*	5q21-q22	Wnt signaling antagonist, cell migration, cell adhesion, transcriptional activation, apoptosis	[37;43;76-82]
BRCA1	*Breast cancer 1, early onset*	17q21	Transcription, DNA repair double-stranded breaks, recombination	[43;76;80;83;84]
BRCA2	*Breast cancer 2, early onset*	13q12.3	DNA repair double-stranded breaks	[43]
CCND2	*Cyclin D2*	12p13	Cell cycle regulation, replication	[34;41;43;80;84;85]
CDH1	*Cadherin 1 type 1, E-cadherin (epithelial)*	16q22.1	Cell adhesion	[37;43;76;79-81;84;86-88]
CDH13	*Cadherin 13, H-cadherin (heart)*	16q24.2-q24.3	Cell adhesion	[89]
CDKN2A	*$p16^{INK4A}$, cyclin-dependent kinase inhibitor 2A*	9p21	Cell cycle regulation	[43;76;77;79;80;84;88]

DAPK1	*Death-associated protein kinase 1*	9q34.1	Apoptosis	[76;79;90]
ESR1	*ERα, estrogen receptor 1*	6q25.1	Gene expression, cellular proliferation, differentiation	[37;43;80;84;87;91;92]
ESR2	*ERβ, estrogen receptor 2*	14q23.2	Gene expression, cellular proliferation, differentiation	[93;94]
FHIT	*Fragile histidine triad gene*	3p14.2	Purine metabolism	[95-99]
GSTP1	*Glutathione S-transferase pi 1*	11q13	Detoxification	[37;76;79-81]
HIC1	*Hypermethylated in cancer 1*	17p13.3	Cellular transcription repressor	[80;100;101]
HOXA5	*Homeobox gene 5*	7p15-14	Gene expression, morphogenesis, differentiation	[102;103]
KLK10	*NES1, kallikrein-related peptidase 10*	19q13.3-q13.4	Tumor suppression	[104;105]
*MGMT**	*O6-methyl-guanine-DNA methyltransferase*	10q26	DNA repair	[106]
MLH1	*hMLH1, mutL homolog 1 colon cancer nonpolyposis type 2 (Escheria coli)*	3p21.3	DNA mismatch repair	[77;107-111]
PGR	*PR, Progesterone receptor*	11q22-q23	Gene expression, cellular proliferation, differentiation	[92;112]
PYCARD	*TMS1, PYD and CARD domain containing, target of methylation-induced silencing 1*	16p12-p11.2	Apoptosis	[113-115]
RARB	*Retinoic acid receptor β*	3p24	Transcription, cellular signaling, limiting cell growth, cellular differentiation	[41;43;80;81;84;88;116;117]
RASSF1	*RAS (RalGDS/AF-6) association domain family member 1*	3p21.3	Cell cycle arrest, apoptosis	[34;41;43;79;81;118-120]
RUNX3	*Runt-related transcription factor 3*	1p36	Cellular transcription	[79;121-124]
SCGB3A1	*HIN1, secretoglobin family 3A member 1, high in normal 1*	5q35-qter	Cellular growth inhibition	[34;41;43;125]
SERPINB5	*Serpin peptidase inhibitor clade B (ovalbumin) member 5, maspin*	18q21.3	Inhibition growth, invasion, and metastatis	[126]
SFN	*Stratifin, 14-3-3- sigma*	1p36.11	Cell cycle regulation	[127;128]
SFRP1	*Secreted frizzled-related protein 1*	8p12-p11.1	Modulator Wnt signaling, cellular growth, differentiation	[129-131]
SOCS1	*Suppressor cytokine signaling 1*	16p13.13	Suppressor cytokine signaling	[94;132]
SYK	*Spleen tyrosine kinase*	9q22	Cellular proliferation, differentiation, survival, phagocytosis	[133;134]
TIMP3	*Tissue inhibitor of metalloproteinase 3*	22q12.3	Inactivation metalloproteinases	[37;76;135;136]
TP53	*Tumor protein 53, transformation-related protein 53*	17p13.1	Cell cycle arrest, apoptosis, senescence, DNA repair, changes in metabolism	[137]
TWIST1	*TWIST homolog of Drosophila 1*	7p21.2	Cell lineage determination, cellular differentiation	[34;41-43;81;84;138]
WIF1	*WNT inhibitory factor 1*	12q14.3	Inhibition Wnt signalling	[139;140]

*The role of DNA promoter hypermethylation of *MGMT* in breast cancer is arbitrary, since other studies show no methylation in breast cancer tissue. [76;79]

With this gel-based assay a distinction of methylated and unmethylated DNA in bisulphite-modified DNA can be made in a fast, cheap and easy way. MSP requires only small quantities of DNA and is sensitive to 0.1% methylated alleles of a given CpG island locus. Furthermore, MSP can be performed on DNA extracted from paraffin embedded tissue. [33] However, MSP cannot provide quantitative levels of methylation and therefore gives a less precise estimation of the methylation level. [19] Because of this issue, real-time methylation-specific PCR methods have been developed. A very sensitive method for quantification of methylation is Quantitative Multiplex Methylation-Specific PCR (QM-MSP), which combines multiplex PCR with Q-MSP. With this method promoter hypermethylation can be accurately detected in small samples for many genes simultaneously with a sensitivity of 1 in 10^4-10^5 copies of DNA. [34] According to the workshop "Towards Clinical Application of Methylated DNA Sequences as Cancer Biomarkers: A Joint National Cancer Institute's Early Detection Research Network and National Institute of Standards and Technology Workshop" quantitative MSP is the best method for the sensitive detection of methylated alleles. [35]

When comparing MS-MLPA, MSP and QM-MSP for a four gene panel (*CCND2, SCGB3A1, RARB, RASSF1*) in samples from invasive breast carcinomas, MSP and QM-MSP appeared to be highly discrepant. About 20% of tumors that showed no methylated band in MSP, gave more than 10% methylation in QM-MSP. Ten percent showed even more than 50% of methylation. In contrast to this, the correlation between QM-MSP and MS-MLPA targeting the same DNA sequence isolated from paraffin embedded tissue was strong (Spearman correlation coefficient 0.67). In a titration experiment MS-MPLA and MSP could detect methylation levels in 10 ng of DNA, while QM-MSP was at least ten-fold more sensitive. Therefore, QM-MSP is to be preferred for analyzing methylation patterns in samples with low amounts of DNA as are present in nipple fluid. [31]

Methylation in Breast Cancer

Profiles of hypermethylation of the CpG islands in tumor suppressor genes are relatively specific to the cancer type. Each tumor type is thereby characterised by a specific, defining DNA "hypermethylome". Such patterns of epigenetic inactivation occur not only in sporadic tumors, but also in inherited cancer syndromes. [15] In Table 1 the most well known tumor suppressor genes affected by DNA promoter hypermethylation in breast cancer are shown. A complete and updated list can be found on the website www.pubmeth.org.

Methylation is an early event in breast carcinogenesis. [36] Hoque et al. showed that aberrant promoter hypermethylation could be detected in both preinvasive and invasive lesions for *APC, CDH1, CTNNB1, TIMP3, ESR1* and *GSTP1*. Compared with normal breast *APC, CHD1*, and *CTNNB1* promoter regions were methylated more frequently in pathologic samples. Invasive tumors had significantly higher methylation levels of *CDH1* compared with preinvasive lesions. [37] However, methylation aberrations do not only exist in (pre)tumor tissue but are also seen in adjacent normal tissue. In a 6 gene panel (*DAPK1*, *TWIST*, *SCGB3A1*, *RASSF1*, *RARB*, *APC*) normal tissue adjacent to breast cancer had higher methylation values than normal tissue in unaffected women for *RASSF1*, *RARB* and *APC*. Methylation of tumor tissue was significantly higher than in normal tissue of the same breast cancer patient, and a correlation was detected between methylation in both tissues. [38] Yan et al. studied DNA methylation of the *RASSF1* promoter in primary breast tumors and adjacent normal tissue. Compared with primary tumors DNA methylation was low in reduction mammoplasty tissue. Normal tissue adjacent to primary tumors had however an intermediate level of methylation. The regions surrounding the core of the tumor were highly methylated and a field of methylation changes extended as far as 4 cm from primary tumors. These changes may explain local recurrence after radical resection, and methylation status of normal tissue adjacent to tumors could therefore be useful in determining risk of local recurrence. [39]

Methylation is common across the different histologic subtypes of breast cancer, although not all studies agree. Lobular and mucinous breast cancer were described to have a higher prevalence of overall hypermethylation compared with ductal cancer, hypermethylation of *BRCA1* was more often found in mucinous cancer [40], and *TWIST1* was less methylated in lobular cancer. [41] In contrast, our own studies did not show differences in methylation between ductal and lobular breast cancer. [42;43] A *BRCA* mutation also leads to differences in methylation levels. Breast cancer patients with a *BRCA1* mutation show less frequently hypermethylation than patients without a *BRCA1* mutation. [43] Flanagan et al. performed a genome wide DNA-methylation profiling in 33 cases of familial breast cancers with a *BRCA1, BRCA2* or *BRCAx* mutation. *BRCA1* tumors had the most dinstinct genome-wide DNA-methylation profiles with lower methylation levels compared to *BRCA2* and *BRCAx* tumors. However, intrinsic subtypes were not predicted by methylation profiles. A significant relation between methylation and copy number was found with a significant number of genes showing loss of heterozygosity and copy number. Besides, many genes showed a copy number gain and increased methylation. [44] Also ethnicity has been suggested to play a role in the prevalence of hypermethylation. Tumor tissue in Korean breast cancer patients younger than 50 years of age showed higher frequencies of hypermethylation at the time of diagnosis compared to women older than 50 years of age. Younger age was also associated with methylation of multiple genes. However, age did not correlate with the prevalence of hypermethylation in Caucasian women with breast cancer. [45] In contrast to this, we found the amount of methylation to increase with the age at which breast cancer develops [43], which had been shown before in other cancer types. [46]

On the other side of the spectrum of the disease, when tumors become invasive and metastasize, hypermethylation also plays a role. Mehrotra et al. investigated hypermethyation of five genes (*CCND2, RARB, TWIST1, RASSF1, SCGB3A1*) of paired primary breast cancer and its metastases to lymph nodes, bone, brain and lung using MSP. In normal tissue no hypermethylation for these genes was detected. In paired samples, lymph nodes tended to have more methylation compared with the primary tumor, with a significant difference for *SCGB3A1*. Also in distant metastatic sites hypermethylation was more frequent, being significantly higher for *SCGB3A1* and *RARB* in all sites. [47] In contrast, using a seven gene panel (*RASSF1, SCGB3A1, CCND2, TWIST, ESR1, APC, RARB*) Wu et al. found the cumulative methylation profiles of primary tumors to parallel their metastases. [48]

Methylation may also be a prognostic and predictive factor. For instance, Paired-like homeodomain transcription factor 2 (*PITX2*) DNA methylation was shown to be associated with early distant metastasis and poor overall survival in uni- and multivariate analysis. [49] Hypermethylation of Phosposerine aminotransferase (*PSAT1*) methylation was correlated with an advantageous clinical outcome and predicted response to tamoxifen treatment in patients with recurrent breast cancer. [50]

In summary, promoter hypermethylation seems to play a role in different stages of breast carcinogenesis and is therefore an interesting detection marker for (early stage) breast cancer. Besides, it seems to be associated with prognosis and response to therapy.

Methylation Detection in Breast Fluids

The breast ductal system can be directly accessed for diagnostic and therapeutic procedures through the nipple. [51] The acquisition of breast ductal fluid by nipple aspiration and ductal lavage are simple procedures to sample breast tissue. Fluid in the mammary ducts is normally produced in small amounts in non-lactating women (Figure 1). [52] The fluid contains breast cells and other components of the mammary microenvironment, including secreted proteins and free DNA. [53] Multiple approaches have been undertaken to analyze this fluid. As cytology turned out to be insufficiently reproducible and sensitive for breast cancer detection [54], alternatives such as proteomics, chromosomal instability, micro satellite instability, LOH and methylation analysis have been investigated in the last decades. [52]

Papanicolaou was the first to describe the retrieval of nipple fluid using mild suction with a breast pump. [55] At this moment nipple aspiration fluid (NAF) is still obtained non-invasively with a breast pump using intermittent vacuum, supported by oxytocin nasal spray (Figure 3). [56] After administration of oxytocin nasal spray, a suction cup is placed over the nipple. Repeated gentle suction by a syringe draws fluid outside the duct to the nipple surface. Fluid droplets are collected by capillary tubes. The procedure is subsequently repeated at the contralateral breast. In a pilot study with 67 healthy female volunteers the feasibility of this procedure was assessed. In 94% of women fluid was obtained from either one of the breasts and in 75% it was possible to collect fluid bilaterally. Obtained volumes ranged from 5 to 100 μl with an average of 2000 ng of DNA (range 500-6800 ng), sufficient for performing methylation assays such as QM-MSP. The procedure was very well tolerated with no reported side effects. About 99% would undergo the procedure again and recommend the procedure to someone else. [56] Moreover, oxytocin-assisted nipple aspiration is feasible in 90% of women at increased risk for breast cancer including women that previously had breast cancer, despite the high frequency of radiotherapy, breast surgery and chemotherapy in this group. [57]

Another way to retrieve luminal fluid from the ductal network is ductal lavage. Ductal lavage collects a more cellular fluid sample from the ductal system utilizing a micro catheter through a saline solution infused first into the breast and then aspirated. [53]. Fine needle aspiration (FNA), a third way to obtain ductal fluid, can be performed in women with a suspicious breast lesion [58-62] or in high-risk women. The latter case is called random periareolar fine needle aspiration (RPFNA), where the fluid is randomly aspirated in the periareolar region. [61;63-66] FNA is an invasive procedure and therefore less suitable as a screening method.

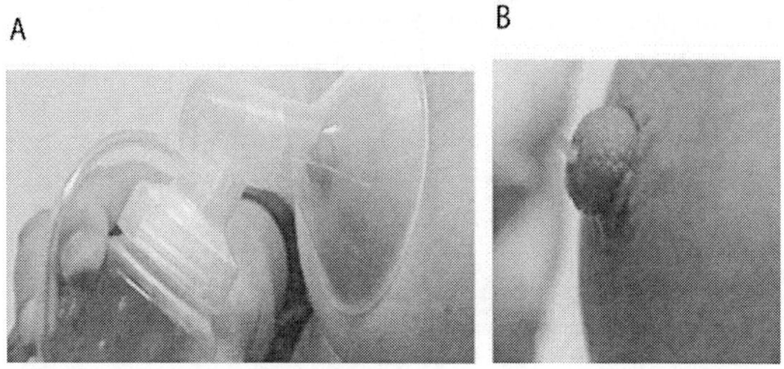

Figure 3. Nipple fluid aspiration. A. Suction cup placed over the nipple, after which intermittent vacuum suction can take place. B. After vacuum suction, nipple fluid is collected by a capillary tube.

Table 2. Studies describing DNA promoter hypermethylation in luminal fluids of the breast.

A. Non-quantitative methylation assays

First author	Year	Methylation assay	Origin fluid	Patients (n)	Genes
Evron [67]	2001	MSP	ROBE fluid DL	IBC (20) DCIS (7) ADH (6) No residual tumor (4) Benign (45) Atypical mild changes (5) Atypical substantial changes (5) Malignant (1)	*CCND2, RARB, TWIST1*
Jeronimo [59]	2003	MSP	FNA	Suspicious mammary lesion (123)	*BRCA1, CDH1, GSTP1, RARB*
Pu [62]	2003	MSP	FNA	IBC (45) DCIS/LCIS (21) Benign (36)	*CCND2, RARB, RASSF1*
Krassenstein* [68]	2004	MSP	NAF	DCIS/IBC (22)	*CDKN2A, DAPK1, GSTP1, $p14^{ARF}$, RARB, RASSF1,*
Bean [65]	2005	MSP	RPFNA	Asymptomatic HR women (38)	*RARB*
Lewis [61]	2005	MSP	FNA RPFNA	IBC (27) Unaffected women (55)	*APC, CCND2, CDH13, RASSF1, RARB*
Bean [63]	2007	MSP	RPFNA	Asymptomatic HR women (61)	*BRCA1*
Bean [64]	2007	MSP	RPFNA	Asymptomatic HR women (86)	*$p14^{ARF}$*
Locke [69]	2007	MSP	DL	Healthy *BRCA1*-carriers (7) Healthy *BRCA2*-carriers (12) Healthy controls (5)	*CCND2, RARB, SCGB3A1, TWIS1T*
Baker [75]	2008	MSP	RPFNA	HR women receiving tamoxifen (18) HR women not receiving tamoxifen (16)	*ESR1*
Vasilatos [66]	2009	MSP	RPFNA	HR women (109)	*BRCA1, ESR1, $p14^{ARF}$, PRA, PRB , RARB, RASSF1, RBP1, SCGB3A1*
Antill [70]	2010	MSP	DL	*BRCA1*-carriers (16) *BRCA2*-carriers (18)	*DKN2A, RARB, RASSF1, TWIST1*

B. Quantitative methylation assays with mean quantifications of methylation %**

First author	Year	Methylation assay	Origin fluid	Patients (n)	*APC* (%)	*BRCA1* (%)	*BRCA2* (%)	*CCND2* (%)	*CDH1*(%)	*CDKN2A* (%)	*ESR1* (%)	*RARB* (%)	*RASSF1* (%)	*SCGB3A1* (%)	*TWIST1* (%)
Fackler [34]	2004	QM-MSP	DL	DCIS/IBC (4) High risk (7)	NA NA	NA NA	NA NA	4.00 0.00	NA NA	NA NA	NA NA	22.25 0.00	12.75 0.06	35.00 0.00	7.75 0.00
Fackler [71]***	2006	QM-MSP	DL	Mastectomy (37) High risk (60)	5.89 0.15	2.77 0.02	0.00 0.01	2.62 0.07	NA NA	0.03 0.00	NA NA	1.12 0.18	8.11 0.21	10.20 0.09	5.83 0.18
Euhus** [73]	2007	QM-MSP	DL	Cancer (34)	4.1	NA	NA	7.8	NA	NA	NA	31.0	6.4	11.4	NA
Euhus [58]****	2008	QM-MSP	PDFNA	IBC (69) Unaffected HR (25) Unaffected LR (70)	****	NA	NA	****	NA	NA	NA	****	****	****	NA
Jeronimo [60]*****	2008	Q-MSP	FNA	IBC (66) Benign (12)	*****	NA	NA	*****	NA	NA	NA	NA	*****	*****	NA
Fackler [72]	2009	QM-MSP	DL	Cancer (7) Papilloma (27) Normal (28)	10.23 1.56 0.28	0.40 2.40 0.00	0.00 0.01 0.05	15.31 0.54 0.53	2.63 3.59 0.05	0.99 0.00 0.00	0.01 0.01 0.02	9.96 1.46 1.40	13.92 3.27 0.29	15.69 1.33 0.15	18.02 0.61 0.35
Zhu [74]	2009	QM-MSP	NAF	Cancer (18)	NA	NA	NA	1.49	NA	0.22	NA	26.14	16.25	NA	NA
			MD**	Cancer (61) Precancer (10) Benign (48)	NA NA NA	NA NA NA	NA NA NA	0.02 0.007 0.013	NA NA NA	0.18 0.17 0.054	NA NA NA	0.02 0.014 0.027	0.90 0.42 0.32	NA NA NA	NA NA NA

Legend

*Krassenstein et al. did not assess the methylation status for each nipple fluid sample for all six genes in the panel together.

**The methylation levels of the ductal lavage samples in the study of Euhus et al., and the ductoscopic samples in the study of Zhu et al. are median percentages.

***Fackler et al. examined 37 ductal lavage samples from women before mastectomy: 27 women (33 ducts) had biopsy proven DCIS or IBC, and 3 women (4 ducts) had no known cancer.

****Euhus et al. did not show quantitative data for the methylation levels in FNA samples, but performed correlation analysis for methylation and patient characteristics.

*****Jeronimo et al. did not show quantitative data for the methylation levels in FNA samples, but performed ROC curve analysis.

ADH: Atypical ductal hyperplasia, DCIS: Ductal carcinoma in situ, DL: Ductal lavage, FNA: Fine needle aspiration, HR: High risk, IBC: Invasive breast cancer, LCIS: Lobular carcinoma in situ, LR: Low risk, MD: Mammary ductoscopy, MSP: Methylation-specific PCR, NA: Not available, NAF: Nipple aspiration fluid, PDFNA: Palpation directed fine needle aspiration, Q-MSP: Quantitative methylation-specific PCR, QM-MSP: Quantitative multiplex methylation-specific PCR, ROBE: Routine operative breast endoscopy, RPFNA: Random periareolar fine needle aspiration

Clinical Results on Methylation Detection in Breast Fluid

In this paragraph studies investigating DNA promoter methylation patterns in fluid obtained by NAF, ductal lavage, ductoscopic samples or FNA are discussed. The results are summarized in Table 2.

Evron et al. were the first to describe methylation patterns in ductal fluid. Methylation-specific PCR was performed for the genes *CCND2*, *RARB* and *TWIST1*. Hypermethylation of at least one of these three genes was frequently detected in fluid from mammary ducts with endoscopically visualised carcinomas (17 cases of 20) or ductal carcinoma in situ (2 of 7). In healthy ducts hypermethylation was rarely detected (5 of 45). Two of the women with healthy mammograms in which hypermethylation was found in ductal lavage fluid were subsequently diagnosed with breast cancer. [67]

Krassenstein et al. searched for aberrant promoter hypermethylation in 22 matched specimens of tumor, normal tissue, and nipple aspiration fluid collected from breast cancer patients. The authors used methylation-specific PCR for a panel of six genes, i.e. *GSTP1*, *RARB*, *CDKN2A*, $p14^{ARF}$, *RASSF1* and *DAPK1*. Hypermethylation of one or more genes was found in all 22 tumor specimen. Once an individual tumor was known to be positive for hypermethylation of a gene in the panel, the corresponding nipple fluid was analyzed for hypermethylation of that particular gene. The amount of DNA available from the nipple fluids did not allow screening for all six genes in the panel by MSP, but the authors believed that detecting methylation of one methylated gene in each breast cancer-associated nipple fluid was sufficient for proof of principle. The authors detected hypermethylation of the same gene in 18 of 22 (82%) nipple fluids. In those tumors positive for more than one gene, the promoter hypermethylation pattern was identical in the matched nipple fluid. In contrast, hypermethylation was absent in benign and normal breast tissue and nipple fluid DNA from healthy women. [68]

A few studies particularly examined samples from healthy *BRCA* mutation carriers. Locke et al. attempted to establish whether *BRCA* mutation carriers demonstrate an increased frequency of aberrant promoter hypermethylation in ductal lavage fluid, compared with negative controls not known to have a *BRCA* mutation. Hypermethylation in a panel of four genes (*RARB*, *SCGB3A1*, *TWIST1*, and *CCND2*) was analyzed by methylation-specific PCR in 51 ductal lavage samples from healthy women of known *BRCA* status. *BRCA* mutation carriers were found to have at least one hypermethylated gene in 42% of cases. No hypermethylation was found in samples from the controls. [69]

The second study investigating *BRCA1/2* mutation carriers was prospectively performed by Antill et al. who assessed promoter methylation in a prospective collection of ductal lavage samples from women with a known *BRCA1* or *BRCA2* mutation. Hypermethylation of *CDKN2A*, *RASSF1*, *TWIST1*, and *RARB* was tested using a qualitative, real-time, nested PCR. A total of 168 samples from 93 ducts in 54 breasts were assessed in 34 women: 16 *BRCA1* and 18 *BRCA2* carriers. A median of two ductal lavages was done (range 1-5). Seven women developed breast cancer, including one woman with bilateral disease. Methylation of *CDKN2A* was associated with a known *BRCA1* mutation and with a history of contralateral breast cancer. An association was found between the development of breast cancer on study and *RASSF1* methylation. [70]

The studies mentioned above determined methylation status in a non-quantitative manner. As described previously Fackler et al. developed the QM-MSP technique by which they detected hypermethylated *RASSF1*, *TWIST1*, *CCND2*, *SCGB3A1*, and *RARB* in high-risk women. Samples were obtained by ductal lavage or by irrigation during ductoscopy in four patients with biopsy proven cancer. In six out of seven samples from high-risk women no hypermethylation was detected in the five genes tested. However, one sample had a low level of methylation in *RASSF1*. Samples derived by ductoscopy from two women with invasive carcinoma had a high level of multigene promoter hypermethylation. The samples from women with DCIS lacked detectable promoter hypermethylation. [34] In a subsequent study, the same research group described the QM-MSP results in 37 ductal lavage samples from women undergoing mastectomy. Hypermethylation of a nine gene panel (*RASSF1*, *TWIST1*, *SCGB3A1*, *CCND2*, *RARB*, *APC*, *BRCA1*, *BRCA2*, *CDKN2A*) was correlated to histology and cytology. Cumulative methylation of the genes detected malignancy with a sensitivity of 62% and specificity of 82% and by receiver operating characteristic (ROC) threshold analysis with a sensitivity of 71% and specificity of 83%. QM-MSP doubled the sensitivity of detection of cancer as compared to cytology. [71] In a more recent study these authors tested hypermethylation in women with pathologic nipple discharge undergoing ductoscopy. Ducts with significant lesions were surgically resected (36 ducts in 33 women) and those with minimal findings were not (28 ducts in 16 women). Cells from ducts with significant lesions found during ductoscopy had significantly higher methylation levels than ducts with minimal findings. Besides, cells form ducts with DCIS displayed higher levels of methylation than ducts with benign lesions such as papilloma or ducts with minimal findings during ductoscopy. Cumultative *RASSF1*, *TWIST1*, and SCGB3A1 gene methylation could accurately distinguish between ducts with malignant and benign lesions with a sensitivity of 100% and specificity of 72%, and area under the curve 0.91 according to receiving operating characteristics (ROC) analyses. QM-MSP analysis appeared to be more accurate than cytology for detecting DCIS. Again the addition of QM-MSP improved the detection of malignant lesions, because the positive predictive value of ductoscopy was raised from 19% to 47% by adding QM-MSP. [72]

Other groups have used QM-MSP as well. Euhus et al. obtained 514 ductal lavage samples from 150 women representing a wide range of breast cancer risk. The samples were evaluated cytologically and by QM-MSP for methylation of *CCND2*, *APC*, *SCGB3A1*, *RASSF1*, and *RARB*. Ductal lavage in a breast containing cancer rarely showed cancer cells cytologically. The frequency of hypermethylation was significantly higher in the tumor tissue than the corresponding fluid sample. Perimenopausal state, increased cellularity in the sample, and risk classification according to the Gail risk model predicted methylation of two or more genes in a multivariate analysis. Methylation also increased with age, but this was not statistically significant. Cytology and methylation results did not correlate, suggesting that both analysis methods assess different underlying mechanisms of carcinogenesis. [73]

Finally, Zhu et al. conducted QM-MSP for *RASSF1*, *CCND2*, *CDKN2A*, and *RARB* in 18 tumor, adjacent normal tissue and nipple aspirate fluid samples. All 18 matched samples from cancer containing breasts provided satisfactory PCR signals for all genes. There was increased methylation in the four genes analyzed in tumorous compared to adjacent normal tissue. Methylation was significantly higher in nipple aspirate fluid than adjacent normal tissue for *CDKN2A*, non-significantly higher for *RARB*, but not for *CCND2* and *RASSF1*. The methylation percentage for *CDKN2A* and *RASSF1* in samples obtained by irrigation during ductoscopy was significantly higher in breasts with cancer than in breasts without. An increase in *CDKN2A* methylation occurred in precancerous lesion. From these data it can be concluded that methylation aberrations in tumor tissue can also be found in matched ductal fluid samples. [74]

As described earlier, a more invasive -and therefore less suitable for screening- way to obtain breast fluid is FNA. To complete the overview of methylation detection in breast fluids, studies analyzing methylation in FNA samples are described shortly in the next section. Methylation percentages in fluid obtained by FNA in women with suspicious mammary lesions are concordant between paired benign and malignant lesion. [59;62] Moreover, in 67% of the FNA samples hypermethylation patterns are identical to patterns in the paired malignant tissues. [59] When using a gene panel with *CCND2, RASSF1, APC*, and *SCGB3A1*, specificity is 100% for detecting breast cancer when 3 of 4 genes are methylated. [60] *CCND2* methylation is significantly more found in breast cancer FNA samples compared to benign samples, while hypermethylation of *APC, RARB,* and *RASSF1* in samples of benign tissue is associated with known risk factors for developing breast cancer. [61] The prediction of methylation markers in RPFNA samples is tested in women with cytologic mammary atypia receiving chemoprevention, but *ESR1* methylation did not appear to be a reliable marker to predict persistent atypia in RPFNA 12 months after the start of chemoprevention. [75]

Also in high risk women hypermethylation in fluid obtained by RPFNA is related to the breast cancer risk. [58] Hypermethylation of *RARB* in RPFNA is positively associated with increasing abnormalities found by cytologic examination [65], while methylation of *BRCA1* does not predict atypia in high-risk women. [63] In RPFNA samples of high-risk women hypermethylation of *RARB*, *CDKN2A*, *SCGB3A1*, *PR*, and overall methylation is associated with abnormal cytology. Moreover, hypermethylation of $p14^{ARF}$ in these samples of high-risk women is highly associated with methylation of *RARB, BRCA1*, and *ESR1*. [64] When comparing methylation levels in RPFNA samples from high risk women, women with a *BRCA1/2* mutation had lower frequencies of hypermethylation than non-carriers [66], as was found in tumor tissue. [43]

All the studies described show that detection of DNA promoter hypermethylation in breast fluids is feasible, although comparison is difficult because of different gene panels used in the described studies. [17] Moreover, the presence of hypermethylation in breast fluids is associated with the development of breast cancer. This makes methylation assessment in breast fluid, especially nipple fluid, a promising approach as a new screening method for breast cancer in addition to the current used screening techniques, in particular for high-risk women. [14] However, large studies are needed to prospectively assess the predictive values of (alterations in) methylation status for the presence of breast cancer in early stages. In the University Medical Center Utrecht (UMC Utrecht), The Netherlands, such a prospective study was started in 2008. In this study nipple fluid is aspirated annually in women at high risk for developing breast cancer defined by a *BRCA1/2* mutation or by a breast cancer (family) history. The aim of this study is to address the predictive value of methylation analysis in nipple fluid in the early detection of breast cancer. In this way the real value of methylation assessment in nipple fluid in addition to current screening modalities including physical examination, mammography and MRI, can be determined. This study is expected to expand to other Dutch Centers in the near future.

Conclusion

Nipple fluid could become a valuable source for population-based screening of high-risk women. [52] Currently, very sensitive methylation assays such as QM-MSP are available, that can assess methylation in as little as a few microliters of nipple fluid. Available evidence suggests a strong correlation between methylation in nipple fluid and breast cancer development, but ongoing large prospective studies, like the one that is currently conducted in the UMC Utrecht, The Netherlands, will be needed to prove the real additive value of methylation detection in nipple fluid to current imaging-based screening.

References

[1] Khatib OMN And Modjtabai A. WHO EMRO Technical Publications Series 30: Guidelines For The Early Detection And Screening Of Breast Cancer. 2006. *http://www.emro.who.int/dsaf/dsa696.pdf*

[2] Chen S And Parmigiani G, Meta-Analysis Of BRCA1 And BRCA2 Penetrance. *J.Clin.Oncol.* 25: 1329-1333, 2007.

[3] Brekelmans CT, Seynaeve C, Bartels CC, Tilanus-Linthorst MM, Meijers-Heijboer EJ, Crepin CM, Van Geel AA, Menke M, Verhoog LC, Van Den Ouweland A, Obdeijn IM, And Klijn JG, Effectiveness Of Breast Cancer Surveillance In BRCA1/2 Gene Mutation Carriers And Women With High Familial Risk. *J.Clin.Oncol.* 19: 924-930, 2001.

[4] Ernestos B, Nikolaos P, Koulis G, Eleni R, Konstantinos B, Alexandra G, And Michael K, Increased Chromosomal Radiosensitivity In Women Carrying BRCA1/BRCA2 Mutations Assessed With The G2 Assay. *Int.J.Radiat.Oncol.Biol.Phys.* 76: 1199-1205, 2010.

[5] Berrington De GA, Berg CD, Visvanathan K, And Robson M, Estimated Risk Of Radiation-Induced Breast Cancer From Mammographic Screening For Young BRCA Mutation Carriers. *J.Natl.Cancer Inst.* 101: 205-209, 2009.

[6] Kriege M, Brekelmans CT, Boetes C, Besnard PE, Zonderland HM, Obdeijn IM, Manoliu RA, Kok T, Peterse H, Tilanus-Linthorst MM, Muller SH, Meijer S, Oosterwijk JC, Beex LV, Tollenaar RA, De Koning HJ, Rutgers EJ, And Klijn JG, Efficacy Of MRI And Mammography For Breast-Cancer Screening In Women With A Familial Or Genetic Predisposition. *N.Engl.J.Med.* 351: 427-437, 2004.

[7] Kuhl CK, Schmutzler RK, Leutner CC, Kempe A, Wardelmann E, Hocke A, Maringa M, Pfeifer U, Krebs D, And Schild HH, Breast MR Imaging Screening In 192 Women Proved Or Suspected To Be Carriers Of A Breast Cancer Susceptibility Gene: *Preliminary Results. Radiology* 215: 267-279, 2000.

[8] Meijers-Heijboer H, Van Geel B, Van Putten WL, Henzen-Logmans SC, Seynaeve C, Menke-Pluymers MB, Bartels CC, Verhoog LC, Van Den Ouweland AM, Niermeijer MF, Brekelmans CT, And Klijn JG, Breast Cancer After Prophylactic Bilateral Mastectomy In Women With A BRCA1 Or BRCA2 Mutation. *N.Engl.J.Med.* 345: 159-164, 2001.

[9] Hartmann LC, Schaid DJ, Woods JE, Crotty TP, Myers JL, Arnold PG, Petty PM, Sellers TA, Johnson JL, Mcdonnell SK, Frost MH, And Jenkins RB, Efficacy Of Bilateral Prophylactic Mastectomy In Women With A Family History Of Breast Cancer. *N.Engl.J.Med.* 340: 77-84, 1999.

[10] Eisen A, Rebbeck TR, Wood WC, And Weber BL, Prophylactic Surgery In Women With A Hereditary Predisposition To Breast And Ovarian Cancer. *J.Clin.Oncol.* 18: 1980-1995, 2000.

[11] King BL And Love SM, The Intraductal Approach To The Breast: Raison D'etre. *Breast Cancer Res.* 8: 206, 2006.

[12] Baylin SB And Herman JG, DNA Hypermethylation In Tumorigenesis: Epigenetics Joins Genetics. *Trends Genet.* 16: 168-174, 2000.

[13] Esteller M, Aberrant DNA Methylation As A Cancer-Inducing Mechanism. *Annu.Rev.Pharmacol.Toxicol.* 45: 629-656, 2005.

[14] Suijkerbuijk KPM, Van Diest PJ, And Van Der Wall E, Improving Early Breast Cancer Detection: Focus On Methylation. *Annals Of Oncology*, 2010.

[15] Esteller M, Epigenetics In Cancer. *N.Engl.J.Med.* 358: 1148-1159, 2008.

[16] Herman JG And Baylin SB, Gene Silencing In Cancer In Association With Promoter Hypermethylation. *N.Engl.J.Med.* 349: 2042-2054, 2003.

[17] Brooks J, Cairns P, And Zeleniuch-Jacquotte A, Promoter Methylation And The Detection Of Breast Cancer. *Cancer Causes Control* 20: 1539-1550, 2009.

[18] Schuebel KE, Chen W, Cope L, Glockner SC, Suzuki H, Yi JM, Chan TA, Van Neste L, Van Criekinge W, Van Den Bosch S, Van Engeland M, Ting AH, Jair K, Yu W, Toyota M, Imai K, Ahuja N, Herman JG, And Baylin SB, Comparing The DNA Hypermethylome With Gene Mutations In Human Colorectal Cancer. *Plos.Genet.* 3: 1709-1723, 2007.

[19] Lo PK And Sukumar S, Epigenomics And Breast Cancer. *Pharmacogenomics* 9: 1879-1902, 2008.

[20] Issa JP, Cpg Island Methylator Phenotype In Cancer. *Nat.Rev.Cancer* 4: 988-993, 2004.

[21] Mccabe MT, Brandes JC, And Vertino PM, Cancer DNA Methylation: Molecular Mechanisms And Clinical Implications. *Clin.Cancer Res.* 15: 3927-3937, 2009.

[22] Kristensen LS, Nielsen HM, And Hansen LL, Epigenetics And Cancer Treatment. *Eur.J.Pharmacol.* 625: 131-142, 2009.

[23] Momparler RL, Cancer Epigenetics. *Oncogene* 22: 6479-6483, 2003.

[24] Jones PA And Baylin SB, The Fundamental Role Of Epigenetic Events In Cancer. *Nat.Rev.Genet.* 3: 415-428, 2002.

[25] Stearns V, Zhou Q, And Davidson NE, Epigenetic Regulation As A New Target For Breast Cancer Therapy. *Cancer Invest* 25: 659-665, 2007.

[26] Dworkin AM, Huang TH, And Toland AE, Epigenetic Alterations In The Breast: Implications For Breast Cancer Detection, Prognosis And Treatment. *Semin.Cancer Biol.* 19: 165-171, 2009.

[27] Mulero-Navarro S And Esteller M, Epigenetic Biomarkers For Human Cancer: The Time Is Now. *Crit Rev.Oncol.Hematol.* 68: 1-11, 2008.

[28] Duffy MJ, Napieralski R, Martens JW, Span PN, Spyratos F, Sweep FC, Brunner N, Foekens JA, And Schmitt M, Methylated Genes As New Cancer Biomarkers. *Eur.J.Cancer* 45: 335-346, 2009.

[29] Nygren AO, Ameziane N, Duarte HM, Vijzelaar RN, Waisfisz Q, Hess CJ, Schouten JP, And Errami A, Methylation-Specific MLPA (MS-MLPA): Simultaneous Detection Of Cpg Methylation And Copy Number Changes Of Up To 40 Sequences. *Nucleic Acids Res.* 33: E128, 2005.
[30] Laird PW, The Power And The Promise Of DNA Methylation Markers. *Nat.Rev.Cancer* 3: 253-266, 2003.
[31] Suijkerbuijk KPM, Pan X, Van Der Wall E, Van Diest PJ, And Vooijs M, Comparison Of Different Promoter Methylation Assays In Breast Cancer. *Cell.Oncol.* In Press: 2010.
[32] Frommer M, Mcdonald LE, Millar DS, Collis CM, Watt F, Grigg GW, Molloy PL, And Paul CL, A Genomic Sequencing Protocol That Yields A Positive Display Of 5-Methylcytosine Residues In Individual DNA Strands. *Proc.Natl.Acad.Sci.U.S.A* 89: 1827-1831, 1992.
[33] Herman JG, Graff JR, Myohanen S, Nelkin BD, And Baylin SB, Methylation-Specific PCR: A Novel PCR Assay For Methylation Status Of Cpg Islands. *Proc.Natl.Acad.Sci.U.S.A* 93: 9821-9826, 1996.
[34] Fackler MJ, Mcveigh M, Mehrotra J, Blum MA, Lange J, Lapides A, Garrett E, Argani P, And Sukumar S, Quantitative Multiplex Methylation-Specific PCR Assay For The Detection Of Promoter Hypermethylation In Multiple Genes In Breast Cancer. *Cancer Res.* 64: 4442-4452, 2004.
[35] Kagan J, Srivastava S, Barker PE, Belinsky SA, And Cairns P, Towards Clinical Application Of Methylated DNA Sequences As Cancer Biomarkers: A Joint NCI's EDRN And NIST Workshop On Standards, Methods, Assays, Reagents And Tools. *Cancer Res.* 67: 4545-4549, 2007.
[36] Agrawal A, Murphy RF, And Agrawal DK, DNA Methylation In Breast And Colorectal Cancers. *Mod.Pathol.* 20: 711-721, 2007.
[37] Hoque MO, Prencipe M, Poeta ML, Barbano R, Valori VM, Copetti M, Gallo AP, Brait M, Maiello E, Apicella A, Rossiello R, Zito F, Stefania T, Paradiso A, Carella M, Dallapiccola B, Murgo R, Carosi I, Bisceglia M, Fazio VM, Sidransky D, And Parrella P, Changes In Cpg Islands Promoter Methylation Patterns During Ductal Breast Carcinoma Progression. *Cancer Epidemiol.Biomarkers Prev.* 18: 2694-2700, 2009.
[38] Van Der Auwera I, Bovie C, Svensson C, Trinh XB, Limame R, Van Dam P, Van Laere SJ, Van Marck EA, Dirix LY, And Vermeulen PB, Quantitative Methylation Profiling In Tumor And Matched Morphologically Normal Tissues From Breast Cancer Patients. *BMC.Cancer* 10: 97, 2010.
[39] Yan PS, Venkataramu C, Ibrahim A, Liu JC, Shen RZ, Diaz NM, Centeno B, Weber F, Leu YW, Shapiro CL, Eng C, Yeatman TJ, And Huang TH, Mapping Geographic Zones Of Cancer Risk With Epigenetic Biomarkers In Normal Breast Tissue. *Clin.Cancer Res.* 12: 6626-6636, 2006.
[40] Bae YK, Brown A, Garrett E, Bornman D, Fackler MJ, Sukumar S, Herman JG, And Gabrielson E, Hypermethylation In Histologically Distinct Classes Of Breast Cancer. *Clin.Cancer Res.* 10: 5998-6005, 2004.
[41] Fackler MJ, Mcveigh M, Evron E, Garrett E, Mehrotra J, Polyak K, Sukumar S, And Argani P, DNA Methylation Of RASSF1A, HIN-1, RAR-Beta, Cyclin D2 And Twist In In Situ And Invasive Lobular Breast Carcinoma. *Int.J.Cancer* 107: 970-975, 2003.

[42] Gort EH, Suijkerbuijk KP, Roothaan SM, Raman V, Vooijs M, Van Der Wall E, And Van Diest PJ, Methylation Of The TWIST1 Promoter, TWIST1 Mrna Levels, And Immunohistochemical Expression Of TWIST1 In Breast Cancer. *Cancer Epidemiol.Biomarkers Prev.* 17: 3325-3330, 2008.

[43] Suijkerbuijk KP, Fackler MJ, Sukumar S, Van Gils CH, Van Laar T, Van Der Wall E, Vooijs M, And Van Diest PJ, Methylation Is Less Abundant In BRCA1-Associated Compared With Sporadic Breast Cancer. *Ann.Oncol.* 19: 1870-1874, 2008.

[44] Flanagan JM, Cocciardi S, Waddell N, Johnstone CN, Marsh A, Henderson S, Simpson P, Da Silva L, Khanna K, Lakhani S, Boshoff C, And Chenevix-Trench G, DNA Methylome Of Familial Breast Cancer Identifies Distinct Profiles Defined By Mutation Status. *Am.J.Hum.Genet.* 86: 420-433, 2010.

[45] Lee JS, Lo PK, Fackler MJ, Argani P, Zhang Z, Garrett-Meyer E, And Sukumar S, A Comparative Study Of Korean With Caucasian Breast Cancer Reveals Frequency Of Methylation In Multiple Genes Correlates With Breast Cancer In Young, ER, PR-Negative Breast Cancer In Korean Women. *Cancer Biol.Ther.* 6: 1114-1120, 2007.

[46] Ahuja N, Li Q, Mohan AL, Baylin SB, And Issa JP, Aging And DNA Methylation In Colorectal Mucosa And Cancer. *Cancer Res.* 58: 5489-5494, 1998.

[47] Mehrotra J, Vali M, Mcveigh M, Kominsky SL, Fackler MJ, Lahti-Domenici J, Polyak K, Sacchi N, Garrett-Mayer E, Argani P, And Sukumar S, Very High Frequency Of Hypermethylated Genes In Breast Cancer Metastasis To The Bone, Brain, And Lung. *Clin.Cancer Res.* 10: 3104-3109, 2004.

[48] Wu JM, Fackler MJ, Halushka MK, Molavi DW, Taylor ME, Teo WW, Griffin C, Fetting J, Davidson NE, De Marzo AM, Hicks JL, Chitale D, Ladanyi M, Sukumar S, And Argani P, Heterogeneity Of Breast Cancer Metastases: Comparison Of Therapeutic Target Expression And Promoter Methylation Between Primary Tumors And Their Multifocal Metastases. *Clin.Cancer Res.* 14: 1938-1946, 2008.

[49] Nimmrich I, Sieuwerts AM, Meijer-Van Gelder ME, Schwope I, Bolt-De VJ, Harbeck N, Koenig T, Hartmann O, Kluth A, Dietrich D, Magdolen V, Portengen H, Look MP, Klijn JG, Lesche R, Schmitt M, Maier S, Foekens JA, And Martens JW, DNA Hypermethylation Of PITX2 Is A Marker Of Poor Prognosis In Untreated Lymph Node-Negative Hormone Receptor-Positive Breast Cancer Patients. *Breast Cancer Res.Treat.* 111: 429-437, 2008.

[50] Martens JW, Nimmrich I, Koenig T, Look MP, Harbeck N, Model F, Kluth A, Bolt-De VJ, Sieuwerts AM, Portengen H, Meijer-Van Gelder ME, Piepenbrock C, Olek A, Hofler H, Kiechle M, Klijn JG, Schmitt M, Maier S, And Foekens JA, Association Of DNA Methylation Of Phosphoserine Aminotransferase With Response To Endocrine Therapy In Patients With Recurrent Breast Cancer. *Cancer Res.* 65: 4101-4117, 2005.

[51] Rochman S, Mills D., Kim J., Kuerer H., And Love S. State Of The Science And The Intraductal Approach For Breast Cancer: Proceedings Summary Of The Sixth International Symposium On The Intraductal Approach To Breast Cancer Santa Monica, California, 19-21 February 2009. 3(Suppl 5), I1. 2009. *BMC Proceedings.*

[52] Suijkerbuijk KP, Van Der Wall E, Vooijs M, And Van Diest PJ, Molecular Analysis Of Nipple Fluid For Breast Cancer Screening. *Pathobiology* 75: 149-152, 2008.

[53] Klein PM And Lawrence JA, Lavage And Nipple Aspiration Of Breast Ductal Fluids: A Source Of Biomarkers For Environmental Mutagenesis. *Environ.Mol.Mutagen.* 39: 127-133, 2002.

[54] Johnson-Maddux A, Ashfaq R, Cler L, Naftalis E, Leitch AM, Hoover S, And Euhus DM, Reproducibility Of Cytologic Atypia In Repeat Nipple Duct Lavage. *Cancer* 103: 1129-1136, 2005.

[55] Holmquist DG, And Papanicolaou GN, *The Exfoliative Cytology Of The Mammary Gland During Pregnancy And Lactation.* Ann.N.Y.Acad.Sci. 63: 1422-1435, 1956.

[56] Suijkerbuijk KP, Van Der Wall E, And Van Diest PJ, Oxytocin: Bringing Magic Into Nipple Aspiration. *Ann.Oncol.* 18: 1743-1744, 2007.

[57] Suijkerbuijk KP, Van Der Wall E, Meijrink H, Pan X, Borel Rinkes I, Ausems MG, And Van Diest PJ, Successful Oxytocin-Assisted Nipple Aspiration In Women At Increased Risk For Breast Cancer. *Fam.Cancer* 9(3):321-325, 2010.

[58] Euhus DM, Bu D, Milchgrub S, Xie XJ, Bian A, Leitch AM, And Lewis CM, DNA Methylation In Benign Breast Epithelium In Relation To Age And Breast Cancer Risk. *Cancer Epidemiol.Biomarkers Prev.* 17: 1051-1059, 2008.

[59] Jeronimo C, Costa I, Martins MC, Monteiro P, Lisboa S, Palmeira C, Henrique R, Teixeira MR, And Lopes C, Detection Of Gene Promoter Hypermethylation In Fine Needle Washings From Breast Lesions. *Clin.Cancer Res.* 9: 3413-3417, 2003.

[60] Jeronimo C, Monteiro P, Henrique R, Nis-Ribeiro M, Costa I, Costa VL, Filipe L, Carvalho AL, Hoque MO, Pais I, Leal C, Teixeira MR, And Sidransky D, Quantitative Hypermethylation Of A Small Panel Of Genes Augments The Diagnostic Accuracy In Fine-Needle Aspirate Washings Of Breast Lesions. *Breast Cancer Res.Treat.* 109: 27-34, 2008.

[61] Lewis CM, Cler LR, Bu DW, Zochbauer-Muller S, Milchgrub S, Naftalis EZ, Leitch AM, Minna JD, And Euhus DM, Promoter Hypermethylation In Benign Breast Epithelium In Relation To Predicted Breast Cancer Risk. *Clin.Cancer Res.* 11: 166-172, 2005.

[62] Pu RT, Laitala LE, Alli PM, Fackler MJ, Sukumar S, And Clark DP, Methylation Profiling Of Benign And Malignant Breast Lesions And Its Application To Cytopathology. *Mod.Pathol.* 16: 1095-1101, 2003.

[63] Bean GR, Ibarra DC, Goldenberg VK, Baker JC, Jr., Troch MM, Paisie C, Wilke LG, Yee L, Marcom PK, Kimler BF, Fabian CJ, Zalles CM, Broadwater G, Scott V, And Seewaldt VL, Hypermethylation Of The Breast Cancer-Associated Gene 1 Promoter Does Not Predict Cytologic Atypia Or Correlate With Surrogate End Points Of Breast Cancer Risk. *Cancer Epidemiol.Biomarkers Prev.* 16: 50-56, 2007.

[64] Bean GR, Bryson AD, Pilie PG, Goldenberg V, Baker JC, Jr., Ibarra C, Brander DM, Paisie C, Case NR, Gauthier M, Reynolds PA, Dietze E, Ostrander J, Scott V, Wilke LG, Yee L, Kimler BF, Fabian CJ, Zalles CM, Broadwater G, Tlsty TD, And Seewaldt VL, Morphologically Normal-Appearing Mammary Epithelial Cells Obtained From High-Risk Women Exhibit Methylation Silencing Of INK4a/ARF. *Clin.Cancer Res.* 13: 6834-6841, 2007.

[65] Bean GR, Scott V, Yee L, Ratliff-Daniel B, Troch MM, Seo P, Bowie ML, Marcom PK, Slade J, Kimler BF, Fabian CJ, Zalles CM, Broadwater G, Baker JC, Jr., Wilke LG, And Seewaldt VL, Retinoic Acid Receptor-Beta2 Promoter Methylation In Random Periareolar Fine Needle Aspiration. *Cancer Epidemiol.Biomarkers Prev.* 14: 790-798, 2005.

[66] Vasilatos SN, Broadwater G, Barry WT, Baker JC, Jr., Lem S, Dietze EC, Bean GR, Bryson AD, Pilie PG, Goldenberg V, Skaar D, Paisie C, Torres-Hernandez A, Grant

TL, Wilke LG, Ibarra-Drendall C, Ostrander JH, D'Amato NC, Zalles C, Jirtle R, Weaver VM, And Seewaldt VL, Cpg Island Tumor Suppressor Promoter Methylation In Non-BRCA-Associated Early Mammary Carcinogenesis. *Cancer Epidemiol.Biomarkers* Prev. 18: 901-914, 2009.

[67] Evron E, Dooley WC, Umbricht CB, Rosenthal D, Sacchi N, Gabrielson E, Soito AB, Hung DT, Ljung B, Davidson NE, And Sukumar S, Detection Of Breast Cancer Cells In Ductal Lavage Fluid By Methylation-Specific PCR. *Lancet* 357: 1335-1336, 2001.

[68] Krassenstein R, Sauter E, Dulaimi E, Battagli C, Ehya H, Klein-Szanto A, And Cairns P, Detection Of Breast Cancer In Nipple Aspirate Fluid By Cpg Island Hypermethylation. *Clin.Cancer Res.* 10: 28-32, 2004.

[69] Locke I, Kote-Jarai Z, Fackler MJ, Bancroft E, Osin P, Nerurkar A, Izatt L, Pichert G, Gui GP, And Eeles RA, Gene Promoter Hypermethylation In Ductal Lavage Fluid From Healthy BRCA Gene Mutation Carriers And Mutation-Negative Controls. *Breast Cancer Res.* 9: R20, 2007.

[70] Antill YC, Mitchell G, Johnson SA, Devereux L, Milner A, Di IJ, Lindeman GJ, Kirk J, Phillips KA, And Campbell IG, Gene Methylation In Breast Ductal Fluid From BRCA1 And BRCA2 Mutation Carriers. *Cancer Epidemiol.Biomarkers Prev.* 19: 265-274, 2010.

[71] Fackler MJ, Malone K, Zhang Z, Schilling E, Garrett-Mayer E, Swift-Scanlan T, Lange J, Nayar R, Davidson NE, Khan SA, And Sukumar S, Quantitative Multiplex Methylation-Specific PCR Analysis Doubles Detection Of Tumor Cells In Breast Ductal Fluid. *Clin.Cancer Res.* 12: 3306-3310, 2006.

[72] Fackler MJ, Rivers A, Teo WW, Mangat A, Taylor E, Zhang Z, Goodman S, Argani P, Nayar R, Susnik B, Sukumar S, And Khan SA, Hypermethylated Genes As Biomarkers Of Cancer In Women With Pathologic Nipple Discharge. *Clin.Cancer Res.* 15: 3802-3811, 2009.

[73] Euhus DM, Bu D, Ashfaq R, Xie XJ, Bian A, Leitch AM, And Lewis CM, Atypia And DNA Methylation In Nipple Duct Lavage In Relation To Predicted Breast Cancer Risk. *Cancer Epidemiol.Biomarkers Prev.* 16: 1812-1821, 2007.

[74] Zhu W, Qin W, Hewett JE, And Sauter ER, Quantitative Evaluation Of DNA Hypermethylation In Malignant And Benign Breast Tissue And Fluids. *Int.J.Cancer* 126: 474-482, 2010.

[75] Baker JC, Jr., Ostrander JH, Lem S, Broadwater G, Bean GR, D'Amato NC, Goldenberg VK, Rowell C, Ibarra-Drendall C, Grant T, Pilie PG, Vasilatos SN, Troch MM, Scott V, Wilke LG, Paisie C, Rabiner SM, Torres-Hernandez A, Zalles CM, And Seewaldt VL, ESR1 Promoter Hypermethylation Does Not Predict Atypia In RPFNA Nor Persistent Atypia After 12 Months Tamoxifen Chemoprevention. *Cancer Epidemiol.Biomarkers Prev.* 17: 1884-1890, 2008.

[76] Esteller M, Corn PG, Baylin SB, And Herman JG, A Gene Hypermethylation Profile Of Human Cancer. *Cancer Res.* 61: 3225-3229, 2001.

[77] Esteller M, Fraga MF, Guo M, Garcia-Foncillas J, Hedenfalk I, Godwin AK, Trojan J, Vaurs-Barriere C, Bignon YJ, Ramus S, Benitez J, Caldes T, Akiyama Y, Yuasa Y, Launonen V, Canal MJ, Rodriguez R, Capella G, Peinado MA, Borg A, Aaltonen LA, Ponder BA, Baylin SB, And Herman JG, DNA Methylation Patterns In Hereditary Human Cancers Mimic Sporadic Tumorigenesis. *Hum.Mol.Genet.* 10: 3001-3007, 2001.

[78] Jin Z, Tamura G, Tsuchiya T, Sakata K, Kashiwaba M, Osakabe M, And Motoyama T, Adenomatous Polyposis Coli (APC) Gene Promoter Hypermethylation In Primary Breast Cancers. *Br.J.Cancer* 85: 69-73, 2001.

[79] Park SY, Kim BH, Kim JH, Cho NY, Choi M, Yu EJ, Lee S, And Kang GH, Methylation Profiles Of Cpg Island Loci In Major Types Of Human Cancers. *J.Korean Med.Sci.* 22: 311-317, 2007.

[80] Parrella P, Poeta ML, Gallo AP, Prencipe M, Scintu M, Apicella A, Rossiello R, Liguoro G, Seripa D, Gravina C, Rabitti C, Rinaldi M, Nicol T, Tommasi S, Paradiso A, Schittulli F, Altomare V, And Fazio VM, Nonrandom Distribution Of Aberrant Promoter Methylation Of Cancer-Related Genes In Sporadic Breast Tumors. *Clin.Cancer Res.* 10: 5349-5354, 2004.

[81] Shinozaki M, Hoon DS, Giuliano AE, Hansen NM, Wang HJ, Turner R, And Taback B, Distinct Hypermethylation Profile Of Primary Breast Cancer Is Associated With Sentinel Lymph Node Metastasis. *Clin.Cancer Res.* 11: 2156-2162, 2005.

[82] Virmani AK, Rathi A, Sathyanarayana UG, Padar A, Huang CX, Cunnigham HT, Farinas AJ, Milchgrub S, Euhus DM, Gilcrease M, Herman J, Minna JD, And Gazdar AF, Aberrant Methylation Of The Adenomatous Polyposis Coli (APC) Gene Promoter 1A In Breast And Lung Carcinomas. *Clin.Cancer Res.* 7: 1998-2004, 2001.

[83] Birgisdottir V, Stefansson OA, Bodvarsdottir SK, Hilmarsdottir H, Jonasson JG, And Eyfjord JE, Epigenetic Silencing And Deletion Of The BRCA1 Gene In Sporadic Breast Cancer. *Breast Cancer Res.* 8: R38, 2006.

[84] Li S, Rong M, And Iacopetta B, DNA Hypermethylation In Breast Cancer And Its Association With Clinicopathological Features. *Cancer Lett.* 237: 272-280, 2006.

[85] Evron E, Umbricht CB, Korz D, Raman V, Loeb DM, Niranjan B, Buluwela L, Weitzman SA, Marks J, And Sukumar S, Loss Of Cyclin D2 Expression In The Majority Of Breast Cancers Is Associated With Promoter Hypermethylation. *Cancer Res.* 61: 2782-2787, 2001.

[86] Caldeira JR, Prando EC, Quevedo FC, Neto FA, Rainho CA, And Rogatto SR, CDH1 Promoter Hypermethylation And E-Cadherin Protein Expression In Infiltrating Breast Cancer. *BMC.Cancer* 6: 48, 2006.

[87] Nass SJ, Herman JG, Gabrielson E, Iversen PW, Parl FF, Davidson NE, And Graff JR, Aberrant Methylation Of The Estrogen Receptor And E-Cadherin 5' Cpg Islands Increases With Malignant Progression In Human Breast Cancer. *Cancer Res.* 60: 4346-4348, 2000.

[88] Tao MH, Shields PG, Nie J, Millen A, Ambrosone CB, Edge SB, Krishnan SS, Marian C, Xie B, Winston J, Vito D, Trevisan M, And Freudenheim JL, DNA Hypermethylation And Clinicopathological Features In Breast Cancer: The Western New York Exposures And Breast Cancer (WEB) Study. *Breast Cancer Res.Treat.* 114: 559-568, 2009.

[89] Toyooka KO, Toyooka S, Virmani AK, Sathyanarayana UG, Euhus DM, Gilcrease M, Minna JD, And Gazdar AF, Loss Of Expression And Aberrant Methylation Of The CDH13 (H-Cadherin) Gene In Breast And Lung Carcinomas. *Cancer Res.* 61: 4556-4560, 2001.

[90] Lehmann U, Celikkaya G, Hasemeier B, Langer F, And Kreipe H, Promoter Hypermethylation Of The Death-Associated Protein Kinase Gene In Breast Cancer Is Associated With The Invasive Lobular Subtype. *Cancer Res.* 62: 6634-6638, 2002.

[91] Lapidus RG, Nass SJ, Butash KA, Parl FF, Weitzman SA, Graff JG, Herman JG, And Davidson NE, Mapping Of ER Gene Cpg Island Methylation-Specific Polymerase Chain Reaction. *Cancer Res.* 58: 2515-2519, 1998.

[92] Lapidus RG, Ferguson AT, Ottaviano YL, Parl FF, Smith HS, Weitzman SA, Baylin SB, Issa JP, And Davidson NE, Methylation Of Estrogen And Progesterone Receptor Gene 5' Cpg Islands Correlates With Lack Of Estrogen And Progesterone Receptor Gene Expression In Breast Tumors. *Clin.Cancer Res.* 2: 805-810, 1996.

[93] Rody A, Holtrich U, Solbach C, Kourtis K, Von MG, Engels K, Kissler S, Gatje R, Karn T, And Kaufmann M, Methylation Of Estrogen Receptor Beta Promoter Correlates With Loss Of ER-Beta Expression In Mammary Carcinoma And Is An Early Indication Marker In Premalignant Lesions. *Endocr.Relat Cancer* 12: 903-916, 2005.

[94] Widschwendter M And Jones PA, DNA Methylation And Breast Carcinogenesis. *Oncogene* 21: 5462-5482, 2002.

[95] Iliopoulos D, Guler G, Han SY, Johnston D, Druck T, Mccorkell KA, Palazzo J, Mccue PA, Baffa R, And Huebner K, Fragile Genes As Biomarkers: Epigenetic Control Of WWOX And FHIT In Lung, Breast And Bladder Cancer. *Oncogene* 24: 1625-1633, 2005.

[96] Naqvi RA, Hussain A, Raish M, Noor A, Shahid M, Sarin R, Kukreti H, Khan NJ, Ahmad S, Deo SV, Husain SA, Pasha ST, Basir SF, And Shukla NK, Specific 50'cpg Island Methylation Signatures Of FHIT And P16 Genes And Their Potential Diagnostic Relevance In Indian Breast Cancer Patients. *DNA Cell Biol.* 27: 517-525, 2008.

[97] Raish M, Dhillon VS, Ahmad A, Ansari MA, Mudassar S, Shahid M, Batra V, Gupta P, Das BC, Shukla N, And Husain SA, Promoter Hypermethylation In Tumor Suppressing Genes P16 And FHIT And Their Relationship With Estrogen Receptor And Progesterone Receptor Status In Breast Cancer Patients From Northern India. *Transl.Oncol.* 2: 264-270, 2009.

[98] Yang Q, Nakamura M, Nakamura Y, Yoshimura G, Suzuma T, Umemura T, Shimizu Y, Mori I, Sakurai T, And Kakudo K, Two-Hit Inactivation Of FHIT By Loss Of Heterozygosity And Hypermethylation In Breast Cancer. *Clin.Cancer Res.* 8: 2890-2893, 2002.

[99] Zochbauer-Muller S, Fong KM, Maitra A, Lam S, Geradts J, Ashfaq R, Virmani AK, Milchgrub S, Gazdar AF, And Minna JD, 5' Cpg Island Methylation Of The FHIT Gene Is Correlated With Loss Of Gene Expression In Lung And Breast Cancer. *Cancer Res.* 61: 3581-3585, 2001.

[100] Fujii H, Biel MA, Zhou W, Weitzman SA, Baylin SB, And Gabrielson E, Methylation Of The HIC-1 Candidate Tumor Suppressor Gene In Human Breast Cancer. *Oncogene* 16: 2159-2164, 1998.

[101] Nicoll G, Crichton DN, Mcdowell HE, Kernohan N, Hupp TR, And Thompson AM, Expression Of The Hypermethylated In Cancer Gene (HIC-1) Is Associated With Good Outcome In Human Breast Cancer. *Br.J.Cancer* 85: 1878-1882, 2001.

[102] Bagadi SA, Prasad CP, Kaur J, Srivastava A, Prashad R, Gupta SD, And Ralhan R, Clinical Significance Of Promoter Hypermethylation Of RASSF1A, Rarbeta2, BRCA1 And HOXA5 In Breast Cancers Of Indian Patients. *Life Sci.* 82: 1288-1292, 2008.

[103] Raman V, Martensen SA, Reisman D, Evron E, Odenwald WF, Jaffee E, Marks J, And Sukumar S, Compromised HOXA5 Function Can Limit P53 Expression In Human Breast Tumours. *Nature* 405: 974-978, 2000.

[104] Kioulafa M, Kaklamanis L, Stathopoulos E, Mavroudis D, Georgoulias V, And Lianidou ES, Kallikrein 10 (KLK10) Methylation As A Novel Prognostic Biomarker In Early Breast Cancer. *Ann.Oncol.* 20: 1020-1025, 2009.

[105] Li B, Goyal J, Dhar S, Dimri G, Evron E, Sukumar S, Wazer DE, And Band V, Cpg Methylation As A Basis For Breast Tumor-Specific Loss Of NES1/Kallikrein 10 Expression. *Cancer Res.* 61: 8014-8021, 2001.

[106] Munot K, Bell SM, Lane S, Horgan K, Hanby AM, And Speirs V, Pattern Of Expression Of Genes Linked To Epigenetic Silencing In Human Breast Cancer. *Hum.Pathol.* 37: 989-999, 2006.

[107] Karray-Chouayekh S, Trifa F, Khabir A, Boujelbane N, Sellami-Boudawara T, Daoud J, Frikha M, Gargouri A, And Mokdad-Gargouri R, Clinical Significance Of Epigenetic Inactivation Of Hmlh1 And BRCA1 In Tunisian Patients With Invasive Breast Carcinoma. *J.Biomed.Biotechno*l. 2009: 369129, 2009.

[108] Murata H, Khattar NH, Kang Y, Gu L, And Li GM, Genetic And Epigenetic Modification Of Mismatch Repair Genes Hmsh2 And Hmlh1 In Sporadic Breast Cancer With Microsatellite Instability. *Oncogene* 21: 5696-5703, 2002.

[109] Murata H, Khattar NH, Gu L, And Li GM, Roles Of Mismatch Repair Proteins Hmsh2 And Hmlh1 In The Development Of Sporadic Breast Cancer. *Cancer Lett.* 223: 143-150, 2005.

[110] Naqvi RA, Hussain A, Deo SS, Kukreti H, Chauhan M, Sarin R, Saxena A, Asim M, Shukla NK, Husain SA, Pasha ST, And Basir SF, Hypermethylation Analysis Of Mismatch Repair Genes (Hmlh1 And Hmsh2) In Locally Advanced Breast Cancers In Indian Women. *Hum.Pathol.* 39: 672-680, 2008.

[111] Sinha S, Singh RK, Alam N, Roy A, Roychoudhury S, And Panda CK, Frequent Alterations Of Hmlh1 And RBSP3/HYA22 At Chromosomal 3p22.3 Region In Early And Late-Onset Breast Carcinoma: Clinical And Prognostic Significance. *Cancer Sci.* 99: 1984-1991, 2008.

[112] Mccormack O, Chung WY, Fitzpatrick P, Cooke F, Flynn B, Harrison M, Fox E, Gallagher E, Mcgoldrick A, Dervan PA, Mccann A, And Kerin MJ, Progesterone Receptor B (PRB) Promoter Hypermethylation In Sporadic Breast Cancer: Progesterone Receptor B Hypermethylation In Breast Cancer. *Breast Cancer Res.Treat.* 111: 45-53, 2008.

[113] Conway KE, Mcconnell BB, Bowring CE, Donald CD, Warren ST, And Vertino PM, TMS1, A Novel Proapoptotic Caspase Recruitment Domain Protein, Is A Target Of Methylation-Induced Gene Silencing In Human Breast Cancers. *Cancer Res.* 60: 6236-6242, 2000.

[114] Levine JJ, Stimson-Crider KM, And Vertino PM, Effects Of Methylation On Expression Of TMS1/ASC In Human Breast Cancer Cells. *Oncogene* 22: 3475-3488, 2003.

[115] Virmani A, Rathi A, Sugio K, Sathyanarayana UG, Toyooka S, Kischel FC, Tonk V, Padar A, Takahashi T, Roth JA, Euhus DM, Minna JD, And Gazdar AF, Aberrant Methylation Of TMS1 In Small Cell, Non Small Cell Lung Cancer And Breast Cancer. *Int.J.Cancer* 106: 198-204, 2003.

[116] Sirchia SM, Ferguson AT, Sironi E, Subramanyan S, Orlandi R, Sukumar S, And Sacchi N, Evidence Of Epigenetic Changes Affecting The Chromatin State Of The

Retinoic Acid Receptor Beta2 Promoter In Breast Cancer Cells. *Oncogene* 19: 1556-1563, 2000.

[117] Widschwendter M, Berger J, Hermann M, Muller HM, Amberger A, Zeschnigk M, Widschwendter A, Abendstein B, Zeimet AG, Daxenbichler G, And Marth C, Methylation And Silencing Of The Retinoic Acid Receptor-Beta2 Gene In Breast Cancer. *J.Natl.Cancer Inst.* 92: 826-832, 2000.

[118] Agathanggelou A, Honorio S, Macartney DP, Martinez A, Dallol A, Rader J, Fullwood P, Chauhan A, Walker R, Shaw JA, Hosoe S, Lerman MI, Minna JD, Maher ER, And Latif F, Methylation Associated Inactivation Of RASSF1A From Region 3p21.3 In Lung, Breast And Ovarian Tumours. *Oncogene* 20: 1509-1518, 2001.

[119] Burbee DG, Forgacs E, Zochbauer-Muller S, Shivakumar L, Fong K, Gao B, Randle D, Kondo M, Virmani A, Bader S, Sekido Y, Latif F, Milchgrub S, Toyooka S, Gazdar AF, Lerman MI, Zabarovsky E, White M, And Minna JD, Epigenetic Inactivation Of RASSF1A In Lung And Breast Cancers And Malignant Phenotype Suppression. *J.Natl.Cancer Inst.* 93: 691-699, 2001.

[120] Dammann R, Yang G, And Pfeifer GP, Hypermethylation Of The Cpg Island Of Ras Association Domain Family 1A (RASSF1A), A Putative Tumor Suppressor Gene From The 3p21.3 Locus, Occurs In A Large Percentage Of Human Breast Cancers. *Cancer Res.* 61: 3105-3109, 2001.

[121] Hwang KT, Han W, Bae JY, Hwang SE, Shin HJ, Lee JE, Kim SW, Min HJ, And Noh DY, Downregulation Of The RUNX3 Gene By Promoter Hypermethylation And Hemizygous Deletion In Breast Cancer. *J.Korean Med.Sci.* 22 Suppl: S24-S31, 2007.

[122] Jiang Y, Tong D, Lou G, Zhang Y, And Geng J, Expression Of RUNX3 Gene, Methylation Status And Clinicopathological Significance In Breast Cancer And Breast Cancer Cell Lines. *Pathobiology* 75: 244-251, 2008.

[123] Lau QC, Raja E, Salto-Tellez M, Liu Q, Ito K, Inoue M, Putti TC, Loh M, Ko TK, Huang C, Bhalla KN, Zhu T, Ito Y, And Sukumar S, RUNX3 Is Frequently Inactivated By Dual Mechanisms Of Protein Mislocalization And Promoter Hypermethylation In Breast Cancer. *Cancer Res.* 66: 6512-6520, 2006.

[124] Subramaniam MM, Chan JY, Soong R, Ito K, Ito Y, Yeoh KG, Salto-Tellez M, And Putti TC, RUNX3 Inactivation By Frequent Promoter Hypermethylation And Protein Mislocalization Constitute An Early Event In Breast Cancer Progression. *Breast Cancer Res.Treat.* 113: 113-121, 2009.

[125] Krop IE, Sgroi D, Porter DA, Lunetta KL, Levangie R, Seth P, Kaelin CM, Rhei E, Bosenberg M, Schnitt S, Marks JR, Pagon Z, Belina D, Razumovic J, And Polyak K, HIN-1, A Putative Cytokine Highly Expressed In Normal But Not Cancerous Mammary Epithelial Cells. *Proc.Natl.Acad.Sci.U.S.A* 98: 9796-9801, 2001.

[126] Futscher BW, O'Meara MM, Kim CJ, Rennels MA, Lu D, Gruman LM, Seftor RE, Hendrix MJ, And Domann FE, Aberrant Methylation Of The Maspin Promoter Is An Early Event In Human Breast Cancer. *Neoplasia.* 6: 380-389, 2004.

[127] Ferguson AT, Evron E, Umbricht CB, Pandita TK, Chan TA, Hermeking H, Marks JR, Lambers AR, Futreal PA, Stampfer MR, And Sukumar S, High Frequency Of Hypermethylation At The 14-3-3 Sigma Locus Leads To Gene Silencing In Breast Cancer. *Proc.Natl.Acad.Sci.*U.S.A 97: 6049-6054, 2000.

[128] Umbricht CB, Evron E, Gabrielson E, Ferguson A, Marks J, And Sukumar S, Hypermethylation Of 14-3-3 Sigma (Stratifin) Is An Early Event In Breast Cancer. *Oncogene* 20: 3348-3353, 2001.

[129] Lo PK, Mehrotra J, D'Costa A, Fackler MJ, Garrett-Mayer E, Argani P, And Sukumar S, Epigenetic Suppression Of Secreted Frizzled Related Protein 1 (SFRP1) Expression In Human Breast Cancer. *Cancer Biol.Ther.* 5: 281-286, 2006.

[130] Suzuki H, Toyota M, Carraway H, Gabrielson E, Ohmura T, Fujikane T, Nishikawa N, Sogabe Y, Nojima M, Sonoda T, Mori M, Hirata K, Imai K, Shinomura Y, Baylin SB, And Tokino T, Frequent Epigenetic Inactivation Of Wnt Antagonist Genes In Breast Cancer. *Br.J.Cancer* 98: 1147-1156, 2008.

[131] Veeck J, Niederacher D, An H, Klopocki E, Wiesmann F, Betz B, Galm O, Camara O, Durst M, Kristiansen G, Huszka C, Knuchel R, And Dahl E, Aberrant Methylation Of The Wnt Antagonist SFRP1 In Breast Cancer Is Associated With Unfavourable Prognosis. *Oncogene* 25: 3479-3488, 2006.

[132] Sutherland KD, Lindeman GJ, Choong DY, Wittlin S, Brentzell L, Phillips W, Campbell IG, And Visvader JE, Differential Hypermethylation Of SOCS Genes In Ovarian And Breast Carcinomas. *Oncogene* 23: 7726-7733, 2004.

[133] Yuan Y, Mendez R, Sahin A, And Dai JL, Hypermethylation Leads To Silencing Of The SYK Gene In Human Breast Cancer. *Cancer Res.* 61: 5558-5561, 2001.

[134] Yuan Y, Liu H, Sahin A, And Dai JL, Reactivation Of SYK Expression By Inhibition Of DNA Methylation Suppresses Breast Cancer Cell Invasiveness. *Int.J.Cancer* 113: 654-659, 2005.

[135] Bachman KE, Herman JG, Corn PG, Merlo A, Costello JF, Cavenee WK, Baylin SB, And Graff JR, Methylation-Associated Silencing Of The Tissue Inhibitor Of Metalloproteinase-3 Gene Suggest A Suppressor Role In Kidney, Brain, And Other Human Cancers. *Cancer Res.* 59: 798-802, 1999.

[136] Lui EL, Loo WT, Zhu L, Cheung MN, And Chow LW, DNA Hypermethylation Of TIMP3 Gene In Invasive Breast Ductal Carcinoma. *Biomed.Pharmacother.* 59 Suppl 2: S363-S365, 2005.

[137] Kang JH, Kim SJ, Noh DY, Park IA, Choe KJ, Yoo OJ, And Kang HS, Methylation In The P53 Promoter Is A Supplementary Route To Breast Carcinogenesis: Correlation Between Cpg Methylation In The P53 Promoter And The Mutation Of The P53 Gene In The Progression From Ductal Carcinoma In Situ To Invasive Ductal Carcinoma. *Lab Invest* 81: 573-579, 2001.

[138] Martin TA, Goyal A, Watkins G, And Jiang WG, Expression Of The Transcription Factors Snail, Slug, And Twist And Their Clinical Significance In Human Breast Cancer. *Ann.Surg.Oncol.* 12: 488-496, 2005.

[139] Ai L, Tao Q, Zhong S, Fields CR, Kim WJ, Lee MW, Cui Y, Brown KD, And Robertson KD, Inactivation Of Wnt Inhibitory Factor-1 (WIF1) Expression By Epigenetic Silencing Is A Common Event In Breast Cancer. *Carcinogenesis* 27: 1341-1348, 2006.

[140] Veeck J, Wild PJ, Fuchs T, Schuffler PJ, Hartmann A, Knuchel R, And Dahl E, Prognostic Relevance Of Wnt-Inhibitory Factor-1 (WIF1) And Dickkopf-3 (DKK3) Promoter Methylation In Human Breast Cancer. *BMC.Cancer* 9: 217, 2009.
[141] Suijkerbuijk KP, Van Der Wall E, Van Laar T, Vooijs M, And Van Diest PJ, Epigenetic Processes In Malignant Transformation: The Role Of DNA Methylation In Cancer Development. *Ned.Tijdschr.Geneeskd.* 151: 907-913, 2007.

In: Tumor Suppressors
Editor: Susan D. Nguyen

ISBN: 978-1-61761-986-1

Chapter 4

Rab GTPases as Potential Tumor Suppressors

Christelle En Lin Chua, Yishan Lim, Ee Ling Ng and Bor Luen Tang [*] *

Department of Biochemistry, Yong Loo Lin School of Medicine, National University of Singapore, 8 Medical Drive, Singapore 117597, Singapore

Abstract

The Ras-associated binding (Rab) family of small GTPases serves as molecular switches in regulating vesicular membrane traffic in all eukaryotic cells. Although not conventionally categorized as oncogenes or tumor suppressors, aberrant expressions of several members of the Rab family in cancer tissues have nonetheless been noted. Recent findings have highlighted the potential of certain Rab family members acting both as oncogenic drivers, as well as tumor suppressors. Rab25's expression status, for example, could be an important determinant of progression and aggressiveness of breast and ovarian cancers. Paradoxically, its over-expression could also be tumor-suppressive. In general, deregulation of Rab expression could perturb proliferative or survival signaling pathways through spatial and temporal changes in growth factor receptor traffic and associated signaling. Furthermore, aberrant expression of Rabs may affect the modulation of the dynamics of cell adhesion components (such as integrins) and the cytoskeleton. This may in turn affect cancer cell migration, invasion and metastasis. Finally, deregulation of Rabs that are important in the differentiation of progenitor cells may impair differentiation and enhance tumorigenesis. We discuss in this chapter recent findings implicating Rabs in a variety of human cancers, and explore in particular, plausible mechanisms of how Rabs could be tumor-suppressive.

Keywords: cancer metastasis, endocytosis, Rabs, tumor suppressor

* (Correspondance: Phone: 65-6516-1040; Fax: 65-6779-1453; Email: bor_luen_tang@nuhs.edu.sg; bchtbl@nus.edu.sg).

Introduction – The Rab Family of Small GTPases

The *RABs*, numbering more than 70 genes and with multiple splice variants of each, are the largest subfamily of the Ras superfamily of small GTPases (Zerial and McBride, 2001; Stenmark, 2009; Lee et al., 2009). Rab family members are key regulators of cellular membrane traffic in both the exocytic (or secretory) and endocytic pathways. They act as molecular switches, flipping between an "on" and an "off" state, depending on changes in their guanine nucleotide binding status. In their GTP-bound form, Rabs are active and mediate a transport carrier's engagement of specific effector molecules that would facilitate the carrier's trafficking, docking and fusion. Nascent, cytosolic Rabs are subjected to C-terminal geranylgeranylation by Rab **g**enanyl**g**eranyl **t**ransferase (Rab GGT) with the aid of **R**ab **e**scort **p**rotein (REP), which facilitates its membrane attachment (Goody et al., 2005). **G**uanine nucleotide **d**issociation **i**nhibitors (GDIs), on the other hand, interacts with the isoprenylated C-terminus of Rabs and could extract GDP-bound Rabs from membranes, thus blocking GDP dissociation and keeping these Rabs cytosolic (Pfeffer et al., 1995; Seabra and Wasmeier, 2004). As illustrated in Figure 1, the guanine nucleotide-binding status of a Rab protein is modulated by its **g**uanine nucleotide **e**xchange **f**actor (GEF) and **G**TPase **a**ctivating **p**rotein (GAP) (Bos et al., 2007; Nottingham and Pfeffer, 2009; Rivera-Molina and Novick, 2009). Rab GEFs activate Rabs by promoting GDP to GTP exchange. Rab GAPs, on the other hand, inactivate GTP-bound Rabs by drastically enhancing their weak intrinsic GTPase activity, thus accelerating the conversion of active Rabs to the inactive, GDP-bound state. The relative expression levels and localized availabilities of the GEFs and GAPs, as influenced by upstream signals and protein-protein interaction networks, collectively define the spatial and temporal activities of Rabs.

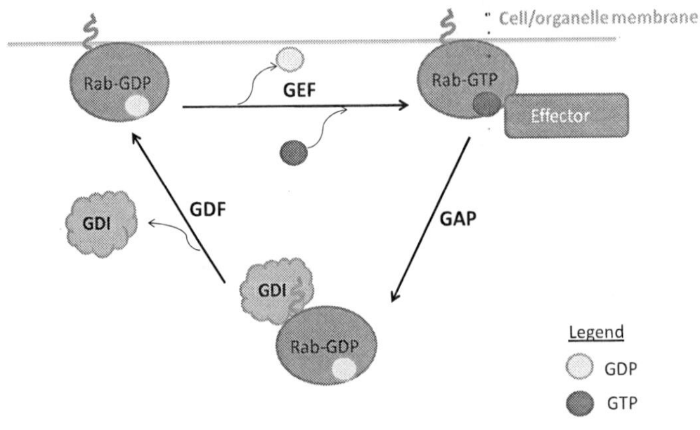

Figure 1. Schematic diagram depicting the Rab cycle.

Guanine nucleotide dissociation inhibitors (GDIs) associate with cytosolic GDP-bound Rabs, and serve to mask the isoprenyl anchor of the Rab GTPase. Membrane attachment of Rab proteins requires the function of a GDI displacement factor (GDF) that dissociates the GDI–Rab complex, thereby allowing the prenyl anchor to be inserted into the membrane. Rabs' membrane association and recruitment of specific downstream effectors are regulated by proteins which modulate its guanine nucleotide binding status (Guanine nucleotide exchange factors, GEFs and GTPase activating proteins, GAPs).

The cellular functions of Rab proteins are brought about by a myriad of effector proteins, which Rabs engage when activated (Grosshans et al., 2006), and which facilitate processes like motor protein-mediated vesicle transport, docking or fusion. Both microtubule-dependent (such as Rabkinesin-6 interacting with Rab6 (Echard et al., 1998)) and actin-dependent (such as myosin Va being recruited by Rab27A to melanosomes via melanophilin (Strom et al., 2002)) motor proteins are known to be Rab effectors. Transport carrier or vesicle docking at the target membranes of the exocytic and endocytic pathways are mediated by Rab-activated tethering complexes (Sztul and Lupashin, 2006) such as p115/GM130 (Allan et al., 2000), the **tra**nsport **p**rotein **p**article (TRAPP) complex (Sacher et al., 2008), and the **e**arly **e**ndosomal **a**ntigen 1 (EEA1) (Christoforidis et al., 1999). Rab-associated regulatory complexes also play tissue or cell type-specific roles in membrane traffic. The neuronal RIM1α/Munc13/α-liprins complex, for example, interacts with Rab3A, a synaptic-vesicle-specific protein, to regulate synaptic vesicle exocytosis (Schoch et al., 2002).

Mutations in Rab and its downstream effectors are known to result in hereditary diseases (Seabra et al., 2002; Corbeel and Freson, 2008), the most prominent of which are those associated with Rab27. Rab27A mutations cause Griscelli Syndrome type II (Ménasché et al., 2000), while Griscelli Syndrome types I and III are caused by mutations in the genes encoding the Rab27-interacting actin motor myosinVa and melanophilin (Van Gele et al., 2009). Mutations in Rab7 precipitate the hereditary peripheral neuropathy Charcot-Marie-Tooth disease type IIB (Verhoeven et al., 2003). Mutations in proteins that regulate Rab activity could also underlie genetic disorders such as X-linked mental retardations (mutations in Rab GDI1 (D'Adamo et al., 1998), choroideremia (deficiency in Rab GGT (Seabra et al., 1993)), and Warburg Micro syndrome (deficiency in Rab3GAP (Aligianis et al., 2005)).

In contrast, the connection between Rabs and human malignancies had been vague. The *RAS* genes (*H-RAS*, *K-RAS* and *N-RAS*) are prototypic oncogenes (DeNicola and Tuveson, 2009). Members of two other Ras-related subfamilies, Ral (Bodemann and White, 2008) and Rho (Gómez del Pulgar et al., 2005), have also been clearly implicated in tumorigenesis. However, implications of involvement of Rab family members in human cancers have been limited until recent advances made by high-throughput, high resolution microarray profiling and array-based comparative genome hybridization (aCGH) technologies. These technological advances have allowed quicker and more thorough interrogation of the cancer genome, revealing more subtle genetic aberrance in cancer cells and tissues. In the ensuing paragraphs of this chapter, we highlight the implicated roles of various Rabs in human cancers, and discuss possible mechanisms by which Rabs could be tumor-suppressive.

Changes in Rab Expression Levels Have Been Noted in Multiple Human Cancers

Deregulated expression of several Rabs have been shown in multiple cancer tissues (Cheng et al., 2005; Chia and Tang, 2009), and reports of these are collated and summarized in Table 1. The **e**ndoplasmic **r**eticulum (ER)-Golgi traffic regulator Rab1A is elevated in tongue squamous cell carcinomas and their premalignant lesions (Shimada et al., 2005), while Rab2 is often found elevated in peripheral lymphocytes of patients with hematopoietic and solid tumors (Culine et al., 1992; Culine et al., 1994). Brain-enriched Rab3A is likewise elevated in cancers of the nervous system and neuroendocrine cells (Culine et al., 1992), as well as insulinoma tissue (Lankat-Buttgereit et al., 1994). Changes in Rab5 levels have been documented in multiple cancer types. Elevated levels of Rab5 correlated with the degree of malignancy and metastatic potential of human lung adenocarcinoma (Yu et al., 1999).

Table 1. A summary of Rabs with known expression level changes in human cancer

Rabs	Subcellular localization/known trafficking function	Implication in human cancer	Reference
Rab1	*ERGIC/ER-Golgi traffic	Elevated in tongue squamous cell carcinomas	Shimada et al., 2005
Rab2	*ERGIC/ER-Golgi traffic	Elevated in peripheral lymphocytes of some cancer patients	Culine et al., 1992; Culine et al., 1994
Rab3	Synaptic vesicles, presynaptic plasma membrane/synaptic vesicle exocytosis	Elevated in cancers of the nervous system and neuroendocrine cells (eg insulinomas)	Culine et al., 1994; Lankat-Buttgereit et al., 1994
Rab5	Early endosome/endosomal fusion and endosomal traffic	Elevated in adenocarcinoma, hepatocellular carcinoma and thyroid adenoma	Yu et al., 1999; Croizet-Berger et al., 2002; Fukui et al., 2007;
Rab5B	Early endosome/endosomal traffic	Decreased in highly metastatic melanoma	Lütcke et al., 1994
Rab7	Late endosome/endosome-lysosome traffic	Elevated in thyroid adenoma	Croizet-Berger et al., 2002
Rab20	Apical endosome in polarized epithelial cells/endosomal traffic	Elevated in pancreatic carcinoma	Amillet et al., 2006
Rab22B/Rab31	Golgi/TGN/TGN-endosome traffic	Elevated in certain breast cancer samples	Kotzsch et al., 2008
Rab23	Plasma membrane, endosome/neural development	1.Elevated in hepatocellular carcinoma and gastric cancer samples 2.Downregulated in malignant follicular thyroid carcinoma (FTC)	Liu et al., 2007; Kim et al., 2007; Hou et al., 2008; Denning et al., 2007
**Rab25	Endosome, plasma membrane autophagosomes, nucleus/endocytic recycling	1.Elevated in prostate, interstitial, ovarian and breast cancers 2.Decreased in breast cancer cell lines and samples	Cheng et al., 2004; Cheng et al., Cheng et al. (in press)
Rab-like protein 1 (RBEL1)	???	Elevated in breast cancer samples	Montalbano et al., 2007

*ERGIC – ER-Golgi intermediate compartment

**It should be noted that there is also some evidence (discussed in text) connecting the homologous Rab11s to cancer. In particular Rab25 and Rab11s share the same effector Rab coupling protein (RCP), which is now noted as an oncogene.

Rab5A expression was also shown to be higher in hepatocellular carcinoma (HCC) tissue compared to non-tumorous tissues (Fukui et al., 2007). Rab5A and Rab7 (a late endosomal Rab) are upregulated in autonomous thyroid adenomas compared to quiescent surrounding tissues (Croizet-Berger et al., 2002). However, an earlier report has indicated that the expression level of another Rab5 isoform, Rab5B, was lower in the more highly metastatic melanoma cells (Lütcke et al., 1994). The endocytic Rab20 is found to be upregulated in multiple stages of pancreatic neoplasia (Amillet et al., 2006). A recently identified rab-like small GTPase, Rab-like protein 1 (RBEL1), is found to be overexpressed in about two thirds of primary breast cancer samples examined (Montalbano et al., 2007).

Rab22B/31 is upregulated in breast tumor samples with high expression of an uPA receptor splice variant (uPAR-del4/5), and may be associated with a worse metastasis-free survival endpoint in patients (Kotzsch et al., 2008). The levels of Rab23 are elevated in hepatocellular carcinoma cell lines and tissues (Liu et al., 2007), as well as in atrophic gastritis and intestinal metaplasia (Kim et al., 2007). It is also identified as one of the genes focally amplified in the gastric cancer cell line Hs746T, and its elevated expression is significantly associated with diffuse-type compared to the intestinal-type gastric cancer (Hou et al., 2008). In contrast, a gene expression analysis study found Rab23 to be downregulated in follicular thyroid carcinoma as compared to benign follicular adenoma tissue samples (Denning et al., 2007). Both Rab22B/31 and Rab23 shall be discussed further below as we explore the plausible mechanisms of their pathologically relevant actions in tumor cells.

Rab25, which is enriched in epithelial cells, is perhaps the only Rab family member whose association with human cancer is best documented, with clear evidence for it being a driver of oncogenesis. Rab25 plays important pathogenic roles especially in epithelial cancers, and appears to be a key determinant of aggressiveness observed in ovarian and breast cancers (Cheng et al., 2004). However, Rab25 has also been shown to act like a tumor suppressor (Cheng et al., 2006; Cheng et al., 2009). The role and mechanism of action of Rab25 shall also be discussed in more detail below.

It is interesting to note that thus far, most associations between Rabs and cancers pertain to transcript and/or protein elevations or reductions (presumably resulting from genomic amplifications or deletions), and not mutations. More extensive efforts in the future could uncover Rab mutations, such as constitutively active or inactive mutants, that might directly influence its role in cancer. In the following sections, we shall explore how aberrant levels of Rab expression could contribute to tumorigenecity, or conversely be tumor suppressive.

Changes in Rab Levels and Activity Could Influence Trafficking of Growth Factor Receptors and their Mitogenic Signaling

Oncogenic proteins and tumor supressors typically affect aspects of cellular signaling and impinge on regulation of proliferation, growth and death. Could Rabs have similar effects when their levels are deregulated? One obvious way by which changes in Rabs' expression levels could affect cell growth and proliferation is through their influence on the trafficking itinerary of growth factor receptors, thereby influencing their signaling processes (Figure 2).

This notion would appear to be particularly applicable to Rabs controlling the endocytic itineraries of the various membrane receptors of mitogenic ligands, such as the **e**pidermal **g**rowth **f**actor **r**eceptor (EGFR) and other members of the ErbB family (Ceresa, 2006; Mosesson et al., 2008).

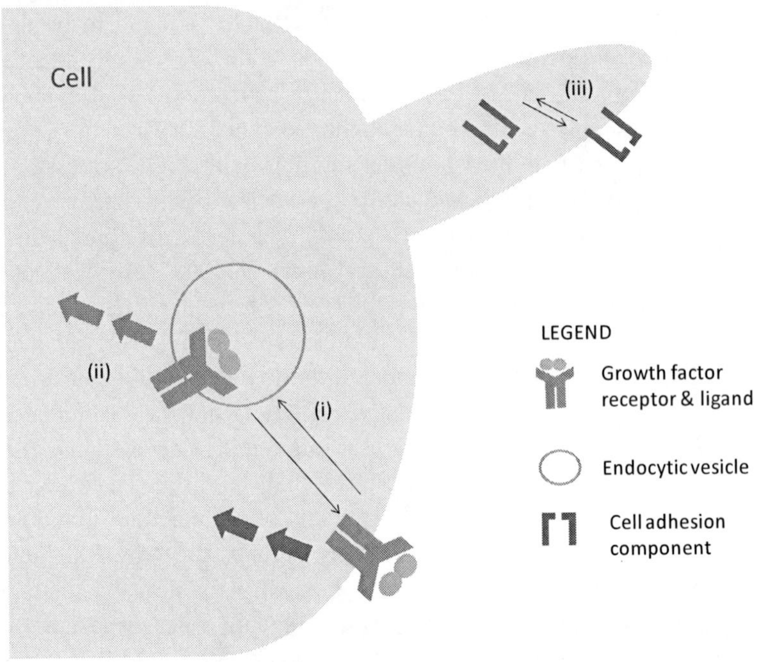

Figure 2. Generalized and hypothetical situations in which Rabs may be tumorigenic or tumor suppressive.

GTP-bound Rab regulates endocytosis and endocytic trafficking of growth factor receptors (i), and changes in levels and activity of certain Rabs may change the strength and duration of growth factor receptor-ligand complex from signaling endosomes, which is qualitatively different from signaling from the cell surface (represented by green and red block arrows, respectively) (ii), leading to enhanced cell proliferation and survival. In some cases (such as that of Rab25), enhanced modulation of the dynamics of cell adhesion components (such as integrin) by elevated levels of Rabs may enhance filopodia formation, tumor invasion and metastasis (iii). Rabs may also play a role in mediating the signaling involved in differentiation and proliferation (not shown in figure).

In fact, many tumors are known to have increased activities of receptor tyrosine kinases, either through aberrant over-expression or constitutive activation resulting from regulation-impairing mutations (Blume-Jensen and Hunter, 2001; Bache et al., 2004). Internalized EGF ligand-receptor complexes continue to signal from intracellular endosomal compartments, and this intracellular signaling differs quantitatively and qualitatively from that at the cell surface, as the association of the EGFR with different signaling adaptors is compartment specific (Balbis et al., 2007). The endosomal Rab5 (Dinneen and Ceresa, 2004) and Rab7 (Ceresa and Bahr, 2006) mutants have been shown to influence EGFR signaling and degradation at different stages of the endocytic route. Somatic gene amplication, or deletion of endocytic Rabs, could plausibly enhance or prolong mitogenic EGFR signaling in ways that could contribute to tumorigenesis. It should also be noted that other than EGFR, receptor tyrosine kinases such as the platelet-derived growth factor receptor (Wang et al., 2004), fibroblast growth factor receptors (Wiedłocha and Sørensen, 2004) and the neurotrophin receptors

(Moises et al., 2007) also exhibit endocytic trafficking-modulated intracellular compartmental signaling. All these could therefore be potentially influenced by aberrant Rab expressions.

Furthermore, aberrant influences on EGFR signaling need not result solely from those Rab proteins that are directly essential to EGFR's endocytic itinerary. Any Rab whose over-expression or deletion could perturb the flow of endocytic traffic, could potentially influence EGFR signaling, perhaps in a cell or tissue specific manner. One such example would be Rab22B/31, a TGN-localized Rab (Rodriguez-Gabin et al., 2001; Ng et al., 2007) which was recently shown to play a role in EGFR trafficking in A431 cells (Ng et al., 2009). Interestingly, silencing of Rab22B/31 (and its putative GEF GAPex-5) delayed EGFR traffic into late endosomes. This delay enhanced EGFR signaling, as indicated by an increase in cell proliferation rate. Conversely, over-expression of Rab22B/31 attenuated A431 cell proliferation. These results suggest that Rab22B/31 has potential tumor suppressive properties that could be manifested in a cell and/or tissue type-dependent manner. This may appear to be in direct contrast to aforementioned evidence that Rab22B/31 is upregulated in breast tumor samples. In the former case, however, it was unclear if Rab22B/31 is an oncogenic driver.

Another noteworthy point to make is that molecules downstream of growth factor receptors could regulate Rab activities, which could in turn influence growth factor receptor trafficking. Phosphatidylinositol 3 (PI3)-kinase is downstream of multiple growth factor signaling pathways, and is, not surprisingly, a major contributor to tumorigenesis of various cancers (Samuels and Ericson, 2006; Vogt et al., 2007). Mutations of both the regulatory and catalytic subunits of PI3-kinase have been implicated in cancer. Of particular interest here is that the regulatory p85 subunit of PI3-kinase has a breakpoint cluster region homology domain with sequence homology to GAPs, and indeed has GAP activity towards certain members of the Rho and Rab family (such as Rab4 and Rab5) (Chamberlain et al., 2004). A point mutant (p85-R274A) which lacks the GAP activity, but not PI3-kinase function, could transform non-malignant NIH3T3 fibroblasts and confers upon these cells the capacity to form tumors in nude mice (Chamberlain et al., 2008). Disruption of the RabGAP activity of p85 may therefore result in cellular transformation due to its inability to modulate Rab or Rho GTPase activities. Interestingly, co-expression of the Rab5 GTP-binding deficient mutant (Rab5-S34N) could actually reverse the transformed phenotype induced by p85-R274A. This attests to the existence of an intricate web of connections between Rabs and growth factor receptor trafficking and signaling, and the notion that deregulation of Rab activity could contribute to oncogenesis.

Changes in Rab Levels and Activity Could Affect Cancer Cell Migration and Invasion

Another important aspect of oncogenesis is heightened cell motility, and cancer cells are particularly motile and invasive. Rabs could in fact play important roles in this motility (Tang and Ng, 2009). As mentioned earlier, Rab25 has a prominent cancer-associated role in epithelial tissues. Cheng et al. identified *RAB25* as the most markedly elevated gene in the chromosome 1q22 amplicon of advanced epithelial ovarian cancers, and Rab25 expression was shown to be higher in late stage tumors than early stage cancers (Cheng et al., 2004). Cell biological analysis indicated that Rab25 over-expression resulted in a marked increase in transformed phenotypes, with elevations in Akt phosphorylation. Rab25 over-expressing ovarian cancer cells formed tumors in nude mice much more efficiently compared to parent cells, although Rab25 over-expressing, non-tumorigenic immortalized ovarian epithelial cells did not. Increased Rab25 over-expression itself therefore appears insufficient for tumor initiation, but it increases the tumor growth and aggressiveness of already transformed tumor cells.

Later studies have shed light on how high levels of Rab25 could enhance growth and aggressiveness of epithelial tumors. Rab25 belongs to the Rab11 subfamily (Rab11A, Rab11B and Rab25), and is enriched in organs with epithelial cells, such as the gastrointestinal mucosa, lung, and kidney (Goldenring et al., 1993). The Rab11 family members have general and presumably overlapping roles in endocytic recycling pathways. Rab25 is associated with the apical recycling system and regulates apical endocytosis and transcytosis (Wang et al., 2000). In this regard, it is not unexpected that Rab25 is responsible for mediating the trafficking of proteins involved in cell migration. In fact, Rab25 was found to interact both *in vitro* and *in vivo* with α5β1 integrin (Caswell et al., 2007). Rab25 over-expression augmented cancer cell invasion through a 3-dimensional matrix in a manner that is enhanced by fibronectin, and could be specifically blocked by antibodies against the α5 or the β1 integrin subunit, as well as the α5β1-binding site in fibronectin. Rab25 apparently slowed the overall speed, but enhanced the persistence of cell migration on the matrix through the extension of pseudopods. In Rab25 over-expressing cells, vesicles containing both Rab25 and α5β1 accumulated and colocalized at the pseudopodal tips. Photoactivation and time-lapse observation showed that these vesicles are in fact responsible for delivering α5β1 to the plasma membrane of pseudopodal tips. Rab25 expression thus appears to sustain the availability of a distal pseudopodal α5β1 pool via a plasma membrane recycling mechanism. This α5β1 pool in turn presumably stabilizes the pseudopods and provides robustness and persistence to cell invasion.

The preceding discussions indicate that deregulation of Rab levels and activity could affect cancer cell migration and invasion. There is, in fact, a connection between integrin recycling and the growth factor receptor trafficking that was discussed in the previous section. A recent report suggests that the **Rab11-f**amily **i**nteracting **p**rotein 1 (Rab11-FIP1) (or **R**ab **c**oupling **p**rotein, RCP), a Rab11 effector, could, under certain circumstances, interact with both α5β1 integrin and EGFR, and mediate their coordinated recycling in a manner which increases downstream signaling and AKT phosphorylation (Caswell et al., 2008). Rab11A has been previously shown to be increased in mammary ductal carcinoma compared to normal ducts (Palmieri et al., 2006). Overexpression of wild type Rab11A increased, while a S25N dominant-negative mutant delayed, EGFR recycling, and inhibited proliferation and anchorage-dependent growth of a breast cancer cell line MCF10A (Palmieri et al., 2006). Recycling of multiple factors mediated by Rab11 family members and their effectors (such as RCP) could therefore collectively contribute to tumorigenesis and tumor progression. In fact, two important recent findings have now confirmed RCP's role in tumorigenesis. Miller and co-workers (Zhang et al., 2009) found high RCP expression in several breast cancer samples corresponding to a common breast cancer-associated 8p11-12 amplicon. RCP over-expression induced anchorage-independent growth in MCF10A immortalized mammary epithelial cells, and enhanced tumorigenicity of multiple breast cancer cell lines. RCP also stimulates **e**xtracellular signal-**r**egulated **k**inases (ERK) and the activation of H-RAS and RAS mutations are common in epithelial cancers. As activated H-RAS is also endosomally localized and could be immunoprecipitated by RCP, there is an apparent interaction between the two molecules. In another report, Vousden's group (Muller et al., 2009) reported that certain mutants of the tumor suppressor p53 have a gain-of-function effect in promoting invasion and metastasis through enhanced integrin and EGFR trafficking, apparently acting by binding to and inactivating the p53 paralogue p63. Mutant p53 increased $\alpha5\beta1$ integrin and EGFR recycling to the plasma membrane in a manner that is absolutely dependent on RCP. The emerging picture provides an unexpected and exciting connection between deregulated Rab11/Rab25 function with mutant forms of p53.

Further to the above, it is noteworthy that another member of the Rab family, namely Rab35, also participates in endosomal recycling and affects cell migration (Chua et al., 2010). In this connection, it is interesting to note that Rab35 is the most highly upregulated small GTPase when androgen-responsive ovarian cancer cells are stimulated with dihydrotestosterone (Sheach et al., 2009). In fact, 95% of samples in the Newcastle ovarian cancer tissue microarray (TMA) (Wilkinson et al., 2008) is positive for Rab35, although the staining showed no significant correlation with cancer staging and survival. Rab35 has been shown recently to interact with fascin (Zhang et al., 2009), an actin bundling protein (Kureishy et al., 2002). Fascin has important roles in cell adhesion and motility (Adams, 2004), and has been extensively implicated in a variety of human cancers. Its upregulation in a variety of human carcinomas, as well as its functional potential as a driver of oncogenic activities, has led to proposals of its potential as a biomarker or therapeutic target (Hashimoto et al., 2005). Although not yet demonstrated as such, it is conceivable that deregulation of Rab35 levels could lead to untimely and undesirable activities of fascin, which could in turn influence cancer cell adhesion and migration.

Rab25 as a Tumor Suppressor

From the preceding discussions, it is clear that Rabs, although not usually considered oncogenes or tumor suppressors, could affect the proliferation, survival and invasiveness of cancer cells when their levels are changed. In most of the cases described thus far, levels of the various Rabs are elevated, and not decreased, in the respective cancer tissues. It is, however, conceivable that Rabs' influence on cell proliferation and migration could go both ways. A prominent example is the documented loss of Rab25 expression in some breast cancer cell lines and breast cancer tissues from patients (Cheng et al., 2006). Exogenous over-expression of Rab25 in the RAO-3 breast cancer line (mammary epithelial cells immortalized with telomerase and transformed with RAS Q61L mutant), reversed transformation-associated phenotypes such as anchorage-dependent growth. The authors found that three out of the four breast cancer cell lines with a loss of Rab25 expression also had H-Ras or K-Ras mutations and noted that the GTP-binding site sequence of Rab25 is different from that of other Rab proteins, but identical to the GTP-binding site of the oncogenic Ras Q61L mutant. The same authors have also recently provided evidence that Rab25 enhances apoptosis and suppresses angiogenesis and invasion by modulating vascular endothelial growth factor-A (VEGF-A) and VEGF receptor-1 (VEGFR-1) expression, mechanisms that are particularly prominent in hormone-insensitive breast cancer lines (Cheng et al., 2009).

How does one reconcile the disparity in the findings above, which suggest that Rab25 could either be a promoter of tumorigenesis or a tumor suppressor in a context-dependent manner? We hypothesize that whether Rab25 acts as a promoter or suppressor in tumor progression depends on the expression status of one of its key effectors, namely RCP. As discussed above, Rab25 could promote not just cell invasion through enhanced $\alpha5\beta1$ recycling, but also mitogenic signaling through increased EGFR recycling by enaging RCP. On the other hand, the anti-tumor activity of Rab25 observed by Rao and colleagues in their Ras mutant-transformed cells could be a consequence of a competition between Ras mutants and Rab25 for a limiting effector molecule like RCP. Over-expression of Rab25 in mutant Ras expressing cells could sequester RCP away from activated Ras, thus reducing its transforming activity in a yet undefined manner. Alternatively, a complex containing RCP, Ras and Rab25 may be less efficient in promoting the transformed phenotype. Therefore, in cells with RCP gene locus amplification and elevated expression, a simultaneous amplification of Rab25 may provide a selective proliferative advantage. On the other hand, for cells with activating Ras mutations but without RCP amplification, a *loss* of Rab25 could also lead to a proliferative advantage. In this regard, it is plausible that any cancer-associated Rab has a context-dependent tumor suppressive potential.

Appropriate Levels of Rab May Be Required to Effect Proper Stem/progenitor Cell Differentiation and Suppress Tumorigenesis

Other than growth factor receptors, aberrant Rab-mediated trafficking of components of signaling pathways during development and cellular differentiation could also be potentially tumorigenic. The Wnt (Fodde and Brabletz, 2007; Polakis, 2007) and Notch (Roy et al., 2007) signaling pathways have been extensively implicated in cancer. It is unclear if Rabs are involved in canonical Wnt signaling, but *Xenopus* Rab40 has been recently shown to participate in the noncanonical Wnt pathway (Lee et al., 2007). Although a firm connection between mammalian Rabs and Notch-mediated tumorigenesis has yet to emerge, *Drosophila* DRab6/Warthog (Purcell and Artavanis-Tsakonas, 1999) and Rab11-mediated recycling of Delta are both involved in fly Notch signaling.

Aberrant signaling of another developmentally important morphogen, sonic hedgehog (Shh), has been implicated in multiple human cancers (Ruiz i Altaba et al., 2002; Katoh and Katoh, 2005; Datta and Datta, 2006; Kayed et al., 2006; Athar et al., 2006; Marino, 2005). Shh signaling during development involves an association with Rab23 activity (Wang et al., 2006). Shh functions as a morphogen at the early neural tube to specify the expression of ventral cell markers. The *open brain (opb)* mutation was first identified as a natural mouse mutation resulting in severe defects in the developing neural tube (Günther et al., 1994). The neural patterning defects of *opb* appear to be opposite to that of *shh*. The *opb* gene acts downstream of *shh*, as *shh* phenotype is at least partially rescued in a *shh/opb* double mutant. Cloning of *opb* revealed that it encodes mouse Rab23 (Eggenschwiler et al., 2001), and recent findings indicate that several nonsense mutations of human Rab23 underlie Carpenter's syndrome (Jenkins et al., 2007), an autosomal recessive disorder with anatomical and physiological deformities. Although Rab23's activity during development appears to antagonize that of Shh (at least in mammals), the exact mechanism underlying this antagonism is unclear at the moment (Wang et al., 2006). Genetic analysis indicates that it does not work directly on membrane receptor components of Shh signaling, but appears to affect unknown factors downstream of Smoothened but upstream of the Gli transcription factors (Eggenschwiler et al., 2006).

In view of the antagonism exhibited by Rab23 for Shh signaling, aberrant expression of Rab23 could potentially contribute to cancers in cells or tissues where Shh signaling plays a key role. Theoretically at least, Rab23 could act like a tumor suppressor, in which its deletion or loss of function could result in pathologically heightened Shh signaling that is tumorigenic. As mentioned earlier, Rab23 levels have been shown to be elevated in hepatocellular carcinoma cell lines and tissues (Liu et al., 2007), atrophic gastritis and intestinal metaplasia (Kim et al., 2007), and *Rab23* is focally amplified in the gastric cancer cell line Hs746T as well as in primary gastric tumors (Hou et al., 2008). In the latter case, Rab23 appears to be an oncogenic driver, and Rab23 silencing reduced the invasive capacity of Hs746T cells (Hou et al., 2008). Since Rab23 is known to antagonize tumorigenic Shh signaling, its contribution to tumorigenesis when upregulated may appear to be counterintuitive at first glance. However, it remains unclear if Shh signaling contributes to the tumor phenotype of Hs746T. Rab23 may have non-Shh signaling related activities that contribute towards tumorigenesis. In view of the postnatal persistence of Rab23 expression in the brain (Guo et al., 2006), it would be interesting to check if Rab23 deletions or changes in expression levels are associated with brain cancers, particularly pediatric medulloblastoma in which aberrant Shh signaling is prominent.

Concluding Remarks

In this short review, we have highlighted evidence in the literature that aberrant expressions of several members of the Rab GTPase family have been associated with human cancer. We further expounded three major plausible mechanisms by which aberrant Rab levels could be tumorigenic or tumor suppressive (see figure 2). Thus far, Rab25 appears to be the only Rab that would qualify as a tumor promoter or a tumor suppressor in the classical sense. However, as discussed, Rabs that influence growth factor receptor trafficking, integrin recycling, or differentiation of progenitor cells could all potentially impinge on cellular proliferation and migration dynamics.

With widespread use of high throughput, high sensitivity genomics approaches, one could expect more associations between aberrant Rab gene expression and human cancers to be revealed. As the underlying mechanisms of Rab-mediated tumorigenesis or tumor suppression are gradually deciphered, Rab expression profiling might be useful in cancer staging and prognosis, and some Rabs might even turn out to be useful novel therapeutic targets.

Acknowledgments

Work on Rab proteins in BLT's laboratory was supported by a grant from the Biomedical Research Council (BMRC) of the Agency for Science, Technology and Research (A*STAR) (08/1/21/19/553). BLT wrote the first draft, CEC improved the draft and drew the figures. YSL and ELN improved the draft. The authors declare no financial conflict of interest.

References

Adams, J.C. (2004). Roles of fascin in cell adhesion and motility. *Curr Opin Cell Biol.* 16,590-596.

Aligianis, I.A., Johnson, C.A., Gissen, P., Chen, D., Hampshire, D., Hoffmann, K. et al. (2005). Mutations of the catalytic subunit of RAB3GAP cause Warburg Micro syndrome. *Nat Genet.* 37,221-223.

Allan, B.B., Moyer, B.D., Balch, W.E. (2000). Rab1 recruitment of p115 into a cis-SNARE complex: programming budding COPII vesicles for fusion. *Science.* 289,444-448.

Amillet, J.M., Ferbus, D., Real, F.X., Antony, C., Muleris, M., Gress, T.M. et al. (2006). Characterization of human Rab20 overexpressed in exocrine pancreatic carcinoma. *Hum Pathol.* 37,256-263.

Athar, M., Tang, X., Lee, J.L., Kopelovich, L., Kim, A.L. (2006). Hedgehog signalling in skin development and cancer. *Exp Dermatol.* 15,667-677.

Bache, K.G., Slagsvold, T., Stenmark, H. (2004). Defective downregulation of receptor tyrosine kinases in cancer. *EMBO J.* 23,2707-2712.

Balbis, A., Parmar, A., Wang, Y., Baquiran, G., Posner, B.I. (2007). Compartmentalization of signaling-competent epidermal growth factor receptors in endosomes. *Endocrinology.* 148,2944-2954.

Blume-Jensen, P., Hunter, T. (2001). Oncogenic kinase signalling. *Nature.* 411,355-365.

Bodemann, B.O., White, M.A. (2008). Ral GTPases and cancer: linchpin support of the tumorigenic platform. *Nat Rev Cancer.* 8,133-140.

Bos, J.L., Rehmann, H., Wittinghofer, A. (2007). GEFs and GAPs: critical elements in the control of small G proteins. *Cell.* 129,865-877.

Caswell, P.T., Chan, M., Lindsay, A.J., McCaffrey, M.W., Boettiger, D., Norman, J.C. et al. (2008). Rab-coupling protein coordinates recycling of alpha5beta1 integrin and EGFR1 to promote cell migration in 3D microenvironments. *J Cell Biol.* 183,143-155.

Caswell, P.T., Spence, H.J., Parsons, M., White, D.P., Clark, K., Cheng, K.W. et al. (2007). Rab25 associates with alpha5beta1 integrin to promote invasive migration in 3D microenvironments. *Dev Cell.* 13,496-510.

Ceresa, B.P. (2006). Regulation of EGFR endocytic trafficking by rab proteins. *Histol Histopathol.* 21,987-993.

Ceresa, B.P., Bahr, S.J. (2006). rab7 activity affects epidermal growth factor:epidermal growth factor receptor degradation by regulating endocytic trafficking from the late endosome. *J Biol Chem.* 281,1099-1106.

Chamberlain, M.D., Berry, T.R., Pastor, M.C., Anderson, D.H. (2004). The p85alpha subunit of phosphatidylinositol 3'-kinase binds to and stimulates the GTPase activity of Rab proteins. *J Biol Chem.* 279,48607-48614.

Chamberlain, M.D., Chan, T., Oberg, J.C., Hawrysh, A.D., James, K.M., Saxena, A. et al. (2008). Disrupted RabGAP function of the p85 subunit of phosphatidylinositol 3-kinase results in cell transformation. *J Biol Chem.* 283,15861-15868.

Cheng, J.M., Ding, M., Aribi, A., Shah, P., Rao, K. (2006). Loss of RAB25 expression in breast cancer. *Int J Cancer.* 118,2957-2964.

Cheng, J.M., Volk, L., Janaki, D.K.M., Vyakaranam, S., Ran, S., Rao, K.A. et al. (2009). Tumor suppressor function of Rab25 in triple negative breast cancer. *Int J Cancer.*

Cheng, K.W., Lahad, J.P., Kuo, W.L., Lapuk, A., Yamada, K., Auersperg, N. et al. (2004). The RAB25 small GTPase determines aggressiveness of ovarian and breast cancers. *Nat Med.* 10,1251-1256.

Cheng, K.W., Lahad, J.P., Gray, J.W., Mills, G.B. (2005). Emerging role of RAB GTPases in cancer and human disease. *Cancer Res.* 65,2516-2519.

Chia, W.J., Tang, B.L. (2009). Emerging roles for Rab family GTPases in human cancer. *Biochim Biophys Acta.* 1795,110-116.

Christoforidis, S., McBride, H.M., Burgoyne, R.D., Zerial, M. (1999). The Rab5 effector EEA1 is a core component of endosome docking. *Nature.* 397,621-625.

Chua, C.E.L., Lim, Y.S., Tang, B.L. (2010). Rab35--a vesicular traffic-regulating small GTPase with actin modulating roles. *FEBS Lett.* 584,1-6.

Corbeel, L., Freson, K. (2008). Rab proteins and Rab-associated proteins: major actors in the mechanism of protein-trafficking disorders. *Eur J Pediatr.* 167,723-729.

Croizet-Berger, K., Daumerie, C., Couvreur, M., Courtoy, P.J., van den Hove, M.F. (2002). The endocytic catalysts, Rab5a and Rab7, are tandem regulators of thyroid hormone production. *Proc Natl Acad Sci U S A.* 99,8277-8282.

Culine, S., Honore, N., Closson, V., Droz, J.P., Extra, J.M., Marty, M. et al. (1994). A small GTP-binding protein is frequently overexpressed in peripheral blood mononuclear cells from patients with solid tumours. *Eur J Cancer.* 30A,670-674.

Culine, S., Honoré, N., Tavitian, A., Olofsson, B. (1992). Overexpression of the ras-related rab2 gene product in peripheral blood mononuclear cells from patients with hematological and solid neoplasms. *Cancer Res.* 52,3083-3088.

Culine, S., Rousseau-Merck, M.F., Honoré, N., Nezelof, C., Olofsson, B. (1992). Specific expression of the ras-related rab3A gene in human normal and malignant neuroendocrine cells. *Cancer.* 70,2552-2556.

D'Adamo, P., Menegon, A., Lo Nigro, C., Grasso, M., Gulisano, M., Tamanini, F. et al. (1998). Mutations in GDI1 are responsible for X-linked non-specific mental retardation. *Nat Genet.* 19,134-139.

Datta, S., Datta, M.W. (2006). Sonic Hedgehog signaling in advanced prostate cancer. *Cell Mol Life Sci.* 63,435-448.

DeNicola, G.M., Tuveson, D.A. (2009). RAS in cellular transformation and senescence. *Eur J Cancer.* 45 Suppl 1,211-216.

Denning, K.M., Smyth, P.C., Cahill, S.F., Finn S.P., Conlon, E., Li, J.H., Flavin, R.J., Aherne, S.T., Guenther, S.M., Ferlinz, A., O'Leary, J.J., Sheils, O.M. (2007). A molecular expression signature distinguishing follicular lesions in thyroid carcinoma using preamplification RT-PCR in archival samples. *Modern Pathology.* 20,1095-1102

Dinneen, J.L., Ceresa, B.P. (2004). Continual expression of Rab5(Q79L) causes a ligand-independent EGFR internalization and diminishes EGFR activity. *Traffic.* 5,606-615.

Echard, A., Jollivet, F., Martinez, O., Lacapère, J.J., Rousselet, A., Janoueix-Lerosey, I. et al. (1998). Interaction of a Golgi-associated kinesin-like protein with Rab6. *Science.* 279,580-585.

Eggenschwiler, J.T., Espinoza, E., Anderson, K.V. (2001). Rab23 is an essential negative regulator of the mouse Sonic hedgehog signalling pathway. *Nature.* 412,194-198.

Eggenschwiler, J.T., Bulgakov, O.V., Qin, J., Li, T., Anderson, K.V. (2006). Mouse Rab23 regulates hedgehog signaling from smoothened to Gli proteins. *Dev Biol.* 290,1-12.

Fodde, R., Brabletz, T. (2007). Wnt/beta-catenin signaling in cancer stemness and malignant behavior. *Curr Opin Cell Biol.* 19,150-158.

Fukui, K., Tamura, S., Wada, A., Kamada, Y., Igura, T., Kiso, S. et al. (2007). Expression of Rab5a in hepatocellular carcinoma: Possible involvement in epidermal growth factor signaling. *Hepatology research : the official journal of the Japan Society of Hepatology.* 37,957-965.

Goldenring, J.R., Shen, K.R., Vaughan, H.D., Modlin, I.M. (1993). Identification of a small GTP-binding protein, Rab25, expressed in the gastrointestinal mucosa, kidney, and lung. *J Biol Chem.* 268,18419-18422.

Goody, R.S., Rak, A., Alexandrov, K. (2005). The structural and mechanistic basis for recycling of Rab proteins between membrane compartments. *Cell Mol Life Sci.* 62,1657-1670.

Grosshans, B.L., Ortiz, D., Novick, P. (2006). Rabs and their effectors: achieving specificity in membrane traffic. *Proc Natl Acad Sci U S A.* 103,11821-11827.

Guo, A., Wang, T., Ng, E.L., Aulia, S., Chong, K.H., Teng, F.Y.H. et al. (2006). Open brain gene product Rab23: expression pattern in the adult mouse brain and functional characterization. *J Neurosci Res.* 83,1118-1127.

Gómez del Pulgar, T., Benitah, S.A., Valerón, P.F., Espina, C., Lacal, J.C. (2005). Rho GTPase expression in tumourigenesis: evidence for a significant link. *Bioessays.* 27,602-613.

Günther, T., Struwe, M., Aguzzi, A., Schughart, K. (1994). Open brain, a new mouse mutant with severe neural tube defects, shows altered gene expression patterns in the developing spinal cord. *Development.* 120,3119-3130.

Hashimoto, Y., Skacel, M., Adams, J.C. (2005). Roles of fascin in human carcinoma motility and signaling: prospects for a novel biomarker? *Int J Biochem Cell Biol.* 37,1787-1804.

Hou, Q., Wu, Y.H., Grabsch, H., Zhu, Y., Leong, S.H., Ganesan, K. et al. (2008). Integrative genomics identifies RAB23 as an invasion mediator gene in diffuse-type gastric cancer. *Cancer Res.* 68,4623-4630.

Jenkins, D., Seelow, D., Jehee, F.S., Perlyn, C.A., Alonso, L.G., Bueno, D.F. et al. (2007). RAB23 mutations in Carpenter syndrome imply an unexpected role for hedgehog signaling in cranial-suture development and obesity. *Am J Hum Genet.* 80,1162-1170.

Katoh, Y., Katoh, M. (2005). Hedgehog signaling pathway and gastric cancer. *Cancer Biol Ther.* 4,1050-1054.

Kayed, H., Kleeff, J., Osman, T., Keleg, S., Büchler, M.W., Friess, H. et al. (2006). Hedgehog signaling in the normal and diseased pancreas. *Pancreas.* 32,119-129.

Kim, K.R., Oh, S.Y., Park, U.C., Wang, J.H., Lee, J.D., Kweon, H.J. et al. (2007). [Gene expression profiling using oligonucleotide microarray in atrophic gastritis and intestinal metaplasia]. *Korean J Gastroenterol.* 49,209-224.

Kotzsch, M., Sieuwerts, A.M., Grosser, M., Meye, A., Fuessel, S., Meijer-van Gelder, M.E. et al. (2008). Urokinase receptor splice variant uPAR-del4/5-associated gene expression in breast cancer: identification of rab31 as an independent prognostic factor. *Breast Cancer Res Treat.* 111,229-240.

Kureishy, N., Sapountzi, V., Prag, S., Anilkumar, N., Adams, J.C. (2002). Fascins, and their roles in cell structure and function. *Bioessays.* 24,350-361.

Lankat-Buttgereit, B., Fehmann, H.C., Hering, B.J., Bretzel, R.G., Göke, B. (1994). Expression of the ras-related rab3a gene in human insulinomas and normal human pancreatic islets. *Pancreas.* 9,434-438.

Lee, M.T.G., Mishra, A., Lambright, D.G. (2009). Structural mechanisms for regulation of membrane traffic by rab GTPases. *Traffic.* 10,1377-1389.

Lee, R.H.K., Iioka, H., Ohashi, M., Iemura, S.I., Natsume, T., Kinoshita, N. et al. (2007). XRab40 and XCullin5 form a ubiquitin ligase complex essential for the noncanonical Wnt pathway. *EMBO J.* 26,3592-3606.

Liu, Y.J., Wang, Q., Li, W., Huang, X.H., Zhen, M.C., Huang, S.H. et al. (2007). Rab23 is a potential biological target for treating hepatocellular carcinoma. *World J Gastroenterol.* 13,1010-1017.

Lütcke, A., Parton, R.G., Murphy, C., Olkkonen, V.M., Dupree, P., Valencia, A. et al. (1994). Cloning and subcellular localization of novel rab proteins reveals polarized and cell type-specific expression. *J Cell Sci.* 107 (Pt 12),3437-3448.

Marino, S. (2005). Medulloblastoma: developmental mechanisms out of control. *Trends Mol Med.* 11,17-22.

Moises, T., Dreier, A., Flohr, S., Esser, M., Brauers, E., Reiss, K. et al. (2007). Tracking TrkA's trafficking: NGF receptor trafficking controls NGF receptor signaling. *Mol Neurobiol.* 35,151-159.

Montalbano, J., Jin, W., Sheikh, M.S., Huang, Y. (2007). RBEL1 is a novel gene that encodes a nucleocytoplasmic Ras superfamily GTP-binding protein and is overexpressed in breast cancer. *J Biol Chem.* 282,37640-37649.

Mosesson, Y., Mills, G.B., Yarden, Y. (2008). Derailed endocytosis: an emerging feature of cancer. *Nat Rev Cancer.* 8,835-850.

Muller PA, Caswell PT, Doyle B, Iwanicki MP, Tan EH, Karim S et al. (2009). Mutant p53 Drives Invasion by Promoting Integrin Recycling. *Cell.* 139,1327-1341.

Ménasché, G., Pastural, E., Feldmann, J., Certain, S., Ersoy, F., Dupuis, S. et al. (2000). Mutations in RAB27A cause Griscelli syndrome associated with haemophagocytic syndrome. *Nat Genet.* 25,173-176.

Ng, E.L., Ng, J.J., Liang, F., Tang, B.L. (2009). Rab22B is expressed in the CNS astroglia lineage and plays a role in epidermal growth factor receptor trafficking in A431 cells. *J Cell Physiol.* 221,716-728.

Ng, E.L., Wang, Y., Tang, B.L. (2007). Rab22B's role in trans-Golgi network membrane dynamics. *Biochem Biophys Res Commun.* 361,751-757.

Nottingham, R.M., Pfeffer, S.R. (2009). Defining the boundaries: Rab GEFs and GAPs. *Proc Natl Acad Sci U S A.* 106,14185-14186.

Palmieri, D., Bouadis, A., Ronchetti, R., Merino, M.J., Steeg, P.S. (2006). Rab11a differentially modulates epidermal growth factor-induced proliferation and motility in immortal breast cells. *Breast Cancer Res Treat.* 100,127-137.

Pfeffer, S.R., Dirac-Svejstrup, A.B., Soldati, T. (1995). Rab GDP dissociation inhibitor: putting rab GTPases in the right place. *J Biol Chem.* 270,17057-17059.

Polakis, P. (2007). The many ways of Wnt in cancer. *Curr Opin Genet Dev.* 17,45-51.

Purcell, K., Artavanis-Tsakonas, S. (1999). The developmental role of warthog, the notch modifier encoding Drab6. *J Cell Biol.* 146,731-740.

Rivera-Molina, F.E., Novick, P.J. (2009). A Rab GAP cascade defines the boundary between two Rab GTPases on the secretory pathway. *Proc Natl Acad Sci U S A.* 106,14408-14413.

Rodriguez-Gabin, A.G., Cammer, M., Almazan, G., Charron, M., Larocca, J.N. (2001). Role of rRAB22b, an oligodendrocyte protein, in regulation of transport of vesicles from trans Golgi to endocytic compartments. *J Neurosci Res.* 66,1149-1160.

Roy, M., Pear, W.S., Aster, J.C. (2007). The multifaceted role of Notch in cancer. *Curr Opin Genet Dev.* 17,52-59.

Ruiz i Altaba, A., Sánchez, P., Dahmane, N. (2002). Gli and hedgehog in cancer: tumours, embryos and stem cells. *Nat Rev Cancer.* 2,361-372.

Sacher, M., Kim, Y.G., Lavie, A., Oh, B.H., Segev, N. (2008). The TRAPP complex: insights into its architecture and function. *Traffic.* 9,2032-2042.

Samuels, Y., Ericson, K. (2006). Oncogenic PI3K and its role in cancer. *Curr Opin Oncol.* 18,77-82.

Schoch, S., Castillo, P.E., Jo, T., Mukherjee, K., Geppert, M., Wang, Y. et al. (2002). RIM1alpha forms a protein scaffold for regulating neurotransmitter release at the active zone. *Nature.* 415,321-326.

Seabra, M.C., Brown, M.S., Goldstein, J.L. (1993). Retinal degeneration in choroideremia: deficiency of rab geranylgeranyl transferase. *Science.* 259,377-381.

Seabra, M.C., Mules, E.H., Hume, A.N. (2002). Rab GTPases, intracellular traffic and disease. *Trends Mol Med.* 8,23-30.

Seabra, M.C., Wasmeier, C. (2004). Controlling the location and activation of Rab GTPases. *Curr Opin Cell Biol.* 16,451-457.

Sheach, L.A., Adeney, E.M., Kucukmetin, A., Wilkinson, S.J., Fisher, A.D., Elattar, A. et al. (2009). Androgen-related expression of G-proteins in ovarian cancer. *Br J Cancer.* 101,498-503.

Shimada, K., Uzawa, K., Kato, M., Endo, Y., Shiiba, M., Bukawa, H. et al. (2005). Aberrant expression of RAB1A in human tongue cancer. *Br J Cancer.* 92,1915-1921.

Stenmark, H. (2009). Rab GTPases as coordinators of vesicle traffic. *Nat Rev Mol Cell Biol.* 10,513-525.

Strom, M., Hume, A.N., Tarafder, A.K., Barkagianni, E., Seabra, M.C. (2002). A family of Rab27-binding proteins. Melanophilin links Rab27a and myosin Va function in melanosome transport. *J Biol Chem.* 277,25423-25430.

Sztul, E., Lupashin, V. (2006). Role of tethering factors in secretory membrane traffic. *Am J Physiol Cell Physiol.* 290,C11-C26.

Tang, B.L., Ng, E.L. (2009). Rabs and cancer cell motility. *Cell Motil Cytoskeleton.* 66,365-370.

Van Gele, M., Dynoodt, P., Lambert, J. (2009). Griscelli syndrome: a model system to study vesicular trafficking. *Pigment cell & melanoma research.* 22,268-282.

Verhoeven, K., De Jonghe, P., Coen, K., Verpoorten, N., Auer-Grumbach, M., Kwon, J.M. et al. (2003). Mutations in the small GTP-ase late endosomal protein RAB7 cause Charcot-Marie-Tooth type 2B neuropathy. *Am J Hum Genet.* 72,722-727.

Vogt, P.K., Kang, S., Elsliger, M.A., Gymnopoulos, M. (2007). Cancer-specific mutations in phosphatidylinositol 3-kinase. *Trends Biochem Sci.* 32,342-349.

Wang, X., Kumar, R., Navarre, J., Casanova, J.E., Goldenring, J.R. (2000). Regulation of vesicle trafficking in madin-darby canine kidney cells by Rab11a and Rab25. *J Biol Chem.* 275,29138-29146.

Wang, Y., Ng, E.L., Tang, B.L. (2006). Rab23: what exactly does it traffic? *Traffic.* 7,746-750.

Wang, Y., Pennock, S.D., Chen, X., Kazlauskas, A., Wang, Z. (2004). Platelet-derived growth factor receptor-mediated signal transduction from endosomes. *J Biol Chem.* 279,8038-8046.

Wiedłocha, A., Sørensen, V. (2004). Signaling, internalization, and intracellular activity of fibroblast growth factor. *Curr Top Microbiol Immunol.* 286,45-79.

Wilkinson, S.J., Kucukmetin, A., Cross, P., Darby, S., Gnanapragasam, V.J., Calvert, A.H. et al. (2008). Expression of gonadotrophin releasing hormone receptor I is a favorable prognostic factor in epithelial ovarian cancer. *Hum Pathol.* 39,1197-1204.

Yu, L., Hui-chen, F., Chen, Y., Zou, R., Yan, S., Chun-xiang, L. et al. (1999). Differential expression of RAB5A in human lung adenocarcinoma cells with different metastasis potential. *Clin Exp Metastasis.* 17,213-219.

Zerial, M., McBride, H. (2001). Rab proteins as membrane organizers. *Nat Rev Mol Cell Biol.* 2,107-117.

Zhang, J., Liu, X., Datta, A., Govindarajan, K., Tam, W.L., Han, J. et al. (2009). RCP is a human breast cancer-promoting gene with Ras-activating function. *J Clin Invest.* 119,2171-2183.

Zhang, J., Fonovic, M., Suyama, K., Bogyo, M., Scott, M.P. (2009). Rab35 controls actin bundling by recruiting fascin as an effector protein. *Science.* 325,1250-1254.

In: Tumor Suppressors
Editor: Susan D. Nguyen

ISBN: 978-1-61761-986-1

Chapter 5

Regulation of Neutrophil Function by Tumor Suppressor PTEN

Subhanjan Mondal and Hongbo R. Luo*
Department of Pathology, Harvard Medical School;
Department of Lab Medicine, The Stem Cell program, Joint Program in Transfusion Medicine, Children's Hospital Boston;
Dana-Farber/Harvard Cancer Center, MA USA

Introduction

PTEN

Identification of the first tumor supressor RB1, or the retinoblastoma gene laid the groundwork for identification of other tumor supressor genes. Over the years genetic evidences implied that at least one factor in chromosome 10 is an important tumor supressor. Partial or complete loss of chromosome 10 led to prostrate, bladder or brain cancer and when wild type chromosone 10 was reintroduced in glioblastoma cell lines it reduced the ability of these cells to form tumors in nude mice. Later through LOH analysis it was identified that the region 10q23 is the most common region of loss of chromosome 10 in prostrate cancer. Further analysis revealed that protein involved in these cancer is a protein tyrosine phosphatase with a large region homologus to chick tensin and was thus named PTEN standing for phosphatsase and tensin homolog deleted on chromosome 10. Following years unfolded that PTEN regulates the PI3K pathway by acting as a 3' phosphatase converting the product of PI3K, PtdIns(3,4,5)P3 to PtdIns(4,5,)P2.

PTEN was initially thought to encode a protein tyrosine phosphatase (PTP), based on sequence identity with PTP superfamily proteins, having a highly conserved Cys-x_5-Arg (Cx_5R) active-site motif that is a hallmark of PTP family proteins (Fauman and Saper, 1996). But PTEN showed extremely poor protein phosphatase activity when tested against a number

* Address correspondence to: Hongbo R. Luo, Karp Family Research Building, Room 10214, 1 Blackfan Circle, Boston, MA 02115, Phone: 617-919-2303, Fax: 617-730-0885. E-mail: Hongbo.Luo@childrens.harvard.edu

of phosphorylated artificial protein and peptide substrates. PTEN showed weak activity towards acidic peptides indicating its preference for negatively charged substrates (Myers et al., 1997). Subsequently it was identified that PTEN could specifically dephosphorylate the D3 position of inositol ring of phosphatidylinositol (3,4,5) triphosphate (PtdIns(3,4,5)P3), which is highly acidic. The same study showed overexpression of PTEN dramatically reduces cellular PtdIns(3,4,5)P3 levls, thus confirming that PTEN acts as a phosphatase for PtdIns(3,4,5)P3 in vivo (Maehama and Dixon, 1998). PtdIns(3,4,5)P3 plays a major role as a second messenger to regulate cell survival, proliferation, cell migration and cytoskeletal reorganization through activation of Ser/Thr kinase PDK1 and Akt (Fruman et al., 1998; Rameh et al., 1997). Overexpression of PTEN was also shown to down-regulate activity of Akt and PTEN-deficient mouse embryonic fibroblast showed a higher levels of PtdIns(3,4,5)P3 and Akt activity indicating PTEN acts to regulate PtdIns(3,4,5)P3-mediated signaling by metabolizing PtdIns(3,4,5)P3 to PtdIns(4,5)P2 (Stambolic et al., 2000; Sun et al., 1999).

Mammalian PTEN proteins are conserved and encodes a protein of 40-50 Kda size, consisting of an N-terminal phosphatase domain and a C-terminal C2 domain. C2 domains are present in a number of proteins that are involved in phospholipid-mediated intracellular signaling or phospholipid metabolism indicating that C2 domains may facilitate phospholipid targeting (Rizo and Sudhof, 1998). The phosphatase domain of PTEN has significant identity with members of the PTP superfamily including the invariant Cx_5R motif in the active site. Within the phosphatase domain is a large region homologous to cytoskeletal proteins tensin and auxillin. The N-terminal region of several PTEN homologs including mammalian PTEN contains a putative consensus PtdIns(4,5)P2-binding motif (Lys/Arg-x4-Lys/Arg-x-Lys/Arg-Lys/Arg), which is commonly found in actin regulatory proteins. The extreme C-terminal end contains two PEST homology regions and a consensus PDZ-binding region which may facilitate protein-protein interaction.

Although PTEN acts primarily as a lipid phosphatase by acting on the inositol ring of PtdIns(3,4,5)P3 some reports suggest that it may act as a dual-specificty phosphatase by acting on phosphorylated protein substrates. Denaturated focal adhesion kinase (FAK) can be dephosphorylated by PTEN invitro and overexpression of PTEN in mammalian cells decreases fibronectin-induced tyrosine phosphorylation of FAK. It was also shown that FAK and PTEN can interact with each other and the interaction is favored upon FAK phosphorylation. Tyrosine-phosphorylated Shc also binds to PTEN and can be dephosphorylated by PTEN (Gu et al., 1998; Tamura et al., 1999; Tamura et al., 1998).

PTEN as a Tumor Suppressor

Numerous mutations and deletions have been found in the PTEN gene in tumor tissues and cancer cell lines, indicating the strong correlation between loss of PTEN function and cancer. PTEN is the most frequent gene mutated in kidney and uterine endometrial carcinomas (45%) and also to a great degree in glioblastomas (24%), breast cancer, lung cancer, colon cancer and melanoma (Li et al., 1997; Risinger et al., 1997; Risinger et al., 1998; Steck et al., 1997). Mutations include nonsense, missense, frameshift, deletion or insertion mutations. The most common mutations in gliobastoma are missense mutations at codons for Arg15 and Arg173. Mutation of Arg15 to either Ser (R15S) or Ile (R15I) lies in the conserved region associated with binding to phospholipid and thus results in the loss of the lipid phosphatase activity (Maehama et al., 2001). In addition, PTEN germline mutations are associated with other pathologies including Cowden syndrome and releted diseases Bannayan-Zonana syndrome, Lhermitte-duclos disease, Proteus and Proteus-like syndrome, all rare autosomal dominant diseases charecterized by developmental disorders, neurological defects, multiple hamartomas and increased risk of breast, thyroid and endometrial cancers (Liaw et al., 1997; Marsh et al., 1997; Tsou et al., 1997). Three of the four germline mutations identified in Cowden and bannayan-Zonana syndrome affects codons Arg130, Arg233 and Arg 335. It is also relevant that in Cowdens disease Gly129 changed to Glu is also noticed. This G129E mutation specifically alters the lipid phosphatase activity of PTEN, which suggests that Cowden disease may result from a failure to dephosphorylate PtdIns(3,4,5)P3(Myers et al., 1998).

Homozygous deletion of PTEN results in embryonic lethality in mice. Mice with PTEN deletion and mutations are highly susceptable to tumor induction and conditional knockout of PTEN leads to neoplasia in multiple organs such as mammary glands, skin, prostrate (Di Cristofano et al., 1998; Podsypanina et al., 1999). PTEN+/- nice shows enlargement of auxillary and several other lymph nodes and spleenomegaly and enlargement of thymus have also been observed. Lymphocytes isolated from PTEN+/- mice are insensitive to Fas-mediated apoptosis, which is required for elimination of autoreactive lymphocytes during development. This results in autoimmunity in these mice with high levels of serum immunoglobulins and high titres of antibodies against single-stranded DNA (Di Cristofano et al., 1999).

PtdIns(3,4,5)P3-mediated Signaling in Neutrophils

Inositol phospholipid (phosphoinositide), phosphatidylinositol 3, 4, 5 trisphosphate (PtdIns(3,4,5)P3), is a major secondary messenger in cells. It exerts its function by mediating protein translocation via binding to their pleckstrin homolog (PH)-domains. A subset of PH-domains, including those in Btk, Protein kinase B (PKB)/Akt, PLC-γ, Gab1, PDK1 and Grp1, drive membrane translocation of their host proteins through specific, high-affinity recognition of PtdIns(3,4,5)P3 (Cantley, 2002; Cantrell, 2001). This membrane translocation is crucial for these proteins to fulfill their functions in PtdIns(3,4,5)P3 mediated cellular processes such as cell survival, proliferation, growth, differentiation, polarization, chemotaxis, cytoskeletal rearrangement, and membrane trafficking (Brunet et al., 2001; Corvera and Czech, 1998; Downward, 1998; Hemmings, 1997; Rickert et al., 2000; Rodgers and Theibert, 2002; Shi et al., 2003). While PtdIns(3,4,5)P3 is synthesized by the enzyme PI3 kinase (PI3K), its level can also be regulated by PTEN, a phosphatidylinositol 3'-phosphatase (Maehama and Dixon, 1999). Since PTEN degrades PtdIns(3,4,5)P3 to PtdIns(4,5)P2, it emerged as an ideal candidate for modulating PtdIns(3,4,5)P3 signaling.

Neutrophils are short-lived, multi-lobed cells of the myeloid lineage with a primary role in host defence, immune regulation and regulation of inflammation (innate immunity). Several features of neutrophils make them a key player in innate immunity, they are ameboid in nature that allow them to rapidly migrate to sites of inflammation by chemotaxis, engulf and clear foreign bodies by phagocytosis, generation of reactive oxygen species secretion of granule components and production of proinflammatory cytokines. In this respect, signaling trough PtdIns(3,4,5)P3 regulates several aspects of neutrophil functions like cell survival and growth, cell adhesion, chemotaxis, cytoskeletal reorganization, generation of reactive oxygen species (ROS). As a consequence of the importance of PtdIns(3,4,5)P3 signaling, regulators of PtdIns(3,4,5)P3 signaling become important. Loss of PTEN correlates with enhanced and prolonged Akt phosphorylation, actin polymerization and superoxide production, indicating that PTEN is a negative regulator of multiple responses to extracellular stimuli. It is noteworthy that PtdIns(3,4,5)P3 signal can be negatively regulated by other factors such as SHIP (SH2-containing inositol 5'-phosphatase (Di Cristofano and Pandolfi, 2000; Rauh et al., 2003) and InsP3KB (Jia et al., 2008a; Jia et al., 2008b; Jia et al., 2007). Thus, neutrophil functions may also be negatively regulated by manipulating these pathways. The review will focus on regulation of neutrophil functions by tumor supressor PTEN.

Role of PTEN in Chemotactic Migration

There is substantial evidence of the role of PtdIns(3,4,5)P3 signaling in cell migration by regulating the cytoskeleton. Stimulation of migratory cells with chemoattractants which is regulated through G-protein coupled receptor (GPCR) signaling leads to localization and activation of PI3K at the leading edge where it catalyses transient formation of PtdIns(3,4,5)P3. This subsequently leads to reorganization of the actin cytoskeleton and formation of the pseudopod and cell migration. F-actin reorganization is mediated by the action of PtdIns(3,4,5)P3 by recruiting PH domain proteins which include exchange factors for Rac GTPases. Activation of the Rac GTPases leads to activation of SCAR(WAVE) and WASP proteins that leads to massive F-actin polymerization.

PTEN has been implicated in chemotactic migration. It was recently reported that PTEN's intracellular localization and activity can be regulated by chemoattractants in both Dictyostelium discoideum (Funamoto et al., 2002; Iijima and Devreotes, 2002) and neutrophils (Li et al., 2005; Li et al., 2003). In chemoattractant-stimulated *Dictyostelium*, PI3K is localized at the front of the chemotaxing cells and PTEN is excluded from the cell front and localized at the uropod (cell back). It was believed that this reciprocal front/back localization of PI3K and PTEN confines PtdIns(3,4,5)P3 production to the leading edge of the cell and thereby mediates directional actin polymerization, pseudopod formation and chemotaxis (Funamoto et al., 2002; Iijima et al., 2002). Chemoattractant stimulation of PTEN$^{-/-}$ Dictyostelium results in an enhanced and prolonged PtdIns(3,4,5)P3 production and actin polymerization, leading to defects of polarity and directional sensing. A similar uropod localization of PTEN has also been reported in chemoattractant stimulated neutrophils (Li et al., 2005; Li et al., 2003). However, it appears that loss of PTEN does not have a significant effect on directional migration of neutrophils (Subramanian et al., 2007). Hence, there is clearly a different role for PTEN in direction sensing of neutrophils and Dictyostelium. Interestingly, neutrophils isolated from mice carrying a "knockin" allele of PI3Kgamma showed GPCR-uncoupled PtdIns(3,4,5)P3 accumulation. These Mutant leukocytes displayed much severe impairment in directional cell migration in response to chemoattractants. Stimulated mutant macrophages did not polarize PtdIns(3,4,5)P3. In these cells chemoattractant-elicited Rac activation was shortened due to enhanced PI3K-dependent activation of RacGAPs (Costa et al., 2007).

Since a homozygous PTEN knockout is embryonic lethal, the role of PTEN in neutrophils was investigated using a myeloid-specific PTEN knockout mouse (Subramanian et al., 2007; Zhu et al., 2006). Chemoattractant stimulation of PTEN$^{-/-}$ mouse neutrophils results in increased PtdIns(3,4,5)P3 synthesis, characterized by phosphorylation of downstream effector Akt. Consistently, PTEN$^{-/-}$ neutrophils displayed more exaggerated and sustained F-actin polymerization than WT neutrophils. PTEN$^{-/-}$ neutrophils were found to be more sensitive to chemoattractant stimulation. For the same dose of chemoattractant, more PTEN$^{-/-}$ neutrophils ruffled, extended pseudopods and polarized in comparison to WT neutrophils, suggesting that PTEN$^{-/-}$ neutrophils were more capable of mitigating the threshold required for transition from basal to activated state (Subramanian et al., 2007). PtdIns(3,4,5)P3 signaling is a critical regulator of NADPH oxidase-mediated ROS production in neutrophils. Consistent with the elevated PtdIns(3,4,5)P3 signaling in the PTEN null neutrophils, these cells produced nearly three times more superoxide than WT neutrophils. Although the superoxide production was transient in both PTEN$^{-/-}$ and WT neutrophils, PTEN$^{-/-}$ exhibited a more sustained response. At saturating concentrations of chemoattractant, the maximal response observed in both WT and PTEN$^{-/-}$ was similar, showing that both populations were equally capable of generating superoxide. However, even at these high chemoattractant concentrations, the prolonged response was still apparent in the PTEN$^{-/-}$ neutrophils. The difference in superoxide production could not be observed when cells were stimulated with phorbol myristate acetate (PMA), indicating that PTEN's effect on superoxide production was G-protein coupled receptor (GPCR) mediated (Subramanian et al., 2007).

The ultimate stage of cancer progression is the gain of an invasive or metastatic property. The role of PTEN and activation of Akt in this process is being unraveled. In addition to the regulation of cell motility and cell migration by Akt and PTEN in tumor cells, the tumor cells need to alter it cell adhesion properties so that it can detach from the surrounding cells. Tumor cells also increase the expression and activation of extracellular proteases that degrades the extracellular matrix. HT1080 fibroblastic cell line a highly metastatic cell type showed high levels of Akt activation and enrichment of akt at the leading edge during cell migration. These cells also exhibited a high level of expression of matrix metalloproteinase 9 (MMP-9) (Kim et al., 2001). MMPs are zinc-dependent proteinases that degrades the extracellular matrix like collagen and basement membrane and promotes tumor cell invasion and metastasis. Increased expression of MMPs expecially MMP2, MMP-7, MMP-9 have been correlated with progression and metastasis of cancer. Neutrophil migration which is amoeboid in nature, allows the cells to change shape and deform during migration towards a chemoattractant and in this way differs in some aspects to fibroblastic cell migration through tissues where cells are not that flexible, thus a role of MMP in neutrophil migration is not as curtail as for a metastasizing cell.

Role of PTEN in Neutrophil Survival and Apoptosis

The PtdIns(3,4,5)P3 signaling mediates cell survival, proliferation and aging of cells and organisms by its actions through Akt activation (Coffer et al., 1998). Akt is recruited to the membrane by PtdIns(3,4,5)P3 where it is activated by phosphorylation at Ser473 and Thr308 residues by PDK1 which itself is a phosphoinositide dependent protein kinase regulated by PtdIns(3,4,5)P3. Constitutive activation and phosphorylation of Akt was observed in numerous cancer cell lines (glioblastomas, prostrate cancers, breast cancer) that carry a nonfunctional PTEN gene. In some cells overexpression of PTEN rescued the Akt phosphorylation and activity. Activated Akt phosphorylates several downstram effector molecules to activate or inhibit specific signaling cascades. The proapoptotic factor Bad is a phosphorylated by Akt. When unphosphorylated it associateses with Bcl-2 to generate an apoptotic signal, upon phosphorylation by Akt the association is inhibited, thus inhibiting cells to undergo apoptosis (Datta et al., 1997; del Peso et al., 1997). Akt also phosphorylates GSK3β and $p70^{S6K}$, which mediates antiapoptotic signaling (Coffer et al., 1998). Mouse embryonic fibroblasts lacking PTEN are highly resistant to apoptotic stimuli like UV radiation, heat treatment, osmotic shock, TNF-α (Stambolic et al., 1998). Consistent with this T and B cells from $PTEN^{+/-}$ mice show reduced apoptosis upon stimulation with Fas and CD3ε (Di Cristofano et al., 1999). In addition to regulation of apoptosis, PTEN also regulated cell proliferation by regulating cell cycle. Loss of PTEN activates Akt which then regulates the cell cycle dependent kinase (CDK) inhibitor $p27^{Kip}$. $p27^{Kip}$ inhibits the CDK2/cyclinE activity, which is required for entry into S phase. Overexpression of PTEN leads to higher expression of $p27^{Kip}$ and thus results in cell cycle arrest in G1 phase (Cheney et al., 1999; Li and Sun, 1998; Sun et al., 1999). Akt was shown to increase the transcription of c-Myc which is a strong promoter of cell cycle progression and causes cells to exit from G0 and proliferate. The tumor supressor Rb was also identified as a target of Akt. In its dephosphorylated state Rb binds to and inactivates downstream proteins like c-Myc and EF2 required for cell cycle progression (Paramio et al., 1999). Upon phosphorylation of Rb by Akt this interaction and the inhibition is lost and allows cell proliferation.

In neutrophils two main pathways of regulate apoptosis, a death receptor pathway triggered by Fas, TNFα and TNF-related apoptosis inducing ligand (TRAIL) and the other a mitochondrial pathway stimulated by stress such as UV, growth factor deprivation and chemotherapeutic drugs. The nonconventional mechanisms of cell death include death by formation of neutrophil extracellular traps and by autophagic cell death. The term apoptosis is used to define a pattern of cell death characterized by cell shrinkage, nuclear chromatin condensation and subsequent DNA fragmentation to nucleosomal fragments and exposure of phosphatidylseine on the outer leaflet of the plasma membrane. All of these changes require the activity of caspase (cystineyl aspartate protease) family proteins (Kroemer et al., 2009; Pop and Salvesen, 2009). Thirteen caspases have been identified in humans and seven of them are required for apoptosis. Caspases have been classified according to their role as initiators (3,6,7) and effectors (2,8,9,10) which induces apoptosis by cleaving cellular components. A distinct class of proinflammatory-caspases (1,4,5,11,12) mediate cleavage of pro form of inflammatory cytokines IL-1β and IL-18 resulting in initiation of inflammation (Scott and Saleh, 2007). During apoptosis mitochondrial cytochrome c is release in the cytoplasm which then interacts with Apaf-1, this complex can then bind to procaspase 9 and cleave it and activate it which then activates the "executioner" caspases 3 and 7. Akt phosphorylates procaspase 9 and renders it resistant to processing and thus activation of the caspases (Cardone et al., 1998; Cohen, 1997). Akt also phosphorylates and inactivates the Forkhead transcription factors like FKHR1. When unphosphorylated FKHR1 is present in the nucleus inducing transcription of various cell-death related genes like FasL (Fas ligand). Upon phosphorylation by Akt it cannot enter the nucleus and thereby losing its transcriptional activity (Brunet et al., 1999).

PTEN also acts as a negative regulator of neutrophil survival. Neutrophils normally have a very short life-span and readily undergo spontaneous programmed cell death (apoptosis). This death program needs to be well controlled to maintain the normal neutrophil count. Constitutive neutrophil death is associated with upregulation of death signaling and down-regulation of survival signaling (Luo and Loison, 2008). Deactivation of PtdIns(3,4,5)P3/Akt signaling has been identified as a key event in neutrophil spontaneous death. The activity of Protein kinase B (PKB)/Akt decreases dramatically during the course of neutrophil death. Both PI3 kinase and Akt inhibitors enhance neutrophil death. Neutrophils depleted of PTEN live much longer than wild-type neutrophils (Zhu et al., 2006). Similar results were detected in SHIP-null neutrophils in which PtdIns(3,4,5)P3 pathway is also up-regulated (Liu et al., 1999). These results are also consistent with previous reports that neutrophil apoptosis is enhanced in PI3Kγ deficient mice, where Akt activity is reduced (Webb et al., 2000; Yang et al., 2003).

Neutrophil extracellular trap (NETosis) is a novel neutrophil cell death mechanism triggered by neutrophil activation that leads to release of chromatin material and granule proteins forming webs that can trap a variety of pathogens like bacteria, fungi and parasites. The granular proteins associating with the NETs like MPO, PR3, neutrophil elastase provide high local concentrations of antimicrobial proteins for killing pathogens. This pathway of neutrophil cell death depends on reactive oxygen species (ROS) as neutrophils from patients with chronic ganulomatous disease (CGD) fails to produce NETs (Brinkmann and Zychlinsky, 2007; Fuchs et al., 2007). The role of PtdIns(3,4,5)P3 in this cell death pathway remains to be explored.

Role of PTEN in Inflammation

The role of PtdIns(3,4,5)P3 and PTEN in infection and inflammation was examined using several animal models. A number of studies demonstrated that blocking the kinase activity of PI3K leads to impaired neutrophil recruitment to inflammatory sites in vivo (Camps et al., 2005; Heit et al., 2008; Hirsch et al., 2000; Liu et al., 2007; Puri et al., 2004; Puri et al., 2005; Sasaki et al., 2000; Smith et al., 2006). On the other hand, elevation of PtdIns(3,4,5)P3 signaling via depleting PTEN enhances cell mobility (Gao et al., 2005; Kwak et al., 2003; Lacalle et al., 2004; Liliental et al., 2000; Tamura et al., 1998). Neutrophil recruitment to inflamed peritoneal cavity is significantly elevated in the PTEN knockout mice (Subramanian et al., 2007). Neutrophil migration through blood-vessel wall is a complex process which can be divided into four discrete phases: capture and rolling, activation, arrest or firm adhesion, and diapedesis or transmigration from circulation across endothelium into tissues. PtdIns(3,4,5)P3 is a major downstream target of intergrin and chemokine receptor, and has been implicated in multiple steps in leukocyte trafficking. Smith et al. recently showed that disruption of PI3Kγ, one of the PI3 kinases mediating GPCR signaling, interferes with integrin bond strengthening. PI3Kγ null mice showed an 80% reduction in CXCL1 (KC)-induced leukocyte adhesion in venules of mouse cremaster muscle (Smith et al., 2006). Similar inhibition of tight adhesion was also observed when leukocyte transmigration from cremaster venules was induced with MIP-2 (Liu et al., 2007). Unexpectedly, we didn't observe elevated leukocyte adhesion when the PtdIns(3,4,5)P3 signaling was enhanced via PTEN depletion, suggesting that PtdIns(3,4,5)P3 signaling is essential for stimuli-elicited cell adhesion, but not a limiting step for inducing elevated adhesion (Sarraj et al., 2009). The enhanced neutrophil recruitment in the cremaster muscle in response to different stimuli is like due to faster neutrophil movement in the vascular bed, across the vascular endothelial wall, and in the muscle tissue. Neutrophil rolling influx, rolling speed, and the number of firmly adherent neutrophils were not altered in the PTEN KO mice. Thus, PTEN is a negative regulator in neutrophil trafficking and the enhanced neutrophil recruitment in PTEN KO mice is mainly caused by augmented transendothelial migration (Sarraj et al., 2009).

Disruption of PTEN also enhances neutrophil function in a bacterial pneumonia model (Li et al., 2009). In myeloid-specific PTEN knockout mice, the recruitment of neutrophils to the inflamed lungs is significantly augmented. In addition, depleting PTEN significantly delays the apoptotic death of the recruited neutrophils. Enhanced neutrophil function leads to more severe pulmonary edema and increases mortality rate when bacterial pneumonia is induced in normal non-neutropenic mice. Nevertheless, this becomes less of a concern in neutropenic mice in whom the number of neutrophils is dramatically reduced and the release of noxious compounds, such as oxidants, proteinases, and DNA, by neutrophils is also minimal. The direct cause of neutropenia-related pneumonia is the lack of neutrophils in the infected lungs to clear the invading bacteria. When the dose of E.coli is in a range that can be handled by the host innate immune system, the enhanced neutrophil accumulation and the augmented bacteria-killing capability in the PTEN knockout mice can lead to faster resolution/alleviation of lung inflammation under neutropenic condition. Consequently, the increased bacteria-clearance capability and less severe inflammation in the PTEN null mice results in a much increased survival rate of bacteria-challenged neutropenic mice (Li et al., 2009).

NFκB is a transcription factor which induces the expression of several genes including proinflammatory gene (INFg, TNF, IL-6, IL-1b, IL-12 etc), caspase inhibitors (c-IAP1 and c-IAP2), survival genes (Bcl-2 family member Bfl-1) and matrix metalloproteinases (MMP-9). Expression of proinflammatory genes by NFκB has been well documented. NFκB binds to IκB and is sequestered in the cytoplasm. Upon phosphorylation of IκB by IKKalpha and IKKbeta, IκB is degraded and NFκB can enter the nucleus where it can induce transcription of its target genes (Ghosh and Hayden, 2008). Akt does not phosphorylated NFkB directly but activates it indirectly, exact mechanisms of which is still unknown (Kane et al., 1999; Ozes et al., 1999; Romashkova and Makarov, 1999). Disruption of PTEN resulted in elevated proinflammatory cytokine production in inflamed lungs. Bronchealveolar lavage collected from wild type and PTEN depleted mice after intratracheal instillation of bacteria showed elevated levels of proinflammatory cytokines and chemokines KC, MIP2, TNF-a, IL-6, IL-1b. Macrophages from brocheoalveloar lavage also showed elevated proinflammatory cytokine production upon stimulation with LPS (Li et al., 2009).

PTEN can clearly negatively regulate various neutrophil functions. Why do neutrophils need such a negative regulator? Neutrophil activation is essential for the killing and clearance of pathogens. However, hyper-activation of neutrophils can also damage the surrounding tissues, leading to acute inflammation. Neutrophils encounter various signals that can potentially elicit their responses. More than 50 chemokines have been identified in human and many of them are present in blood or tissues persistently. However, neutrophils will not chemotax or generate superoxide in response to a chemoattractant stimulation unless the stimulation is strong and stable enough, indicating the presence of cellular inhibitory factors that can suppress the positive signals elicited by a weak or unstable chemoattractant stimuli (Foxman et al., 1997; Zigmond, 1989). These intracellular inhibitors establish a threshold for neutrophil responses. Neutrophils respond only when they receive a stimulation that can overcome the negative effect of the inhibitors. PTEN null neutrophils display a more enhanced sensitivity to chemoattractant stimulation, suggesting PTEN might be one such inhibitory regulator. Since more neutrophils are recruited to the sites of inflammation in the PTEN knockout mice, PTEN and other components in PtdIns(3,4,5)P3 signaling pathway may be utilized as therapeutic targets for modulating neutrophil responses, which need to be enhanced to facilitate their pathogen killing capability and suppressed to aid the resolution of inflammation.

Regulation of PTEN Function

The role of PTEN as a 3'-phosphatase for phosphatase is confirmed from numerous studies, but mechanisms which regulate PTEN activity itself is been poorly understood. PTEN contains a number of protein domains and motifs such as the N-terminal phosphoinositide binding motif, C2 domain, PDZ-binding site and the PEST sequences, that can facilitate protein-protein interaction and this might be a possible mechanism of PTEN regulation in cells. It has been demonstrated that PTEN can be upregulated by early growth related transcription factor (EGR1) by binding to the promoter region of PTEN. It was also shown that other transcriptional factors PPARγ, p53, SREBP and activating transcription factor 2 (ATF2) can also upregulate PTEN expression by binding to its promoter region (Patel et al., 2001; Shen et al., 2006; Teresi et al., 2008). Phosphorylation of the C-termional residues Ser380, Thr382 and Thr383 results in a six-fold increase in the half-life of PTEN, suggesting that phosphorylation may be a mechanism of regulating PTEN activity (Vazquez et al., 2000). PTEN activity is also regulated by oxidation and acetylation. In addition to posttranslational modifications PTEN can also be regulated at the transcriptional level. PTEN mRNA expression is significantly reduced by treatment with TGF-β and leads to activation of Akt (Li and Sun, 1997). Recent studies have shown involvement of microRNAs (miRNA) in the process, TGF-β induced miR-216a and miR-217, both of which target PTEN, thus inhibition of PTEN activates Akt by TGF-β (Kato et al., 2009). It has also been shown that miR-19a, miR-21 and miR-214 targets the 3'untranslated region of PTEN leading to inhibition of PTEN translation. Interestingly expression of miR-19a and miR-21 was elevated in Cowdens disease (Meng et al., 2006; Olive et al., 2009; Pezzolesi et al., 2008; Yang et al., 2008).

References

Brinkmann, V., and Zychlinsky, A. (2007). Beneficial suicide: why neutrophils die to make NETs. *Nat Rev Microbiol 5*, 577-582.

Brunet, A., Bonni, A., Zigmond, M.J., Lin, M.Z., Juo, P., Hu, L.S., Anderson, M.J., Arden, K.C., Blenis, J., and Greenberg, M.E. (1999). Akt promotes cell survival by phosphorylating and inhibiting a Forkhead transcription factor. *Cell 96*, 857-868.

Brunet, A., Datta, S.R., and Greenberg, M.E. (2001). Transcription-dependent and -independent control of neuronal survival by the PI3K-Akt signaling pathway. *Curr Opin Neurobiol 11*, 297-305.

Camps, M., Ruckle, T., Ji, H., Ardissone, V., Rintelen, F., Shaw, J., Ferrandi, C., Chabert, C., Gillieron, C., Francon, B., *et al.* (2005). Blockade of PI3Kgamma suppresses joint inflammation and damage in mouse models of rheumatoid arthritis. *Nat Med 11*, 936-943.

Cantley, L.C. (2002). The phosphoinositide 3-kinase pathway. *Science 296*, 1655-1657.

Cantrell, D.A. (2001). Phosphoinositide 3-kinase signalling pathways. *J Cell Sci 114*, 1439-1445.

Cardone, M.H., Roy, N., Stennicke, H.R., Salvesen, G.S., Franke, T.F., Stanbridge, E., Frisch, S., and Reed, J.C. (1998). Regulation of cell death protease caspase-9 by phosphorylation. *Science 282*, 1318-1321.

Cheney, I.W., Neuteboom, S.T., Vaillancourt, M.T., Ramachandra, M., and Bookstein, R. (1999). Adenovirus-mediated gene transfer of MMAC1/PTEN to glioblastoma cells inhibits S phase entry by the recruitment of p27Kip1 into cyclin E/CDK2 complexes. *Cancer Res 59*, 2318-2323.

Coffer, P.J., Jin, J., and Woodgett, J.R. (1998). Protein kinase B (c-Akt): a multifunctional mediator of phosphatidylinositol 3-kinase activation. *Biochem J 335 (Pt 1)*, 1-13.

Cohen, G.M. (1997). Caspases: the executioners of apoptosis. *Biochem* J *326 (Pt 1)*, 1-16.

Corvera, S., and Czech, M.P. (1998). Direct targets of phosphoinositide 3-kinase products in membrane traffic and signal transduction. *Trends Cell Biol 8*, 442-446.

Costa, C., Barberis, L., Ambrogio, C., Manazza, A.D., Patrucco, E., Azzolino, O., Neilsen, P.O., Ciraolo, E., Altruda, F., Prestwich, G.D., *et al.* (2007). Negative feedback regulation of Rac in leukocytes from mice expressing a constitutively active phosphatidylinositol 3-kinase gamma. *Proc Natl Acad Sci USA 104*, 14354-14359.

Datta, S.R., Dudek, H., Tao, X., Masters, S., Fu, H., Gotoh, Y., and Greenberg, M.E. (1997). Akt phosphorylation of BAD couples survival signals to the cell-intrinsic death machinery. *Cell 91*, 231-241.

del Peso, L., Gonzalez-Garcia, M., Page, C., Herrera, R., and Nunez, G. (1997). Interleukin-3-induced phosphorylation of BAD through the protein kinase Akt. *Science 278*, 687-689.

Di Cristofano, A., Kotsi, P., Peng, Y.F., Cordon-Cardo, C., Elkon, K.B., and Pandolfi, P.P. (1999). Impaired Fas response and autoimmunity in Pten+/- mice. *Science 285*, 2122-2125.

Di Cristofano, A., and Pandolfi, P.P. (2000). The multiple roles of PTEN in tumor suppression. *Cell 100*, 387-390.

Di Cristofano, A., Pesce, B., Cordon-Cardo, C., and Pandolfi, P.P. (1998). Pten is essential for embryonic development and tumour suppression. *Nat Genet 19*, 348-355.

Downward, J. (1998). Mechanisms and consequences of activation of protein kinase B/Akt. *Curr Opin Cell Biol 10*, 262-267.

Fauman, E.B., and Saper, M.A. (1996). Structure and function of the protein tyrosine phosphatases. *Trends Biochem Sci 21*, 413-417.

Foxman, E.F., Campbell, J.J., and Butcher, E.C. (1997). Multistep navigation and the combinatorial control of leukocyte chemotaxis. *J Cell Biol 139*, 1349-1360.

Fruman, D.A., Meyers, R.E., and Cantley, L.C. (1998). Phosphoinositide kinases. *Annu Rev Biochem 67*, 481-507.

Fuchs, T.A., Abed, U., Goosmann, C., Hurwitz, R., Schulze, I., Wahn, V., Weinrauch, Y., Brinkmann, V., and Zychlinsky, A. (2007). Novel cell death program leads to neutrophil extracellular traps. *J Cell Biol 176*, 231-241.

Funamoto, S., Meili, R., Lee, S., Parry, L., and Firtel, R.A. (2002). Spatial and temporal regulation of 3-phosphoinositides by PI 3-kinase and PTEN mediates chemotaxis. *Cell 109*, 611-623.

Gao, P., Wange, R.L., Zhang, N., Oppenheim, J.J., and Howard, O.M. (2005). Negative regulation of CXCR4-mediated chemotaxis by the lipid phosphatase activity of tumor suppressor PTEN. *Blood 106*, 2619-2626.

Ghosh, S., and Hayden, M.S. (2008). New regulators of NF-kappaB in inflammation. *Nat Rev Immunol 8*, 837-848.

Gu, J., Tamura, M., and Yamada, K.M. (1998). Tumor suppressor PTEN inhibits integrin- and growth factor-mediated mitogen-activated protein (MAP) kinase signaling pathways. *J Cell Biol 143*, 1375-1383.

Heit, B., Liu, L., Colarusso, P., Puri, K.D., and Kubes, P. (2008). PI3K accelerates, but is not required for, neutrophil chemotaxis to fMLP. *J Cell Sci 121*, 205-214.

Hemmings, B.A. (1997). PtdIns(3,4,5)P3 gets its message across. *Science 277*, 534.

Hirsch, E., Katanaev, V.L., Garlanda, C., Azzolino, O., Pirola, L., Silengo, L., Sozzani, S., Mantovani, A., Altruda, F., and Wymann, M.P. (2000). Central role for G protein-coupled phosphoinositide 3-kinase gamma in inflammation. *Science 287*, 1049-1053.

Iijima, M., and Devreotes, P. (2002). Tumor suppressor PTEN mediates sensing of chemoattractant gradients. *Cell 109*, 599-610.

Iijima, M., Huang, Y.E., and Devreotes, P. (2002). Temporal and spatial regulation of chemotaxis. *Dev Cell 3*, 469-478.

Jia, Y., Loison, F., Hattori, H., Li, Y., Erneux, C., Park, S.Y., Gao, C., Chai, L., Silberstein, L.E., Schurmans, S., *et al.* (2008a). Inositol trisphosphate 3-kinase B (InsP3KB) as a physiological modulator of myelopoiesis. *Proc Natl Acad Sci USA 105*, 4739-4744.

Jia, Y., Schurmans, S., and Luo, H.R. (2008b). Regulation of innate immunity by inositol 1,3,4,5-tetrakisphosphate. *Cell Cycle 7*, 2803-2808.

Jia, Y., Subrahmanyam, K.K., Erneux, C., Pouillon, V., Hattori, H., Jo, H., You, J., Zhu, D., Schurmans, S., and Luo, H.R. (2007). Inositol 1,3,4,5-tetrakisphosphate negatively regulates PtdIns(3,4,5)P3 signaling in neutrophils. *Immunity 27*, 453-467.

Kane, L.P., Shapiro, V.S., Stokoe, D., and Weiss, A. (1999). Induction of NF-kappaB by the Akt/PKB kinase. *Curr Biol 9*, 601-604.

Kato, M., Putta, S., Wang, M., Yuan, H., Lanting, L., Nair, I., Gunn, A., Nakagawa, Y., Shimano, H., Todorov, I., *et al.* (2009). TGF-beta activates Akt kinase through a microRNA-dependent amplifying circuit targeting PTEN. *Nat Cell Biol 11*, 881-889.

Kim, D., Kim, S., Koh, H., Yoon, S.O., Chung, A.S., Cho, K.S., and Chung, J. (2001). Akt/PKB promotes cancer cell invasion via increased motility and metalloproteinase production. *FASEB J 15*, 1953-1962.

Kroemer, G., Galluzzi, L., Vandenabeele, P., Abrams, J., Alnemri, E.S., Baehrecke, E.H., Blagosklonny, M.V., El-Deiry, W.S., Golstein, P., Green, D.R., *et al.* (2009). Classification of cell death: recommendations of the Nomenclature Committee on Cell Death 2009. *Cell Death Differ 16*, 3-11.

Kwak, Y.G., Song, C.H., Yi, H.K., Hwang, P.H., Kim, J.S., Lee, K.S., and Lee, Y.C. (2003). Involvement of PTEN in airway hyperresponsiveness and inflammation in bronchial asthma. *J Clin Invest 111*, 1083-1092.

Lacalle, R.A., Gomez-Mouton, C., Barber, D.F., Jimenez-Baranda, S., Mira, E., Martinez, A.C., Carrera, A.C., and Manes, S. (2004). PTEN regulates motility but not directionality during leukocyte chemotaxis. *J Cell Sci 117*, 6207-6215.

Li, D.M., and Sun, H. (1997). TEP1, encoded by a candidate tumor suppressor locus, is a novel protein tyrosine phosphatase regulated by transforming growth factor beta. *Cancer Res 57*, 2124-2129.

Li, D.M., and Sun, H. (1998). PTEN/MMAC1/TEP1 suppresses the tumorigenicity and induces G1 cell cycle arrest in human glioblastoma cells. Proc Natl Acad Sci USA *95*, 15406-15411.

Li, J., Yen, C., Liaw, D., Podsypanina, K., Bose, S., Wang, S.I., Puc, J., Miliaresis, C., Rodgers, L., McCombie, R., *et al.* (1997). PTEN, a putative protein tyrosine phosphatase gene mutated in human brain, breast, and prostate cancer. *Science 275*, 1943-1947.

Li, Y., Jia, Y., Pichavant, M., Loison, F., Sarraj, B., Kasorn, A., You, J., Robson, B.E., Umetsu, D.T., Mizgerd, J.P., *et al.* (2009). Targeted deletion of tumor suppressor PTEN augments neutrophil function and enhances host defense in neutropenia-associated pneumonia. *Blood 113*, 4930-4941.

Li, Z., Dong, X., Wang, Z., Liu, W., Deng, N., Ding, Y., Tang, L., Hla, T., Zeng, R., Li, L., *et al.* (2005). Regulation of PTEN by Rho small GTPases. *Nat Cell Biol 7*, 399-404.

Li, Z., Hannigan, M., Mo, Z., Liu, B., Lu, W., Wu, Y., Smrcka, A.V., Wu, G., Li, L., Liu, M., *et al.* (2003). Directional sensing requires G beta gamma-mediated PAK1 and PIX alpha-dependent activation of Cdc42. *Cell 114*, 215-227.

Liaw, D., Marsh, D.J., Li, J., Dahia, P.L., Wang, S.I., Zheng, Z., Bose, S., Call, K.M., Tsou, H.C., Peacocke, M., *et al.* (1997). Germline mutations of the PTEN gene in Cowden disease, an inherited breast and thyroid cancer syndrome. *Nat Genet 16*, 64-67.

Liliental, J., Moon, S.Y., Lesche, R., Mamillapalli, R., Li, D., Zheng, Y., Sun, H., and Wu, H. (2000). Genetic deletion of the Pten tumor suppressor gene promotes cell motility by activation of Rac1 and Cdc42 GTPases. *Curr Biol 10*, 401-404.

Liu, L., Puri, K.D., Penninger, J.M., and Kubes, P. (2007). Leukocyte PI3Kgamma and PI3Kdelta have temporally distinct roles for leukocyte recruitment in vivo. *Blood 110*, 1191-1198.

Liu, Q., Sasaki, T., Kozieradzki, I., Wakeham, A., Itie, A., Dumont, D.J., and Penninger, J.M. (1999). SHIP is a negative regulator of growth factor receptor-mediated PKB/Akt activation and myeloid cell survival. *Genes Dev 13*, 786-791.

Luo, H.R., and Loison, F. (2008). Constitutive neutrophil apoptosis: mechanisms and regulation. *Am J Hematol 83*, 288-295.

Maehama, T., and Dixon, J.E. (1998). The tumor suppressor, PTEN/MMAC1, dephosphorylates the lipid second messenger, phosphatidylinositol 3,4,5-trisphosphate. *J Biol Chem 273*, 13375-13378.

Maehama, T., and Dixon, J.E. (1999). PTEN: a tumour suppressor that functions as a phospholipid phosphatase. *Trends Cell Biol 9*, 125-128.

Maehama, T., Taylor, G.S., and Dixon, J.E. (2001). PTEN and myotubularin: novel phosphoinositide phosphatases. *Annu Rev Biochem 70*, 247-279.

Marsh, D.J., Dahia, P.L., Zheng, Z., Liaw, D., Parsons, R., Gorlin, R.J., and Eng, C. (1997). Germline mutations in PTEN are present in Bannayan-Zonana syndrome. *Nat Genet 16*, 333-334.

Meng, F., Henson, R., Lang, M., Wehbe, H., Maheshwari, S., Mendell, J.T., Jiang, J., Schmittgen, T.D., and Patel, T. (2006). Involvement of human micro-RNA in growth and response to chemotherapy in human cholangiocarcinoma cell lines. *Gastroenterology 130*, 2113-2129.

Myers, M.P., Pass, I., Batty, I.H., Van der Kaay, J., Stolarov, J.P., Hemmings, B.A., Wigler, M.H., Downes, C.P., and Tonks, N.K. (1998). The lipid phosphatase activity of PTEN is critical for its tumor supressor function. *Proc Natl Acad Sci USA 95*, 13513-13518.

Myers, M.P., Stolarov, J.P., Eng, C., Li, J., Wang, S.I., Wigler, M.H., Parsons, R., and Tonks, N.K. (1997). P-TEN, the tumor suppressor from human chromosome 10q23, is a dual-specificity phosphatase. *Proc Natl Acad Sci USA 94*, 9052-9057.

Olive, V., Bennett, M.J., Walker, J.C., Ma, C., Jiang, I., Cordon-Cardo, C., Li, Q.J., Lowe, S.W., Hannon, G.J., and He, L. (2009). miR-19 is a key oncogenic component of mir-17-92. *Genes Dev 23*, 2839-2849.

Ozes, O.N., Mayo, L.D., Gustin, J.A., Pfeffer, S.R., Pfeffer, L.M., and Donner, D.B. (1999). NF-kappaB activation by tumour necrosis factor requires the Akt serine-threonine kinase. *Nature 401*, 82-85.

Paramio, J.M., Navarro, M., Segrelles, C., Gomez-Casero, E., and Jorcano, J.L. (1999). PTEN tumour suppressor is linked to the cell cycle control through the retinoblastoma protein. *Oncogene 18*, 7462-7468.

Patel, L., Pass, I., Coxon, P., Downes, C.P., Smith, S.A., and Macphee, C.H. (2001). Tumor suppressor and anti-inflammatory actions of PPARgamma agonists are mediated via upregulation of PTEN. *Curr Biol 11*, 764-768.

Pezzolesi, M.G., Platzer, P., Waite, K.A., and Eng, C. (2008). Differential expression of PTEN-targeting microRNAs miR-19a and miR-21 in Cowden syndrome. *Am J Hum Genet 82*, 1141-1149.

Podsypanina, K., Ellenson, L.H., Nemes, A., Gu, J., Tamura, M., Yamada, K.M., Cordon-Cardo, C., Catoretti, G., Fisher, P.E., and Parsons, R. (1999). Mutation of Pten/Mmac1 in mice causes neoplasia in multiple organ systems. *Proc Natl Acad Sci USA 96*, 1563-1568.

Pop, C., and Salvesen, G.S. (2009). Human caspases: activation, specificity, and regulation. *J Biol Chem 284*, 21777-21781.

Puri, K.D., Doggett, T.A., Douangpanya, J., Hou, Y., Tino, W.T., Wilson, T., Graf, T., Clayton, E., Turner, M., Hayflick, J.S., *et al.* (2004). Mechanisms and implications of phosphoinositide 3-kinase delta in promoting neutrophil trafficking into inflamed tissue. *Blood 103*, 3448-3456.

Puri, K.D., Doggett, T.A., Huang, C.Y., Douangpanya, J., Hayflick, J.S., Turner, M., Penninger, J., and Diacovo, T.G. (2005). The role of endothelial PI3Kgamma activity in neutrophil trafficking. *Blood 106*, 150-157.

Rameh, L.E., Arvidsson, A., Carraway, K.L., 3rd, Couvillon, A.D., Rathbun, G., Crompton, A., VanRenterghem, B., Czech, M.P., Ravichandran, K.S., Burakoff, S.J., *et al.* (1997). A comparative analysis of the phosphoinositide binding specificity of pleckstrin homology domains. *J Biol Chem 272*, 22059-22066.

Rauh, M.J., Kalesnikoff, J., Hughes, M., Sly, L., Lam, V., and Krystal, G. (2003). Role of Src homology 2-containing-inositol 5'-phosphatase (SHIP) in mast cells and macrophages. *Biochem Soc Trans 31*, 286-291.

Rickert, P., Weiner, O.D., Wang, F., Bourne, H.R., and Servant, G. (2000). Leukocytes navigate by compass: roles of PI3Kgamma and its lipid products. *Trends Cell Biol 10*, 466-473.

Risinger, J.I., Hayes, A.K., Berchuck, A., and Barrett, J.C. (1997). PTEN/MMAC1 mutations in endometrial cancers. *Cancer Res 57*, 4736-4738.

Risinger, J.I., Hayes, K., Maxwell, G.L., Carney, M.E., Dodge, R.K., Barrett, J.C., and Berchuck, A. (1998). PTEN mutation in endometrial cancers is associated with favorable clinical and pathologic characteristics. *Clin Cancer Res 4*, 3005-3010.

Rizo, J., and Sudhof, T.C. (1998). C2-domains, structure and function of a universal Ca2+-binding domain. *J Biol Chem 273*, 15879-15882.

Rodgers, E.E., and Theibert, A.B. (2002). Functions of PI 3-kinase in development of the nervous system. *Int J Dev Neurosci 20*, 187-197.

Romashkova, J.A., and Makarov, S.S. (1999). NF-kappaB is a target of AKT in anti-apoptotic PDGF signalling. *Nature 401*, 86-90.

Sarraj, B., Massberg, S., Li, Y., Kasorn, A., Subramanian, K., Loison, F., Silberstein, L.E., von Andrian, U., and Luo, H.R. (2009). Myeloid-specific deletion of tumor suppressor PTEN augments neutrophil transendothelial migration during inflammation. *J Immunol 182*, 7190-7200.

Sasaki, T., Irie-Sasaki, J., Jones, R.G., Oliveira-dos-Santos, A.J., Stanford, W.L., Bolon, B., Wakeham, A., Itie, A., Bouchard, D., Kozieradzki, I., *et al.* (2000). Function of PI3Kgamma in thymocyte development, T cell activation, and neutrophil migration. *Science 287*, 1040-1046.

Scott, A.M., and Saleh, M. (2007). The inflammatory caspases: guardians against infections and sepsis. *Cell Death Differ 14*, 23-31.

Shen, Y.H., Zhang, L., Gan, Y., Wang, X., Wang, J., LeMaire, S.A., Coselli, J.S., and Wang, X.L. (2006). Up-regulation of PTEN (phosphatase and tensin homolog deleted on chromosome ten) mediates p38 MAPK stress signal-induced inhibition of insulin signaling. A cross-talk between stress signaling and insulin signaling in resistin-treated human endothelial cells. *J Biol Chem 281*, 7727-7736.

Shi, S.H., Jan, L.Y., and Jan, Y.N. (2003). Hippocampal Neuronal Polarity Specified by Spatially Localized mPar3/mPar6 and PI 3-Kinase Activity. *Cell 112*, 63-75.

Smith, D.F., Deem, T.L., Bruce, A.C., Reutershan, J., Wu, D., and Ley, K. (2006). Leukocyte phosphoinositide-3 kinase {gamma} is required for chemokine-induced, sustained adhesion under flow in vivo. *J Leukoc Biol 80*, 1491-1499.

Stambolic, V., Suzuki, A., de la Pompa, J.L., Brothers, G.M., Mirtsos, C., Sasaki, T., Ruland, J., Penninger, J.M., Siderovski, D.P., and Mak, T.W. (1998). Negative regulation of PKB/Akt-dependent cell survival by the tumor suppressor PTEN. *Cell 95*, 29-39.

Stambolic, V., Tsao, M.S., Macpherson, D., Suzuki, A., Chapman, W.B., and Mak, T.W. (2000). High incidence of breast and endometrial neoplasia resembling human Cowden syndrome in pten+/- mice. *Cancer Res 60*, 3605-3611.

Steck, P.A., Pershouse, M.A., Jasser, S.A., Yung, W.K., Lin, H., Ligon, A.H., Langford, L.A., Baumgard, M.L., Hattier, T., Davis, T., *et al.* (1997). Identification of a candidate tumour suppressor gene, MMAC1, at chromosome 10q23.3 that is mutated in multiple advanced cancers. *Nat Genet 15*, 356-362.

Subramanian, K.K., Jia, Y., Zhu, D., Simms, B.T., Jo, H., Hattori, H., You, J., Mizgerd, J.P., and Luo, H.R. (2007). Tumor suppressor PTEN is a physiologic suppressor of chemoattractant-mediated neutrophil functions. *Blood 109*, 4028-4037.

Sun, H., Lesche, R., Li, D.M., Liliental, J., Zhang, H., Gao, J., Gavrilova, N., Mueller, B., Liu, X., and Wu, H. (1999). PTEN modulates cell cycle progression and cell survival by regulating phosphatidylinositol 3,4,5,-trisphosphate and Akt/protein kinase B signaling pathway. *Proc Natl Acad Sci USA 96*, 6199-6204.

Tamura, M., Gu, J., Danen, E.H., Takino, T., Miyamoto, S., and Yamada, K.M. (1999). PTEN interactions with focal adhesion kinase and suppression of the extracellular matrix-dependent phosphatidylinositol 3-kinase/Akt cell survival pathway. *J Biol Chem 274*, 20693-20703.

Tamura, M., Gu, J., Matsumoto, K., Aota, S., Parsons, R., and Yamada, K.M. (1998). Inhibition of cell migration, spreading, and focal adhesions by tumor suppressor PTEN. Science *280*, 1614-1617.

Teresi, R.E., Planchon, S.M., Waite, K.A., and Eng, C. (2008). Regulation of the PTEN promoter by statins and SREBP. *Hum Mol Genet 17*, 919-928.

Tsou, H.C., Teng, D.H., Ping, X.L., Brancolini, V., Davis, T., Hu, R., Xie, X.X., Gruener, A.C., Schrager, C.A., Christiano, A.M., *et al.* (1997). The role of MMAC1 mutations in early-onset breast cancer: causative in association with Cowden syndrome and excluded in BRCA1-negative cases. *Am J Hum Genet 61*, 1036-1043.

Vazquez, F., Ramaswamy, S., Nakamura, N., and Sellers, W.R. (2000). Phosphorylation of the PTEN tail regulates protein stability and function. *Mol Cell Biol 20*, 5010-5018.

Webb, P.R., Wang, K.Q., Scheel-Toellner, D., Pongracz, J., Salmon, M., and Lord, J.M. (2000). Regulation of neutrophil apoptosis: a role for protein kinase C and phosphatidylinositol-3-kinase. *Apoptosis 5*, 451-458.

Yang, H., Kong, W., He, L., Zhao, J.J., O'Donnell, J.D., Wang, J., Wenham, R.M., Coppola, D., Kruk, P.A., Nicosia, S.V., *et al.* (2008). MicroRNA expression profiling in human ovarian cancer: miR-214 induces cell survival and cisplatin resistance by targeting PTEN. *Cancer Res 68*, 425-433.

Yang, K.Y., Arcaroli, J., Kupfner, J., Pitts, T.M., Park, J.S., Strasshiem, D., Perng, R.P., and Abraham, E. (2003). Involvement of phosphatidylinositol 3-kinase gamma in neutrophil apoptosis. *Cell Signal 15*, 225-233.

Zhu, D., Hattori, H., Jo, H., Jia, Y., Subramanian, K.K., Loison, F., You, J., Le, Y., Honczarenko, M., Silberstein, L., *et al.* (2006). Deactivation of phosphatidylinositol 3,4,5-trisphosphate/Akt signaling mediates neutrophil spontaneous death. *Proc Natl Acad Sci USA 103*, 14836-14841.

Zigmond, S.H. (1989). Chemotactic response of neutrophils. Am J Respir Cell Mol Biol *1*, 451-453.

In: Tumor Suppressors
Editor: Susan D. Nguyen
ISBN: 978-1-61761-986-1

Chapter 6

Wnt Pathway-Independent Activities of the APC Tumor Suppressor

Jenifer R. Prosperi and Kathleen H. Goss*
Department of Surgery, University of Chicago, Chicago, IL, USA

Abstract

The *adenomatous polyposis coli (APC)* tumor suppressor gene is commonly lost in both inherited and sporadic colorectal cancer and is frequently inactivated in many other human cancers. Moreover, *Apc* deficiency in animal models is sufficient for tumorigenesis in a diverse set of tissue types, demonstrating that APC loss not only correlates with cancer pathogenesis but drives tumor development. Over the last two decades since its identification, much attention has been devoted to deciphering the molecular mechanisms responsible for APC's tumor suppressor activity. The picture that is emerging is one of APC as a 'gatekeeper' of epithelial and tissue homeostasis by serving as a scaffold for multi-protein complexes, including the β-catenin destruction machinery. Although regulation of Wnt signaling by APC through β-catenin degradation has been well studied, separable Wnt-independent functions of APC have been identified. In this review, we will summarize the interaction of APC with junctional and polarity complexes, the cytoskeleton, nuclear proteins and apoptotic factors. Emerging evidence will be presented that supports the importance of these interactions in apical-basal and front-rear polarity, migration, differentiation, DNA replication, mitosis, DNA repair and apoptosis through Wnt pathway-independent mechanisms. The contribution of these processes to tumor development as a result of APC inactivation will be discussed. Lastly, we will address how the uncoupling of these activities from Wnt signaling may provide a therapeutic opportunity for treating APC-deficient cancers. Together, these generally under-appreciated, Wnt-independent aspects of APC function may significantly revise the accepted view of APC-mediated tumor suppression and, importantly, uncover novel strategies for cancer treatment.

* Corresponding Author: Kathleen H. Goss, Ph.D., Department of Surgery, University of Chicago, 5841 South Maryland Ave., Chicago, IL 60637, Phone: 773-702-2990, Fax: 773-834-4546, Email: kgoss@uchicago.edu

Introduction

The autosomal dominant transmission of rare, inherited familial cancers have facilitated the identification of tumor suppressor genes that are also commonly inactivated in sporadic cancers. Not only was a locus on chromosome 5q associated with the inherited colorectal cancer predisposition syndrome, familial adenomatous polyposis (FAP) [1-3], but the gene responsible, *adenomatous polyposis coli* (*APC*), was mapped to 5q21 in 1991 using linkage analysis of FAP kindreds and positional cloning approaches [4-7]. Like other classical tumor suppressors following the "two-hit model", one allele of *APC* is mutated in the germline of FAP individuals and the other is lost during colorectal tumor development. Perhaps more exciting than identifying *APC* as the FAP gene was the finding that *APC* mutation and 5q loss is frequently observed in sporadic colorectal cancers. Although the frequency ranges from approximately 35 to 88% depending on the cohort of tumors and the specific study, *APC* inactivation is the most common genetic alteration observed in colorectal cancers ([8] for review). Further, its alteration occurs early in colon tumor progression such that benign adenomatous polyps and even aberrant crypt foci often carry *APC* mutations [8]. In recent years, APC has also been found to be inactivated by mutation or, more commonly, by transcriptional silencing through promoter methylation in several extra-colonic tumor types, including breast, lung, gastric, head/neck, prostate, pancreatic, liver, bladder, skin, central nervous system, musculoskeletal, gynecological, esophageal, adrenal, thyroid, parathyroid ([9] for review). These data underscore the importance of APC not simply as a colon tumor suppressor but also as a key regulator of tissue homeostasis throughout the body.

The *APC* gene spans over 100 kb in the human genome and includes 15 exons, in addition to some alternatively spliced exons, that produces a 8,500-bp coding sequence. Mutations within *APC*, most of which are nonsense located in the central "mutation cluster region" (MCR) of the coding sequence, typically result in a prematurely truncated protein and subsequent loss of its carboxy-terminus. Other mutations scattered throughout the gene are associated with specific phenotypes, such as attenuated polyposis, or extracolonic manifestations of FAP such as congenital hypertrophy of the pigmented epithelium (CHRPE) or desmoids ([10] for review). In a phenomenon dubbed the "just-right hypothesis", the location of the first mutation is predictive of the second event in both FAP and sporadic tumors (i.e. whether gene deletion or a somatic mutation occurs, and if so, where that mutation occurs) ([8] for review). These patterns of mutation frequencies in cancers suggest that particular functional domains of the APC protein inactivated through mutation may be critical to APC's activity as a tumor suppressor such that their loss provides a selective advantage to tumor cells.

Since the *APC* gene was identified, the picture that has emerged regarding the molecular and cellular activities of the APC protein is one of a large (>300 kDa), multi-functional scaffold that controls diverse biological processes from proliferation to survival, differentiation, migration and polarization. How does one protein coordinate all of these activities? Many clues have surfaced from the identification and characterization of the diverse set of protein partners that bind distinct APC structural domains (**Figure 1**). The first identified and best studied of these is β-catenin, an essential component of the adherens junction complex that controls cell-cell interactions and the major effector of the canonical Wnt signal transduction pathway. Binding of β-catenin to the 15- and 20-amino acid repeats within the central domain of APC (overlapping with the MCR in the gene) facilitates β-catenin degradation through GSK3β-mediated phosphorylation, recognition by the βTrCP E3 ubiquitin ligase and degradation via the proteasome [11-14]. As a component of the β-catenin destruction complex, along with GSK3β, other kinases such as casein kinase 1α and the Axin tumor suppressor, APC is considered a potent inhibitor of the Wnt pathway. In the presence of mutant APC lacking the β-catenin binding domain, or when the pathway is activated by other mechanisms such as Wnt ligand expression, accumulation of β-catenin leads to its nuclear translocation and transcriptional activity by partnering with members of the T-cell factor (TCF)/lymphoid enhancer-binding factor (LEF) family of transcription factors. In many cancers, *APC* mutation is frequently associated with nuclear accumulation of β-catenin ([9] for review). *In vitro* and *in vivo* models have illustrated that APC loss is sufficient for nuclear β-catenin and the transcription of β-catenin/TCF endogenous and synthetic gene targets [15-18], and the β-catenin binding domain of APC is sufficient for tumor suppression [19]. Moreover, specific β-catenin/TCF target genes, such as MMP-7 and c-myc, are necessary and/or sufficient for tumorigenesis in *Apc*-mutant mouse models [20, 21] indicating that regulation of Wnt signaling plays a critical role in APC-mediated tumor suppression.

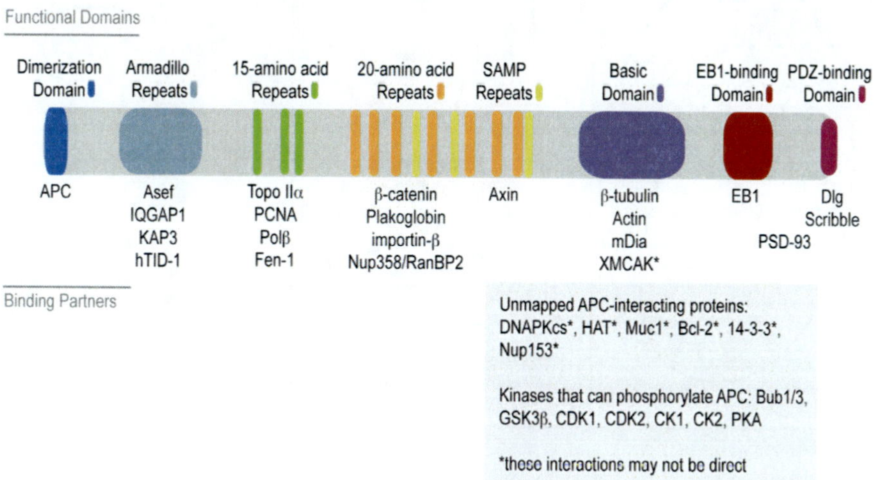

Figure 1. APC is a multifunction scaffolding protein. The characterized domains of APC are illustrated with known binding partners shown below the specific domain with which they interact. Associated APC partners that have not been mapped are listed, as are those kinases demonstated to phosphorylate APC. The proteins labeled with an asterisk (*) are found in immunocomplexes with APC but direct interactions with APC have not been demonstrated.

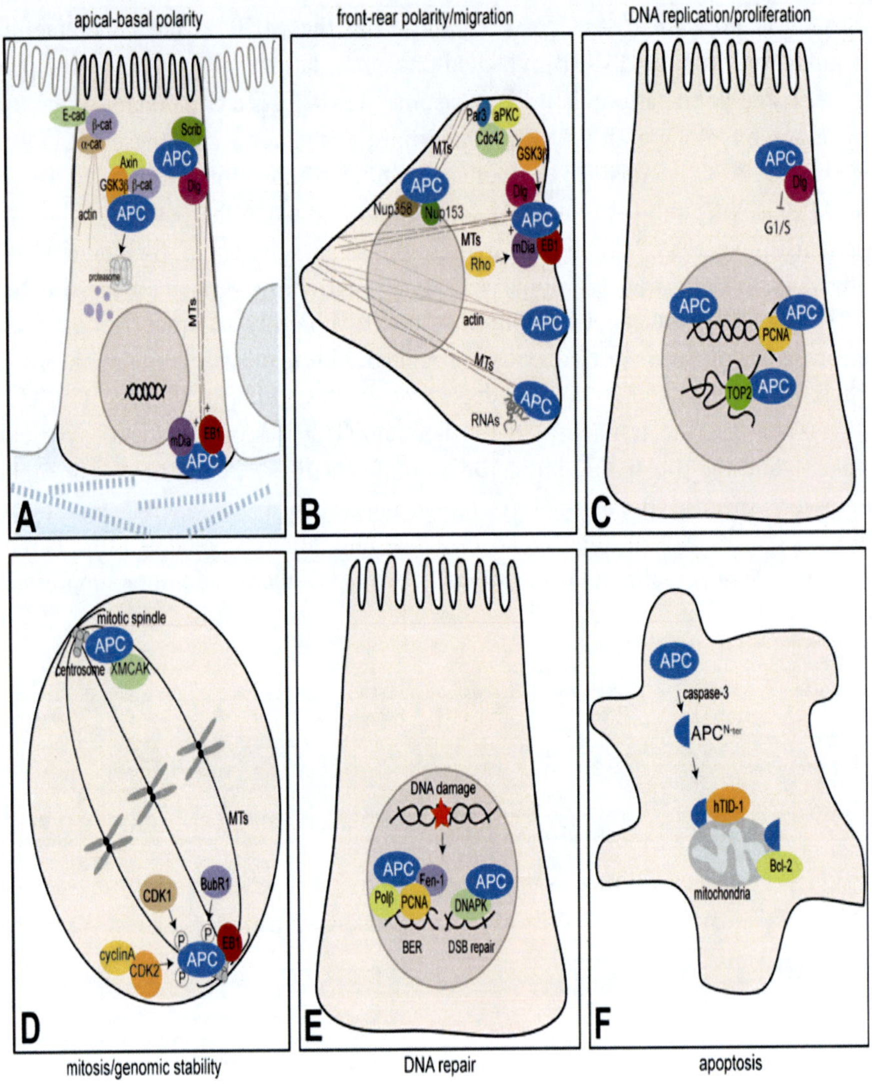

Figure 2. APC impacts numerous cellular processes independent of Wnt pathway regulation. A) APC is implicated in epithelial cell polarity through its interactions with β-catenin at the adherens junction, polarity complex such as Dlg and Scrib, and the plus-ends of microtubules. B) APC is implicated in the polarized region migration through stabilization of microtubule ends at the leading edge, a process that involves mDia, EB1 and Dlg and regulation by Par3/aPKC/Cdc42/GSK3β and Rho. APC binds to the actin cytoskeleton, regulates the polarized transport of RNA along microtubules and interacts with nuclear pore proteins for polarized centrosome orientation. C) APC regulates the G1/S transition indirectly through its association with Dlg and directly by associating with DNA and DNA-associated proteins such as PCNA and TOP2 during DNA replication. D) During mitosis, APC associates with thecentrosome and mitotic spindle, where its interaction with microtubules involves EB1 and XMCAK and is regulated by phosphorylation. E) A nuclear pool of APC modulates base-excision repair (BER) and souble-strand break (DSB) through interactions with DNA and PCNA, Fen-1 and Polβ and DNA protein kinase (DNAPK) catalytic subunit, respectively. F) Caspase-3-mediated cleavage of APC results in release of an amino-terminal fragment ($APC^{N\text{-}ter}$) that promotes apoptosis through its association with hTID-1 and Bcl-2 at the mitochondrial membrane. Details are provided in the text.

The β-catenin destruction complex may be only one of several protein complexes linked by the APC scaffold. In fact, there is accumulating evidence for APC-dependent effects that cannot be explained solely by β-catenin accumulation or transcriptional activation. For example, introduction of exogenous APC into colon cancer cells *in vitro* induces a G1/S-phase cell cycle arrest that can be only partially rescued by a non-degradable mutant of β-catenin [22], and mutant *Apc* alleles that cause profound tumorigenesis do not lead to robust β-catenin stabilization and nuclear accumulation [23, 24]. Moreover, the phenotypes associated with *Apc* loss and β-catenin stabilization or overexpression in hematopoetic stem cells and the mammary gland *in vivo* are not equivalent [24-31]. In this chapter, we will review the molecular interactions of APC that extend beyond β-catenin, including those with components of the cytoskeleton, junctional and polarity complexes, nuclear complexes and apoptosis regulators. The evidence that these associations control various aspects of epithelial and tumor cell biology, including DNA synthesis, replication and repair, mitosis, apical-basal polarization, directed motility, and apoptosis, will be discussed (**Figure 2**). Finally, we will address the profound therapeutic implications of non-Wnt pathway-mediated consequences of APC loss in tumors as the translational medicine field generally moves toward designing targeted and individualized therapies for cancer patients.

Association of APC with Junctional and Polarity Complexes

β-catenin and plakoglobin. When β-catenin was identified as the first known protein partner of APC, other than itself [32], one implication was that APC might be involved in cell-cell interactions and cell migration through β-catenin's well-accepted role at the adherens junction [11]. Not only does APC interact with β-catenin but also its close relative, plakoglobin (also called γ-catenin), a linker protein within the desmosome [33, 34]. Over the subsequent years of studying the interaction between APC and β-catenin, and the key observation that thc APC/β-catenin and β catenin/E-cadherin complexes are mutually exclusive [11, 34, 35], the focus on APC-mediated β-catenin degradation and regulation of the Wnt pathway has largely overshadowed the involvement of APC in cellular adhesion, motility, polarization and morphogenesis. However, there has long been evidence supporting that dysregulation in APC levels is associated with altered cell migration and adhesion, for example. Mice carrying a transgene driving ectopic APC expression in intestinal epithelial cells, one copy of a germline nonsense mutation in *Apc,* designated Apc^{Min}, or conditional knockout of APC in the intestine each displayed altered enterocyte migration along intestinal villi *in vivo* [17, 36, 37]. The tumorigenic potential of SW480 colorectal cancer cells with mutant APC was reduced by APC introduction and accompanied by changes in the localization of adherens junction proteins and tighter cell-cell contacts, altered morphology and reduced cell adhesion [38]. In polarized epithelia *in vitro* and *in vivo*, APC has been localized to both the apical, lateral and basal surfaces depending on the specific model system and context [39-45]. APC localization at cell-cell contacts has been shown to be dependent on β-catenin and E-cadherin, and its phosphorylation by GSK3β and casein kinase I (CKI) shifts the major APC pool to membrane clusters at cell protrusions and promoted cell migration

[46]. The mechanisms by which APC loss modulates cell-cell interactions are unclear but may involve changing the local concentration β-catenin or plakoglobin at cell junctions in addition to regulating β-catenin/TCF target genes specifically implicated in adhesion, such as E-cadherin [47] and CD44 [48], as well as other APC binding partners including the components of polarity complexes or the cytoskeleton.

The Scrib/Dlg/Lgl complex. Epithelial organization and integrity is controlled by cell-cell and cell-matrix interactions as well as complexes that confer the identity of the apical and basolateral membrane domains, such as the Crumbs (CRB)/PALS/PATJ, Par3/Par6/atypical protein kinase C (aPKC) and Scribble/discs large (Dlg)/lethal giant larvae (Lgl) complexes (see [49] for review). The first link of APC to any of these complexes was the isolation of Dlg in a yeast two-hybrid screen using the carboxy-terminus of APC as a "bait" [50]. Dlg1, a PDZ-domain containing tumor suppressor, co-localizes with APC at the basolateral membrane in epithelia *in situ* and in pucta at cell protrusions in glial cells, fibroblasts and subconfluent epithelial cells [50, 51], an observation that is dependent on activation of the Par6/aPKC complex by Cdc42 in astrocytes [52]. In addition to the organizational function of the APC/Dlg complex, overexpression of dominant-negative Dlg1 mutants suppresses the ability of APC to induce a cell cycle arrest, and APC mutants that lack the PDZ-binding carboxy-terminal residues, S/TXV, fail to inhibit proliferation as well as intact APC [53]. The connection to APC may be a common feature of Dlg proteins since Dlg3 (also known as NE-Dlg) also binds to APC [54]. Interestingly, Dlg is required for assembly of the adherens junction and intestinal epithelial cell differentiation [55], effects that might be mediated by APC but also perhaps through an interaction between Dlg and E-cadherin [55] or through APC-independent effects on β-catenin turnover by Dlg [56].

More recent support for the concept that the APC-Dlg interaction at the basolateral membrane is biologically relevant has come from the observation that APC also binds directly to Scribble (Scrib), another PDZ domain-containing component in this basolateral polarity complex, through the S/TXV residues at its carboxy terminus [57]. All three proteins in the Scrib/Dlg/Lgl complex are tumor suppressors and required for polarity, including adherens junction formation (reviewed in [58]). Scrib co-localizes with APC at protrusion ends of migrating epithelial cells and in neuronal cells, like Dlg, and overexpression of the domain of Scrib that binds APC disrupts epithelial polarity [57]. In astrocytes, Scrib controls the recruitment of APC and Dlg to the leading edge to promote cell polarization during migration [59]. Given that APC interacts with both Dlg and Scrib but that Scrib, Dlg and Lgl do not interact directly with each other, it is an attractive possibility that APC serves as the scaffold that brings the complex together or regulates its turnover. An alternative possibility that Scrib is upstream of APC is supported by the demonstration that Scrib depletion disrupts APC localization in polarized intestinal epithelial cells [57]. Because Scrib inhibits the function of the Par3/Par6/aPKC complex to promote the basal domain [60], it is possible that this involves APC since APC also interacts with Par3 to regulate its transport along microtubules [61, 62].

Role in apical-basal polarity of epithelial cells. Evidence for APC regulating aspects of apical-basal polarity and epithelial morphogenesis comes from some non-gastrointestinal model systems. Germline homozygous deletion of *Apc* prevents development past embryonic day 6, consistent with a role for APC in overall epithelial organization [63]. In the mature cochlea, where APC localizes to the plus ends of microtubules at the basal surface of the epithelium, *Apc* mutation results in a reduced number of parallel microtubule arrays, whose organization is essential for epithelial polarization [42]. Studies from our laboratory have demonstrated that altered mammary epithelial polarity and overall integrity appears to underlie the attenuated lobuloavleolar development phenotype observed *Apc*$^{Min/+}$ female mice [41], and APC knockdown in mammary epithelial cells results in altered epithelial morphogenesis in monolayers and in 3D cultures ([41]; J.R.P and K.H.G., unpublished data). Notably, APC is required for the distribution of MUC1, a transmembrane glycoprotein, to the apical membrane of differentiated mammary epithelial cells [41]. This observation is particularly intriguing since MUC1 has been shown to interact with APC [64], and MUC1 mislocalization is frequently observed in cancers [65-67].

Another critical feature of an epithelial organization is symmetric planar cell division. In *Drosophila* neuroepithelial cells, APC is recruited to the adherens junction and is required for symmetric cell division along the planar axis perhaps through positioning the mitotic spindle via its association with microtubules [68]. This role for APC is probably not restricted to polarized epithelial cells as a similar mechanism is likely to be involved in the asymmetric division of Drosophila male germline stem cells [69]. Also at cell-cell junctions in epithelial cells, APC binds to Striatin, a calmodulin-binding protein predominately expressed in the central nervous system, through its armadillo repeats [70]. These two proteins form a complex with ZO-1, a central component of tight junctions, and the interaction of the APC/Striatin complex with the plasma membrane is dependent on an intact actin cytoskeleton [70].

The establishment and maintenance of apical-basal polarity is an essential process during the functional differentiation of all epithelial cells. Recent studies in zebrafish embryos suggest that a role for APC in intestinal differentiation can be uncoupled from β-catenin and involves the transcriptional corepressor carboxy-terminal binding protein 1 (CtBP1) [71]. While CtBP-1 has been previously shown to be impact the transcription of β-catenin/TCF target genes [72], CtBP also interacts with APC to control the expression of enzymes that drive differentiation, including intestinal retinol dehydrogenases [73, 74]. Consistent with these observations in the zebrafish model system, upregulation of CtBP1 in adenomas from FAP patients was accompanied by cytosolic but not nuclear β-catenin [71] suggesting that stabilization of CtBP1, rather than solely β-catenin, by APC may be important in early colorectal tumor development as a result of APC inactivation.

An important unresolved issue is the extent by which APC's action in apical-basal polarity contributes to its tumor suppressive activity. In general, loss of epithelial polarity of and disruption of tissue organization is correlated with more aggressive and advanced cancers ([75, 76] for reviews). Disrupted adherens junction integrity protein localization are frequently observed in cancers [77], and more recently, components of the Scrib/Dlg/Lgl complex have been implicated in cancer. For example, oncogenic viruses, such as human papilloma viruses (HPV) 16 and 18, target components of the Scrib/Dlg/Lgl complex for degradation to disrupt polarity [78]. The basolateral membrane distribution of Dlg and Scrib is significantly perturbed during colorectal cancer progression [79], and Dlg, Scrib and Lgl are mislocalized or downregulated in many other tumor types [76]. Collectively, these data support the concept that APC action in epithelial polarization might be essential to its role in tumor initiation and progression. This hypothesis is also supported by the identification of 14-3-3σ, a multi-functional tumor suppressor implicated in polarity, in a complex with APC [80].

While this idea has important therapeutic implications, it will be necessary to decouple some of these APC activities from Wnt pathway regulation in future work – a difficult task with such a large multi-functional protein.

APC Interaction with the Cytoskeleton

Actin. The localization of APC at the plasma membrane is dependent on interaction with the actin cytoskeleton [44]. APC directly interacts with F-actin through the basic domain in the carboxy-terminal region of APC [81, 82], a region also responsible for direct interactions with microtubules [83]. These data suggest that coordinated regulation of actin and microtubule dynamics may involve APC. Moreover, APC binding to EB1 (a microtubule-binding protein that will be discussed in detail below) blocks the interaction of APC to actin [81]. Recent work demonstrates that APC not only co-localizes with F-actin, but also promotes actin assembly and nucleation [82]. Providing the first molecular hints to how APC controls actin dynamics, it was demonstrated that APC-mediated actin nucleation was through the recruitment of actin monomers by APC rather than the Arp2/3 complex, and the assembly of actin filaments involves the synergistic activity of APC with the formin mDia [82]. Despite some studies showing that APC directly interacts with F-actin through the basic domain, localization of APC to the plasma membrane is primarily mediated through the Arm domain of APC located on the amino-terminal region of APC [82].

Actin effectors. Actin dynamics are tightly controlled by the Rho family of small GTPases and their regulators. APC interacts directly with the APC-stimulated guanine nucleotide exchange factor (Asef)-1 and -2 through its armadillo repeats [84, 85]. Asef-1 functions as a guanine nucleotide exchange factor (GEF) for Rac, which is regulated in the same region as the APC-binding site within Asef-1 [85]; however, APC binding actually activates the GEF activity of Asef-1. The interaction between APC and Asef-1 is critical for maintaining cell morphology and promotes epithelial cell motility [85, 86]. However, in both MDCK epithelial cells and colorectal tumor cells, only truncated, but not full-length, APC cooperates with Asef to induce cell migration [86]. Although Asef-1 does not interact with β-catenin, it is interesting to note that β-catenin can be identified in a complex with APC and Asef-1 [85], suggesting that APC might be a scaffold for this complex in a manner similar to those discussed earlier. Like Asef-1, the association of truncated APC with Asef-2, a GEF specific for both Rac1 and Cdc42, at the amino-terminus of Asef-2 results in enhanced GEF activity and tumor cell migration [84]. As opposed to the single binding domain for APC in Asef-1, it is now appreciated that there are two binding sites for APC in Asef-2, namely the amino-terminal APC binding region and a Src-homology (SH) 3 domain [87].

APC also modulates the actin cytoskeleton through directly binding the actin cross-linking protein IQ motif containing GTPase activating protein (IQGAP1) through its armadillo repeat domain [88]. IQGAP1 is an effector of Rac1 and Cdc42, specifically maintaining the Rho GTPases in an active state [89]. The APC/IQGAP1 complex interacts with Rac1 and Cdc42 to promote cell polarization and migration [88], and binds with the microtubule stabilizing protein, CLIP-170 [88]. IQGAP1 also recruits APC to membrane ruffles, perhaps in a complex with β-catenin and N-cadherin [90]. These findings are particularly interesting, as they imply that the interaction of APC with IQGAP1 may provide a molecular link between the actin and microtubule networks to drive changes in cell morphology and polarized migration.

Microtubules. In addition to β-catenin, one of the first characterized interactions of APC, or carboxy-terminal fragments of APC, was with microtubules using co-localization and *in vitro* studies [91-93]. APC was found to promote microtubule assembly [91] by increasing both the stability and the lifespan of microtubules [94, 95]. To further support the carboxy-terminus of APC, specifically the basic region, as being responsible for microtubule binding [96], it has been shown that microtubule depolymerization from nocodazole treatment causes diffuse APC localization in the cytosol, similar to that observed for truncated APC [93]. The interaction between APC and microtubules is decreased when APC is phosphorylated by GSK3β and protein kinase A (PKA) [94]. Interestingly, phosphorylation of APC by GSK3β strengthens APC's interaction with β-catenin, suggesting that these interactions are differentially regulated, and supporting the existence of mutually exclusive pools of APC with different cellular functions [94].

Microtubule-binding proteins. Despite the ability of APC to directly interact with microtubules, several other binding partners linking APC to microtubules have been identified. One of the best-studied proteins to associate APC with microtubules is end-binding protein 1 (EB1), a plus end binding protein that regulates microtubule polymerization [97]. APC was first found to interact with EB1 through a yeast two-hybrid assay using the carboxy terminus of APC as a "bait" [98]. Since then, the binding domain responsible for the EB1 interaction was mapped not to the basic domain that had been attributed to microtubule association but to the final 170 residues of APC [96]. Despite the fact that the function of EB1 was unknown at the time, subsequent studies showed that EB1 or EB1 homologues are associated with cytosplasmic and spindle microtubules and are required for microtubule stability [99-102]. Specifically, EB1 mutation was found to allow yeast with misaligned spindle to inappropriately advance through the cell cycle [103]. The interaction between APC and EB1 targets APC to microtubule distal ends [96, 104]. APC is required for the ability EB1 to promote microtubule polymerization [97] by cooperating with EB1 to cap the plus ends of microtubules thus preventing exchange of tubulin subunits [105]. Given its importance in microtubule dynamics, it is not surprising that formation of the APC/EB1 complex is tightly regulated. For example, the interaction of APC and EB1 is disrupted by APC phosphorylation by PKA or Cdc2 to prevent microtubule assembly [96, 104]. Interestingly, in SW480 colorectal cancer cells with truncated APC lacking the EB1-binding domain, EB1 remained associated with microtubules [100]. Collectively, these data illustrate that APC's interaction with EB1 plays a key role in microtubule polymerization and stability, although the molecular details still need to be completely elucidated.

Additional APC binding partners regulate the interaction between APC and microtubules. The kinesin superfamly members KAP3 and Kif3 interact with APC to direct its transport to plus ends of microtubules [106]. KAP3 can bind to the APC aminoterminus, in the armadillo repeat region, to target APC to microtubule clusters at cell protrusions and at the leading edge of migrating cells [106]. mDia, a formin protein that stabilizes microtubules, binds the carboxy-terminal domain of APC in a complex with EB1 [105]. Rho-induced stabilization of microtubules by mDia promotes fibroblast motility, and when formation of the complex is inhibited, cell motility is suppressed [105]. The anterograde kinesin, KIF17, was recently shown to participate in localizing APC to the plus ends of microtubules and is required for proper epithelial polarization and morphogenesis [107]. Importin-β, a nuclear pore complex protein, is also implicated in regulating APC-mediated microtubule assembly and spindle integrity [108]. This interaction between APC and importin-β was mapped to the middle region of APC, where importin-β can compete with β-catenin, and within two regions in the carboxy-terminus. Moreover, the interaction is inhibited by RanGTP and diminishes the ability of APC to regulate microtubule assembly but not APC's association with microtubules or EB1 [108]. Lastly, the polarity protein Dlg may also be involved in APC-mediated control of microtubule dynamics as it was shown that Dlg, described above, promotes APC accumulation at plus ends of microtubules and the interaction of microtubules with the plasma membrane [52].

Role in front-rear polarity and directional cell migration. Given that cytoskeleton dynamics dictates cell shape and motility, it is not surprising that APC's role in directional cell migration is tightly linked to its association with the actin and microtubule network. In neuronal and non-neuronal cells of the central nervous system, as well as subconfluent epithelial cells in culture, APC expression is predominantly localized to puncta at the leading edge or ends of cell protrusions [92, 109]. This localization has been shown to be dependent on the microtubule cytoskeleton but not actin [51, 92, 110] and is regulated by phosphorylation [46]. APC loss results in decreased microtubule stability, fewer cell protrusions and reduced cell migration [95, 111]; conversely, APC overexpression induces the formation of cell protrusions [111].

Recent work has illustrated that APC is required for the polarization of migrating astrocytes [110] and that the molecular mechanisms that regulate this activity of APC involve common cytoskeleton modulators. The Rac effector Cdc42, a small Rho GTPase required to polarize the actin and microtubule networks during migration, activates the atypical PKCζ at the leading edge and phosphorylates and inactivates GSK3β. This, in turn, promotes the association of APC with microtubule plus ends as well as the assembly of Dlg-containing puncta at the plasma membrane at the leading edge [52, 110]. Expression of APC mutants lacking more than 800 residues of the carboxy-terminus (encoding the microtubule, EB1, and Dlg/Srib-binding domains) as well as just the PDZ-binding domain (i.e. the last 20 amino acids) severely disrupted centrosome orientation and polarized motility [52, 110]. These data indicate that the interactions of APC with PDZ domain-containing proteins, such as Dlg and Scrib, and are essential for microtubule polarization and directed cell migration. Consistent with these observations, APC is required for the polarity of neuronal progenitors and the response of these cells to polarity maintenance cues during development of the cerebral cortex *in vivo* [112].

Similar mechanisms are likely invoked during neuronal cell migration. Consistent with a role for APC in promoting axon outgrowth, APC is localized to early axons while they are still indistinguishable from dendrites [113]. Localized inactivation of GSK3β by the PI3K and AKT kinases results in APC-mediated regulated of microtubule stability and axon growth [62, 114], perhaps involving the polarized localization of Par3 through an association with APC [62]. Other studies have described AKT-independent inhibition of GSK3β at the tip of the presumptive axon [115], and recent studies demonstrated that the LKB1 polarity kinase also inactivates GSK3β to stabilize APC at the microtubule distal ends to promote forward movement of the centrosome and neuronal motility [116]. This is especially interesting because LKB1 is a Par4 homolog considered to be a master polarity regulator and potent tumor suppressor inactivated in individuals with the inherited cancer syndrome, Peutz-Jeghers ([117] for review). Despite this evidence supporting an important role for APC in neuronal cell polarity and migration, a recent study using neuronal progenitors and neurons, showed that APC was not required for polarity or axon outgrowth [118]. Possible explanations for these discrepancies that warrant further investigation include differences in the model systems or tissues studied, non-specific effects of overexpressing APC mutants and the contribution of Wnt-dependent APC effects.

Recently, APC has been found to associate with Dishevelled (Dvl), activated focal adhesion kinase (FAK) and paxillin at the leading edge in migrating cells to regulate focal adhesion turnover, suggesting that APC can also act to impact cell motility by controlling cell-matrix interactions [119]. This effect might be mediated, in part, by Wnt signaling since FAK is upregulated in the intestinal epithelium in a myc-dependent fashion following *Apc*-depletion *in vivo* [120]. Nevertheless, the biological relevance of this finding is supported by the observation that FAK activity was required for tumorigenesis in *Apc*-mutant mice [120]. Also in migrating cells, a novel function of APC is to transport and localize RNA molecules to cell protrusions [121]. It is known that RNA transport along actin filaments or microtubules is required for its localization at protrusion ends to mediate cell polarity, a process that requires APC perhaps even through a direct APC/RNA interaction [121]. APC also modulates cell migration through its association with two microtubule-binding nuclear pore complex proteins, Nup153 and Nup358. A direct interaction of APC with Nup153 in neurons and fibroblasts promotes the association of microtubules with the nuclear membrane and is essential for centrosome reorganization in migration [122]. In the central region of APC, there is also a binding site for the nucleoporin, Nup358 (also called RanBP2), which regulates the localization of APC to microtubule plus ends at the cell cortex in a kinesin 2-dependent mechanism [123]. RNA interference studies additionally indicate that Nup358 is required for polarized cell migration [123].

Role in mitosis. During mitosis, APC localizes near the centrosomes and is associated with the microtubule-organizing center to maintain chromatin structure [124]. Although it is expressed and phosphorylated throughout the cell cycle, APC is transiently hyperphosphorylated in M-phase [125]. The G2/M-phase cyclin-dependent kinase (cdk) complex, cyclinB/cdk1, co-localizes with APC and phosphorylates its carboxy-terminus [126], an event that regulates its interaction with EB1 in mitosis [96, 97]. The cyclin A/cdk2 complex, which is required for mitotic entry, also associates with APC in G2/M and phosphorylates APC at Ser1360 within the MCR to control anchoring of the spindle to the cell cortex during mitosis [127]. The APC/EB1 complex at the spindle provides stable kinetochore microtubule attachment for proper chromosome alignment, an activity that is also regulated by the BubR1 mitotic checkpoint kinase [128, 129]. APC forms a complex with Bub1 and Bub3 during mitosis at microtubule ends, and phosphorylation of APC by the Bub kinases, after priming by GSK3β phosphorylation, regulates the interaction between microtubules and kinetochores [130].

Underscoring the importance of APC in chromosome segregation and cytokinesis, embryonic stem (ES) cells from *Apc*-mutant mice have severe chromosomal and mitotic spindle defects [131]. Additional studies indicate that depletion of either APC or EB1 results in misorientation and altered stretching of the aligned sister kinetochores to promote missegregation of chromosomes that go undetected by the spindle checkpoint [128, 132, 133]. This is most likely an early consequence of APC loss since normal tissues isolated from an

Apc-mutant mouse models exhibit aneuploidy and severe mitotic defects, including misorientation of spindles and misalignment of chromosomes [133, 134]. Specifically the misorientation of spindles worsens as intestinal tumor development progresses such that heterozygous adenomas show more spindle disorganization than normal tissues, and APC loss of heterozygosity is associated with an even more dramatic phenotype [135]. Loss of APC decreases the interaction of Bub1 with kinetochores and blocks the mitotic checkpoint to promote cells entering G1 with a 4n DNA content [133].

Additional studies indicate that mutant APC proteins act dominantly to interfere with microtubule plus ends and to induce abnormalities in mitosis [136]. Using the *Xenopus* model, deletion of the microtubule-binding region of APC results in a redistribution of microtubules from spindle center to the poles and less tightly assembled microtubules [137]. One possible explanation for this specific spindle defect is that the APC interacts with *Xenopus* mitotic centromere-associated kinesin (XMCAK) at its carboxy-terminus [138]. APC and XMCAK localize to the centromere and kinetochore to regulate chromosomal segregation and spindle assembly, but, interestingly, have opposing roles on microtubules. Moreover, neither protein is required for localization of the other, implying that perhaps there are other components of this complex to regulate spindle microtubule dynamics [138]. It is also possible that APC's amino-terminus, in addition to its carboxy-terminus, be involved in mitosis. Amino-terminal APC mutants advance mitotic exit and inhibit proliferation perhaps due to weakening the microtubules/kinetochore interaction to effect chromosomal stability [139]. To further complicate APC's role in mitosis, β-catenin/TCF-mediated transcription has been implicated in promoting chromosomal instability in APC-mutant cells [140].

The role for APC at the mitotic spindle checkpoint through its interaction with microtubules and microtubule-binding proteins has important therapeutic implications since several chemotherapeutic agents, such as taxanes and vinca alkaloids, work as spindle poisons by disrupting microtubules. Recent work demonstrated that APC-deficient cells *in vivo* are resistant to arrest in response to low but not high levels of Taxol and that this Wnt-independent effect was due to mictrotubule destabilization following Taxol treatment rather than a generalized spindle checkpoint defect [141]. These results are consistent with *in vitro* studies that demonstrated a role for APC in response to lower levels of mitotic arrest caused by nocodozole treatment but no impact of APC loss on high levels of arrest [132, 133]. Collectively, these data indicate that the amount of drug and the threshold necessary for checkpoint engagement is critical for considering treatment options for APC-mutant cancers. Much more work is needed in this area to fully understand the extent by which APC status influences therapuetic response to specific agents.

Association of Apc with Nuclear Proteins

Nuclear factors. In addition its cytosolic and cytoskeletal localization, a nuclear pool of APC has been observed in several normal and tumor cell lines [142, 143]. Characterization of this subcellular fraction suggests that this pool may be regulated by cell density and phosphorylation [144, 145], phase of the cell cycle [146, 147], the LEF-1 transcription factor [148], and the B56 alpha subunit of the protein phosphatase (PP) 2A [148]. Despite the controversy regarding the specificity of nuclear APC localization using certain antibodies

[149], additional data indicate that APC interacts with chromatin under some circumstances. For example, APC has been identified as a co-repressor along with CtBP in chromatin immunoprecipitations at the *c-myc* promoter to inhibit β-catenin/TCF-mediated transcription [150]. Additional studies indicate that the carboxy-terminus of APC associates *in vivo* with euchromatin and preferentially binds *in vitro* to acetylated histone H3 [151]. Collectively, these data indicate that the nuclear pool of APC, although not very abundant compared to the cytosolic fractions [149], may play important roles in DNA metabolism, including transcription, replication and repair.

Role in cell cycle control and DNA replication. There is evidence that APC mediates all phases of the cell cycle, including a direct role in mitosis through its association with the centrosome and microtubules at the mitotic spindle as described above. Loss of APC can modulate cell cycle progression partially through activation of the Wnt/β-catenin pathway. For example, over-expression of APC in colorectal cancer cells with mutant APC results in a G1/S arrest [152], which is only partially rescued by β-catenin [22, 153]. In fibroblasts, the interaction of APC with Dlg is required for the APC-induced G1/S arrest independent of mediating β-catenin degradation [53]. Further studies showed that it is the carboxy-terminal region of APC that is responsible for inhibiting DNA replication. This occurs specifically by direct binding of APC to DNA to inhibit G1/S progression; however, APC phosphorylation by cdk1 and cdk2 relieves this G1/S block [154]. APC does not bind a specific consensus sequence in DNA but, rather, associates with A/T rich sequences [83]. Another nuclear APC protein partner is proliferating cell nuclear antigen (PCNA), which has roles in both DNA replication and repair [155, 156]. It is a marker for G1/S phase of the cell cycle, and is a co-factor of DNA polymerase, assisting in DNA replication. PCNA binding occurs through the 15 amino acid repeat region of APC between residues 1245-1273 where the PCNA-interacting protein (PIP)-like box is located [155]. APC also binds to topoisomerase IIα through the 15 amino acid repeat region to regulate cell cycle progression [157]. Although this region is also important for APC binding to and inducing the degradation of β-catenin, the interaction with topoisomerase IIα appears to be independent of β-catenin binding. Functionally, cells over-expressing the APC fragment responsible for binding topoisomerase IIα exhibit a G2 cell cycle arrest [157].

Additional regulation of APC during proliferation comes from casein kinase 2 (CK2). Not only does CK2 phosphorylate APC to promote its nuclear translocation [145], the interaction of CK2 with APC specifically attenuates CK2 activity to inhibit proliferation [158]. Interestingly, although it is the amino-terminus of APC that binds to CK2, a carboxy-terminal region of APC is required to inhibit CK2 activity, suggesting that full-length APC is required for complete interaction and functional activity of the APC/CK2 complex [158]. Despite all of these findings, there are data showing that APC loss does not impact proliferative rates or the percentage of cells in mitosis [111].

Role in DNA repair. In addition to the evidence that APC influences DNA replication during S-phase, APC is implicated in multiple DNA repair pathways. It interacts with DNA polymerase β (Pol-β) and flap endonuclease 1 (Fen-1) to inhbit both single nucleotide and long-patch base excision repair (SN-BER and LP-BER) [155, 159, 160]. APC interacts with Pol-β through the PIP-like box to inhibit Pol-β activity perhaps through disrupting Lys72, a critical residue for its activity in SN-BER [159]. In double-stranded DNA break repair, APC is induced to the site of damaged DNA and then interacts with the DNA-dependent protein kinase catalytic subunit (DNAPKcs) to enhance the early response to the damage by promoting the phosphorylation of H2AX [151]. Therefore, when APC is lost or mutated, repair is slowed and an accumulation of cells harboring mutations can occur [151]. This role for APC is consistent with its designation as a "gatekeeper" [161], such that its loss early in tumors facilitates the acquisition of subsequent mutations during cancer progression. The interaction of APC with the 14-4-3σ tumor suppressor that is transcriptionally controlled by p53 and involved in the DNA damage response [80] further supports this hypothesis, although the detailed mechanisms need to be elucidated.

Loss or mutation of APC results in cells having increased ability to repair mutated DNA [155]. In LP-BER, APC interacts with Pol-β and Fen-1 to block LP-BER [159, 160]. When APC is lost cells become resistant to treatment with the DNA alkylation agent methylmethane sulfonate (MMS) [162], suggesting that cells with higher levels of APC are more sensitive to chemotherapeutic alkylating agents due to decreased in LP-BER. In other words, APC status could impact therapeutic outcome since those damaged cells with wildtype APC should undergo apoptosis while cells with mutant APC might be able to survive. Interestingly, APC expression is regulated by a variety of alkylating agents, including MMS [163], and carcinogens [164-166].

Association of APC with Apoptosis Regulators

APC cleavage. The amino-terminus of APC appears to have a direct link to apoptosis. It has been observed that caspase 3-induced cleavage of APC occurs during apoptosis, releasing a 90-kDa amino-terminal fragment (residues 1-777) [167-169]. Release of this segment is necessary for apoptosis induced by the full-length APC *in vitro*, and a truncated APC mutant was resistant to cleavage and unable to induce apoptosis [168]. Subsequent characterization of this fragment recently identified the mitochondrial tumor suppressor protein hTID-1 as a direct binding partner, interacting with residues 202-512 of APC [170]. Brocardo et al. [171] confirmed that mitochondrial association of APC was dependent also on the amino-terminus of APC (residues 1-900). Interestingly, this study identified the anti-apoptotic protein Bcl-2 in a complex with APC in the mitochondrial lysate fractions while also suggesting that the effects of APC on apoptosis involved regulating Bcl-2 expression but did not involve β-catenin and its target gene survivin [171]. This latter finding is not entirely surprising given that the β-catenin binding domain does not overlap with this amino-terminal fragment.

Role in apoptosis. APC mutation has long been associated with changes in cellular apoptosis [167, 172, 173]. In fact, inducible introduction of APC into HT-29 colorectal cancer cells, which lack full-length APC protein, significantly increased the baseline level of apoptosis in these cells by approximately 10-fold [174] as well as drug-induced apoptosis [175]. It is likely that part of APC's involvement in apoptosis is due to the regulation of Wnt target genes such as survivin, a member of the inhibitor of apoptosis (IAP) family of pro-survival factors [176]. Suppression of survivin levels upon APC introduction is one potentially important mechanism by which APC modifies the sensitivity to histone deacetylase inhibitor-induced apoptosis in the HT-29 model [175]. However, control of Wnt signaling by APC does not sufficiently explain some of the evidence supporting a role for APC in apoptosis. For example, exogenous full-length, but not mutant, APC induced apoptosis-associated caspase activity in a cell-free *in vitro* assay [177]. The mammary lobuloalveolar development defect in *Apc*$^{Min/+}$ mice is accompanied by a striking increase in apoptosis; yet, there is no evidence for activation of the Wnt pathway in the mammary tissues from these animals or APC-knockdown mammary epithelial cells [41]. Data like these strongly suggest that transcriptional changes mediated by APC expression cannot be exclusively responsible for the effect of APC on apoptosis.

One complication in assessing the role for APC in regulating is apoptosis is that APC mutation or depletion, like APC overexpression, often induces apoptosis. This observation is highly context-dependent and may be due to APC loss in normal cells, as compared to tumor cells, or an indirect consequence of some other change in cell behavior that may induce apoptosis when it cannot be resolved. For example, the induction in apoptosis in mammary epithelial cells from lactating *Apc*$^{Min/+}$ mice may be linked to the significant disruption in epithelial polarization [41]. Acute loss of *Apc* in the adult small intestine epithelium promotes apoptosis but also induces proliferation, and perturbs migration and differentiation [178]. Retinal degeneration in *Apc* fly mutants results from apoptotic cell death and defects in differentiation [179]. It this case, β-catenin depletion is sufficient to rescue the apoptosis but not differentiation phenotype [179], suggesting that these complex phenotypes can be uncoupled under some conditions. Triggering apoptosis in APC-deficient cancers by introducing APC domains or other approaches might prove to be a promising therapeutic strategy, but has not yet been carefully explored despite some exciting recent proof-of-concept studies [180].

Conclusion

The role of APC as a scaffold in normal cells clearly extends beyond the β-catenin destruction complex to facilitate interactions with multiple binding partners in the cytoskeleton, cytosol and nucleus to impact a diverse array of cellular processes. In many ways, this is not surprising given that APC is such a large protein with several protein-protein interaction domains and *APC* mutations are generally found throughout the coding sequence. These functions, while adding layers of complexity to our understanding how this one protein is involved in so different activities in the cell, underscore APC's critical importance and the dramatic impact of its loss on tissue homeostasis and tumorigenesis. Particularly when considering the development of therapies directed at cancers in which *APC* is mutated, underexpressed or transcriptionally silenced, the field has a long way to go in dissecting fully which of those molecular actions are absolutely essential for its tumor suppressive activity. From the data that we have presented it this chapter, it is evident that β-catenin/TCF inhibitors, for example, may not be sufficient for a sustained anti-tumor response in *APC*-mutant cancers. One possibility is that a combination of drugs that target several APC-dependent activities might be necessary for efficacious cancer treatment. Moreover, context, including the cell type, phase of the cell cycle, and differentiation state of the cell, likely contributes significantly to APC action and the downstream effects of its loss. A final consideration is that APC loss has been associated with driving proliferation, disrupting polarity, promoting motility, enhancing survival, causing aneuploidy and altering the response of tumor cells to therapeutic agents, suggesting that APC inactivation can theoretically impact all stages of tumor progression. Despite that APC is implicated in tumor initiation in colorectal cancers, rather than advanced stages, a role for APC inactivation in tumor invasion and metastasis cannot be excluded and warrants further investigation. Taken together, the Wnt-pathway independent activities of the APC might comprise the more uncharacterized functions of this tumor suppressor, but represent a bright future for the field in terms of understanding APC cell biology and the therapeutic opportunities for APC-deficient cancers.

References

[1] Herrera, L;Kakati, S;Gibas, L;Pietrzak, ESandberg, A A. Gardner syndrome in a man with an interstitial deletion of 5q. *Am J Med Genet*, 1986 25, 473-476.

[2] Tanaka, K;Oshimura, M;Kikuchi, R;M., S;Hayashi, TMiyaki, M. Supression of tumorigenicity in human colon cancer cells by introduction of normal chromosome 5 or 18. *Nature*, 1989 349, 340-342.

[3] Leppert, M;Burt, R;Hughes, J P;Samowitz, W;Nakamura, Y;Woodward, S;Gardner, E;Lalouel, J MWhite, R. Genetic analysis of an inherited predisposition to colon cancer in a family with a variable number of adenomatous polyps. *N Engl J Med,* 1990 322, 904-908.

[4] Groden, J;Thliveris, A;Samowitz, W;Carlson, M;Gelbert, L;Albertsen, H;Joslyn, G;Stevens, J;Spirio, L;Robertson, M;Sargeant, L;Krapcho, K;Wolff, E;Burt, R;Hughes, J;Warrington, J;McPherson, J;Wasmuth, J;Le Paslier, D;Abderrahim, H;Cohen, D;Leppert, MWhite, R. Identification and characterization of the familial adenomatous polyposis coli gene. *Cell*, 1991 66, 589-600.

[5] Joslyn, G;Carlson, M;Thliveris, A;Albertsen, H;Gelbert, L;Samowitz, W;Groden, J;Stevens, J;Spirio, L;Robertson, M;Krapcho, K;Sargeant, L;Wolff, E;Burt, R;Hughes, J P;Warrington, J;McPherson, J;Wasmuth, J;Le Paslier, D;Abderrahim, H;Cohen, D;Leppert, MWhite, R. Identification of deletion mutations and three new genes at the familial polyposis locus. *Cell*, 1991 66, 601-613.

[6] Kinzler, K;Nilbert, M C;Su, L-K;Vogelstein, B;Bryan, T M;Levy, D B;Smith, K J;Preisinger, A M;Hedge, P;McKechnie, D;Finniear, R;Markham, A;Groffen, J;Boguski, M S;Altschul, S F;Horii, A;Ando, H;Miyoshi, Y;Miki, Y;Nishisho, INakamura, Y. Identification of FAP locus genes from chromosome 5q21. *Science*, 1991 253, 661-665.

[7] Nishisho, I;Nakamura, Y;Miyoshi, Y;Miki, Y;Ando, H;Horii, A;Koyama, K;Utsunomiya, J;Baba, S;Hedge, P;Markham, A;Krush, A J;Peterson, G;Hamiltom, S R;Nilbert, M C;Levy, D B;Bryan, T M;Preisinger, A M;Smith, K J;Su, L-K;Kinzler, K WVogelstein, B. Mutations of chromosome 5q21 genes in FAP and colorectal cancer patients. *Science*, 1991 253, 665-669.

[8] Segditsas, STomlinson, I. Colorectal cancer and genetic alterations in the Wnt pathway. *Oncogene*, 2006 25, 7531-7537.

[9] Prosperi, J R;Lue, H HGoss, K H. Dysregulation of the WNT Pathway in Solid Tumors. *Targeting the Wnt Pathway in Cancer* (Goss and Kahn, eds), Springer, in press

[10] Lynch, H T;Thorson, A G;McComb, R D;Franklin, B A;Tinley, S TLynch, J F. Familial adenomatous polyposis and extracolonic cancer. *Dig Dis Sci*, 2001 46, 2325-2332.
[11] Rubinfeld, B;Souza, B;Albert, I;Muller, O;Chamberlain, S H;Masiarz, F R;Munemitsu, SPolakis, P. Association of the APC gene product with beta-catenin. Science, 1993 262, 1731-1734.
[12] Rubinfeld, B;Albert, I;Porfiri, E;Fiol, C;Munemitsu, SPolakis, P. Binding of GSK3beta to the APC-beta-catenin complex and regulation of complex assembly. *Science*, 1996 272, 1023-1026.
[13] Easwaran, V;Song, V;Polakis, PByers, S. The ubiquitin-proteasome pathway and serine kinase activity modulate adenomatous polyposis coli protein-mediated regulation of beta-catenin-lymphocyte enhancer-binding factor signaling. *J Biol Chem,* 1999 274, 16641-16645.
[14] Latres, E;Chiaur, D SPagano, M. The human F box protein beta-Trcp associates with the Cul1/Skp1 complex and regulates the stability of beta-catenin. *Oncogene*, 1999 18, 849-854.
[15] Morin, P J;Sparks, A B;Korinek, V;Barker, N;Clevers, H;Vogelstein, BKinzler, K W. Activation of beta-catenin-Tcf signaling in colon cancer by mutations in beta-catenin or APC. *Science*, 1997 275, 1787-1790.
[16] Korinek, V;Barker, N;Morin, P J;van Wichen, D;de Weger, R;Kinzler, K W;Vogelstein, BClevers, H. Constitutive transcriptional activation by a beta-catenin-Tcf complex in APC-/- colon carcinoma. *Science*, 1997 275, 1784-1787.
[17] Sansom, O J;Reed, K R;Hayes, A J;Ireland, H;Brinkmann, H;Newton, I P;Batlle, E;Simon-Assmann, P;Clevers, H;Nathke, I S;Clarke, A RWinton, D J. Loss of Apc in vivo immediately perturbs Wnt signaling, differentiation, and migration. *Genes Dev,* 2004 18, 1385-1390.
[18] Barker, N;Ridgway, R A;van Es, J H;van de Wetering, M;Begthel, H;van den Born, M;Danenberg, E;Clarke, A R;Sansom, O JClevers, H. Crypt stem cells as the cells-of-origin of intestinal cancer. *Nature*, 2009 457, 608-611.
[19] Shih, I M;Yu, J;He, T C;Vogelstein, BKinzler, K W. The beta-catenin binding domain of adenomatous polyposis coli is sufficient for tumor suppression. *Cancer Res*, 2000 60, 1671-1676.
[20] Wilson, C L;Heppner, K J;Labosky, P A;Hogan, B LMatrisian, L M. Intestinal tumorigenesis is suppressed in mice lacking the metalloproteinase matrilysin. *Proc Natl Acad Sci U S A*, 1997 94, 1402-1407.
[21] Sansom, O J;Meniel, V S;Muncan, V;Phesse, T J;Wilkins, J A;Reed, K R;Vass, J K;Athineos, D;Clevers, HClarke, A R. Myc deletion rescues Apc deficiency in the small intestine. *Nature*, 2007 446, 676-679.
[22] Heinen, C D;Goss, K H;Cornelius, J R;Babcock, G F;Knudsen, E S;Kowalik, TGroden, J. The APC tumor suppressor controls entry into S-phase through its ability to regulate the cyclin D/RB pathway. *Gastroenterology*, 2002 123, 751-763.
[23] Pollard, P;Deheragoda, M;Segditsas, S;Lewis, A;Rowan, A;Howarth, K;Willis, L;Nye, E;McCart, A;Mandir, N;Silver, A;Goodlad, R;Stamp, G;Cockman, M;East, P;Spencer-Dene, B;Poulsom, R;Wright, NTomlinson, I. The Apc 1322T mouse develops severe polyposis associated with submaximal nuclear beta-catenin expression. *Gastroenterology*, 2009 136, 2204-2213 e2201-2213.

[24] Gaspar, C;Franken, P;Molenaar, L;Breukel, C;van der Valk, M;Smits, RFodde, R. A targeted constitutive mutation in the APC tumor suppressor gene underlies mammary but not intestinal tumorigenesis. *PLoS Genet*, 2009 5, e1000547.

[25] Qian, Z;Chen, L;Fernald, A A;Williams, B OLe Beau, M M. A critical role for Apc in hematopoietic stem and progenitor cell survival. *J Exp Med,* 2008 205, 2163-2175.

[26] Scheller, M;Huelsken, J;Rosenbauer, F;Taketo, M M;Birchmeier, W;Tenen, D GLeutz, A. Hematopoietic stem cell and multilineage defects generated by constitutive beta-catenin activation. *Nat Immunol*, 2006 7, 1037-1047.

[27] Kirstetter, P;Anderson, K;Porse, B T;Jacobsen, S ENerlov, C. Activation of the canonical Wnt pathway leads to loss of hematopoietic stem cell repopulation and multilineage differentiation block. *Nat Immunol,* 2006 7, 1048-1056.

[28] Gallagher, R C;Hay, T;Meniel, V;Naughton, C;Anderson, T J;Shibata, H;Ito, M;Clevers, H;Noda, T;Sansom, O J;Mason, J OClarke, A R. Inactivation of Apc perturbs mammary development, but only directly results in acanthoma in the context of Tcf-1 deficiency. *Oncogene*, 2002 21, 6446-6457.

[29] Moser, A R;Luongo, C;Gould, K A;McNeley, M K;Shoemaker, A RDove, W F. ApcMin: a mouse model for intestinal and mammary tumorigenesis. *Eur J Cancer*, 1995 31A, 1061-1064.

[30] Michaelson, J SLeder, P. beta-catenin is a downstream effector of Wnt-mediated tumorigenesis in the mammary gland. *Oncogene*, 2001 20, 5093-5099.

[31] Miyoshi, K;Shillingford, J M;Le Provost, F;Gounari, F;Bronson, R;von Boehmer, H;Taketo, M M;Cardiff, R D;Hennighausen, LKhazaie, K. Activation of beta -catenin signaling in differentiated mammary secretory cells induces transdifferentiation into epidermis and squamous metaplasias. *Proc Natl Acad Sci U S A*, 2002 99, 219-224.

[32] Joslyn, G;Richardson, D S;White, RAlber, T. Dimer formation by an N-terminal coiled coil in the APC protein. *Proc Natl Acad Sci USA*, 1993 90, 11109-11113.

[33] Shibata, D;Peinado, M A;Ionov, Y;Malkhosyan, SPerucho, M. Genomic instability in repeated sequences is an early somatic event in colorectal tumorigenesis that persists after transformation. *Nat Genet*, 1994 6, 273-281.

[34] Rubinfeld, B;Souza, B;Albert, I;Munemitsu, SPolakis, P. The APC protein and E-cadherin form similar but independent complexes with alpha-catenin, beta-catenin, and plakoglobin. *Journal of Biological Chemistry*, 1995 270, 5549-5555.

[35] Hulsken, J;Birchmeier, WBehrens, J. E-cadherin and APC compete for the interaction with beta-catenin and the cytoskeleton. *J Cell Biol,* 1994 127, 2061-2069.

[36] Wong, M H;Hermiston, M L;Syder, A JGordon, J I. *Forced expression of the tumor suppressor adenomatosis polyposis coli protein induces disordered cell migration in the intestinal epithelium.* Proc Natl Acad Sci U S A, 1996 93, 9588-9593.

[37] Mahmoud, N N;Boolbol, S K;Bilinski, R T;Martucci, C;Chadburn, ABertagnolli, M M. Apc gene mutation is associated with a dominant-negative effect upon intestinal cell migration. *Cancer Res*, 1997 57, 5045-5050.

[38] Faux, M C;Ross, J L;Meeker, C;Johns, T;Ji, H;Simpson, R J;Layton, M JBurgess, A W. Restoration of full-length adenomatous polyposis coli (APC) protein in a colon cancer cell line enhances cell adhesion. *J Cell Sci,* 2004 117, 427-439.

[39] McCartney, B M;Dierick, H A;Kirkpatrick, C;Moline, M M;Baas, A;Peifer, MBejsovec, A. Drosophila APC2 is a cytoskeletally-associated protein that regulates wingless signaling in the embryonic epidermis. *J Cell Biol,* 1999 146, 1303-1318.

[40] Yu, XBienz, M. Ubiquitous expression of a Drosophila adenomatous polyposis coli homolog and its localization in cortical actin caps. *Mech Dev,* 1999 84, 69-73.

[41] Prosperi, J R;Becher, K R;Willson, T A;Collins, M H;Witte, D PGoss, K H. The APC tumor suppressor is required for epithelial integrity in the mouse mammary gland. *J Cell Physiol,* 2009 220, 319-331.

[42] Mogensen, M M;Tucker, J B;Mackie, J B;Prescott, A RNathke, I S. The adenomatous polyposis coli protein unambiguously localizes to microtubule plus ends and is involved in establishing parallel arrays of microtubule bundles in highly polarized epithelial cells. *J Cell Biol,* 2002 157, 1041-1048.

[43] Reinacher-Schick, AGumbiner, B M. Apical membrane localization of the adenomatous polyposis coli tumor suppressor protein and subcellular distribution of the beta-catenin destruction complex in polarized epithelial cells. *J Cell Biol,* 2001 152, 491-502.

[44] Rosin-Arbesfeld, R;Ihrke, GBienz, M. Actin-dependent membrane association of the APC tumour suppressor in polarized mammalian epithelial cells. *Embo J,* 2001 20, 5929-5939.

[45] Townsley, F MBienz, M. Actin-dependent membrane association of a Drosophila epithelial APC protein and its effect on junctional Armadillo. *Curr Biol,* 2000 10, 1339-1348.

[46] Harris, E SNelson, W J. Adenomatous polyposis coli regulates endothelial cell migration independent of roles in beta-catenin signaling and cell-cell adhesion. *Mol Biol Cell,* 2010 21, 2611-2623.

[47] Jamora, C;DasGupta, R;Kocieniewski, PFuchs, E. Links between signal transduction, transcription and adhesion in epithelial bud development. *Nature*, 2003 422, 317-322.

[48] Wielenga, V J;Smits, R;Korinek, V;Smit, L;Kielman, M;Fodde, R;Clevers, HPals, S T. Expression of CD44 in Apc and Tcf mutant mice implies regulation by the WNT pathway. *Am J Pathol*, 1999 154, 515-523.

[49] Bryant, D MMostov, K E. From cells to organs: building polarized tissue. *Nat Rev Mol Cell Biol,* 2008 9, 887-901.

[50] Matsumine, A;Ogai, A;Senda, T;Okumura, N;Satoh, K;Baeg, G H;Kawahara, T;Kobayashi, S;Okada, M;Toyoshima, KAkiyama, T. Binding of APC to the human homolog of the Drosophila discs large tumor suppressor protein [see comments]. *Science*, 1996 272, 1020-1023.

[51] Iizuka-Kogo, A;Shimomura, ASenda, T. Colocalization of APC and DLG at the tips of cellular protrusions in cultured epithelial cells and its dependency on cytoskeletons. *Histochem Cell Biol,* 2005 123, 67-73.

[52] Etienne-Manneville, S;Manneville, J B;Nicholls, S;Ferenczi, M AHall, A. Cdc42 and Par6-PKCzeta regulate the spatially localized association of Dlg1 and APC to control cell polarization. *J Cell Biol,* 2005 170, 895-901.

[53] Ishidate, T;Matsumine, A;Toyoshima, KAkiyama, T. The APC-hDLG complex negatively regulates cell cycle progression from the G0/G1 to S phase. *Oncogene*, 2000 19, 365-372.

[54] Makino, K;Kuwahara, H;Masuko, N;Nishiyama, Y;Morisaki, T;Sasaki, J;Nakao, M;Kuwano, A;Nakata, M;Ushio, YSaya, H. Cloning and characterization of NE-dlg: a novel human homolog of the Drosophila discs large (dlg) tumor suppressor protein interacts with the APC protein. *Oncogene*, 1997 14, 2425-2433.

[55] Laprise, P;Viel, ARivard, N. Human homolog of disc-large is required for adherens junction assembly and differentiation of human intestinal epithelial cells. *J Biol Chem*, 2004 279, 10157-10166.

[56] Hanada, N;Makino, K;Koga, H;Morisaki, T;Kuwahara, H;Masuko, N;Tabira, Y;Hiraoka, T;Kitamura, N;Kikuchi, ASaya, H. NE-dlg, a mammalian homolog of Drosophila dlg tumor suppressor, induces growth suppression and impairment of cell adhesion: possible involvement of down-regulation of beta-catenin by NE-dlg expression. *Int J Cancer*, 2000 86, 480-488.

[57] Takizawa, S;Nagasaka, K;Nakagawa, S;Yano, T;Nakagawa, K;Yasugi, T;Takeuchi, T;Kanda, T;Huibregtse, J M;Akiyama, TTaketani, Y. Human scribble, a novel tumor suppressor identified as a target of high-risk HPV E6 for ubiquitin-mediated degradation, interacts with adenomatous polyposis coli. *Genes Cells*, 2006 11, 453-464.

[58] Humbert, P O;Grzeschik, N A;Brumby, A M;Galea, R;Elsum, IRichardson, H E. Control of tumourigenesis by the Scribble/Dlg/Lgl polarity module. *Oncogene*, 2008 27, 6888-6907.

[59] Osmani, N;Vitale, N;Borg, J PEtienne-Manneville, S. Scrib controls Cdc42 localization and activity to promote cell polarization during astrocyte migration. *Curr Biol*, 2006 16, 2395-2405.

[60] Dow, L EHumbert, P O. Polarity regulators and the control of epithelial architecture, cell migration, and tumorigenesis. *Int Rev Cytol*, 2007 262, 253-302.

[61] Nishimura, T;Kato, K;Yamaguchi, T;Fukata, Y;Ohno, SKaibuchi, K. Role of the PAR-3-KIF3 complex in the establishment of neuronal polarity. *Nat Cell Biol,* 2004 6, 328-334.

[62] Shi, S H;Cheng, T;Jan, L YJan, Y N. APC and GSK-3beta are involved in mPar3 targeting to the nascent axon and establishment of neuronal polarity. *Curr Biol,* 2004 14, 2025-2032.

[63] Moser, A R;Shoemaker, A R;Connelly, C S;Clipson, L;Gould, K A;Luongo, C;Dove, W F;Siggers, P HGardner, R L. Homozygosity for the Min allele of Apc results in disruption of mouse development prior to gastrulation. *Dev Dyn,* 1995 203, 422-433.

[64] Hattrup, C L;Fernandez-Rodriguez, J;Schroeder, J A;Hansson, G CGendler, S J. MUC1 can interact with adenomatous polyposis coli in breast cancer. *Biochem Biophys Res Commun*, 2004 316, 364-369.

[65] Gendler, S J. MUC1, the renaissance molecule. *J Mammary Gland Biol Neoplasia,* 2001 6, 339-353.

[66] Rahn, J J;Dabbagh, L;Pasdar, MHugh, J C. The importance of MUC1 cellular localization in patients with breast carcinoma: an immunohistologic study of 71 patients and review of the literature. *Cancer*, 2001 91, 1973-1982.

[67] Inagaki, Y;Xu, H;Nakata, M;Seyama, Y;Hasegawa, K;Sugawara, Y;Tang, WKokudo, N. Clinicopathology of sialomucin: MUC1, particularly KL-6 mucin, in gastrointestinal, hepatic and pancreatic cancers. *Biosci Trends*, 2009 3, 220-232.

[68] Lu, B;Roegiers, F;Jan, L YJan, Y N. Adherens junctions inhibit asymmetric division in the Drosophila epithelium. *Nature*, 2001 409, 522-525.

[69] Yamashita, Y M;Jones, D LFuller, M T. Orientation of asymmetric stem cell division by the APC tumor suppressor and centrosome. *Science*, 2003 301, 1547-1550.

[70] Breitman, M;Zilberberg, A;Caspi, MRosin-Arbesfeld, R. The armadillo repeat domain of the APC tumor suppressor protein interacts with Striatin family members. *Biochim Biophys Acta*, 2008 1783, 1792-1802.
[71] Phelps, R A;Chidester, S;Dehghanizadeh, S;Phelps, J;Sandoval, I T;Rai, K;Broadbent, T;Sarkar, S;Burt, R WJones, D A. A two-step model for colon adenoma initiation and progression caused by APC loss. *Cell*, 2009 137, 623-634.
[72] Fang, M;Li, J;Blauwkamp, T;Bhambhani, C;Campbell, NCadigan, K M. C-terminal-binding protein directly activates and represses Wnt transcriptional targets in Drosophila. *Embo J,* 2006 25, 2735-2745.
[73] Hamada, FBienz, M. The APC tumor suppressor binds to C-terminal binding protein to divert nuclear beta-catenin from TCF. *Dev Cell*, 2004 7, 677-685.
[74] Nadauld, L D;Phelps, R;Moore, B C;Eisinger, A;Sandoval, I T;Chidester, S;Peterson, P W;Manos, E J;Sklow, B;Burt, R WJones, D A. Adenomatous polyposis coli control of C-terminal binding protein-1 stability regulates expression of intestinal retinol dehydrogenases. *J Biol Chem*, 2006 281, 37828-37835.
[75] Thiery, J P. Epithelial-mesenchymal transitions in tumour progression. *Nat Rev Cancer*, 2002 2, 442-454.
[76] Huang, LMuthuswamy, S K. Polarity protein alterations in carcinoma: a focus on emerging roles for polarity regulators. *Curr Opin Genet Dev*, 2010 20, 41-50.
[77] Schmalhofer, O;Brabletz, SBrabletz, T. E-cadherin, beta-catenin, and ZEB1 in malignant progression of cancer. *Cancer Metastasis Rev*, 2009 28, 151-166.
[78] Scheffner, MWhitaker, N J. Human papillomavirus-induced carcinogenesis and the ubiquitin-proteasome system. *Semin Cancer Biol,* 2003 13, 59-67.
[79] Gardiol, D;Zacchi, A;Petrera, F;Stanta, GBanks, L. Human discs large and scrib are localized at the same regions in colon mucosa and changes in their expression patterns are correlated with loss of tissue architecture during malignant progression. *Int J Cancer,* 2006 119, 1285-1290.
[80] Benzinger, A;Muster, N;Koch, H B;Yates, J R, 3rdHermeking, H. Targeted proteomic analysis of 14-3-3 sigma, a p53 effector commonly silenced in cancer. Mol Cell Proteomics, 2005 4, 785-795.
[81] Moseley, J B;Bartolini, F;Okada, K;Wen, Y;Gundersen, G GGoode, B L. Regulated binding of adenomatous polyposis coli protein to actin. J Biol Chem, 2007 282, 12661-12668.
[82] Okada, K;Bartolini, F;Deaconescu, A M;Moseley, J B;Dogic, Z;Grigorieff, N;Gundersen, G GGoode, B L. Adenomatous polyposis coli protein nucleates actin assembly and synergizes with the formin mDia1. *J Cell Biol,* 2010 189, 1087-1096.
[83] Deka, J;Kuhlmann, JMuller, O. A domain within the tumor suppressor protein APC shows very similar biochemical properties as the microtubule-associated protein tau. *Eur J Biochem*, 1998 253, 591-597.
[84] Kawasaki, Y;Sagara, M;Shibata, Y;Shirouzu, M;Yokoyama, SAkiyama, T. Identification and characterization of Asef2, a guanine-nucleotide exchange factor specific for Rac1 and Cdc42. *Oncogene*, 2007 26, 7620-7267.
[85] Kawasaki, Y;Senda, T;Ishidate, T;Koyama, R;Morishita, T;Iwayama, Y;Higuchi, OAkiyama, T. Asef, a link between the tumor suppressor APC and G-protein signaling. *Science*, 2000 289, 1194-1197.

[86] Kawasaki, Y;Sato, RAkiyama, T. Mutated APC and Asef are involved in the migration of colorectal tumour cells. *Nat Cell Biol*, 2003 5, 211-215.
[87] 8Hamann, M J;Lubking, C M;Luchini, D NBilladeau, D D. Asef2 functions as a Cdc42 exchange factor and is stimulated by the release of an autoinhibitory module from a concealed C-terminal activation element. *Mol Cell Biol*, 2007 27, 1380-1393.
[88] Watanabe, T;Wang, S;Noritake, J;Sato, K;Fukata, M;Takefuji, M;Nakagawa, M;Izumi, N;Akiyama, TKaibuchi, K. Interaction with IQGAP1 links APC to Rac1, Cdc42, and actin filaments during cell polarization and migration. *Dev Cell*, 2004 7, 871-883.
[89] Tirnauer, J S. A new cytoskeletal connection for APC: linked to actin through IQGAP. *Dev Cell,* 2004 7, 778-780.
[90] Sharma, MHenderson, B R. IQ-domain GTPase-activating protein 1 regulates beta-catenin at membrane ruffles and its role in macropinocytosis of N-cadherin and adenomatous polyposis coli. *J Biol Chem*, 2007 282, 8545-8556.
[91] Munemitsu, S;Souza, B;Muller, O;Albert, I;Rubinfeld, BPolakis, P. The APC gene product associates with microtubules in vivo and promotes their assembly in vitro. *Cancer Res*, 1994 54, 3676-3681.
[92] Nathke, I S;Adams, C L;Polakis, P;Sellin, J HNelson, W J. The adenomatous polyposis coli tumor suppressor protein localizes to plasma membrane sites involved in active cell migration. *J Cell Biol*, 1996 134, 165-179.
[93] Smith, K J;Levy, D B;Maupin, P;Pollard, T D;Vogelstein, BKinzler, K W. Wild-type but not mutant APC associates with the microtubule cytoskeleton. *Cancer Research*, 1994 54, 3672-3675.
[94] Zumbrunn, J;Kinoshita, K;Hyman, A ANathke, I S. Binding of the adenomatous polyposis coli protein to microtubules increases microtubule stability and is regulated by GSK3 beta phosphorylation. *Curr Biol,* 2001 11, 44-49.
[95] Kita, K;Wittmann, T;Nathke, I SWaterman-Storer, C M. Adenomatous polyposis coli on microtubule plus ends in cell extensions can promote microtubule net growth with or without EB1. *Mol Biol Cell,* 2006 17, 2331-2345.
[96] Askham, J M;Moncur, P;Markham, A FMorrison, E E. Regulation and function of the interaction between the APC tumour suppressor protein and EB1. *Oncogene*, 2000 19, 1950-1958.
[97] Nakamura, M;Zhou, X ZLu, K P. Critical role for the EB1 and APC interaction in the regulation of microtubule polymerization. *Curr Biol*, 2001 11, 1062-1067.
[98] Su, L K;Burrell, M;Hill, D E;Gyuris, J;Brent, R;Wiltshire, R;Trent, J;Vogelstein, BKinzler, K W. APC binds to the novel protein EB1. *Cancer Res*, 1995 55, 2972-2977.
[99] Schwartz, K;Richards, KBotstein, D. BIM1 encodes a microtubule-binding protein in yeast. *Mol Biol Cell,* 1997 8, 2677-2691.
[100] Berrueta, L;Kraeft, S K;Tirnauer, J S;Schuyler, S C;Chen, L B;Hill, D E;Pellman, DBierer, B E. The adenomatous polyposis coli-binding protein EB1 is associated with cytoplasmic and spindle microtubules. *Proc Natl Acad Sci USA*, 1998 95, 10596-10601.
[101] Juwana, J P;Henderikx, P;Mischo, A;Wadle, A;Fadle, N;Gerlach, K;Arends, J W;Hoogenboom, H;Pfreundschuh, MRenner, C. EB/RP gene family encodes tubulin binding proteins. *Int J Cancer,* 1999 81, 275-284.
[102] Morrison, E E;Wardleworth, B N;Askham, J M;Markham, A FMeredith, D M. EB1, a protein which interacts with the APC tumour suppressor, is associated with the microtubule cytoskeleton throughout the cell cycle. *Oncogene*, 1998 17, 3471-3477.

[103] Muhua, L;Adames, N R;Murphy, M D;Shields, C RCooper, J A. A cytokinesis checkpoint requiring the yeast homologue of an APC-binding protein. *Nature*, 1998 393, 487-491.

[104] Mimori-Kiyosue, Y;Shiina, NTsukita, S. The dynamic behavior of the APC-binding protein EB1 on the distal ends of microtubules. *Curr Biol,* 2000 10, 865-868.

[105] Wen, Y;Eng, C H;Schmoranzer, J;Cabrera-Poch, N;Morris, E J;Chen, M;Wallar, B J;Alberts, A SGundersen, G G. EB1 and APC bind to mDia to stabilize microtubules downstream of Rho and promote cell migration. *Nat Cell Biol,* 2004 6, 820-830.

[106] Jimbo, T;Kawasaki, Y;Koyama, R;Sato, R;Takada, S;Haraguchi, KAkiyama, T. Identification of a link between the tumour suppressor APC and the kinesin superfamily. *Nat Cell Biol,* 2002 4, 323-327.

[107] Jaulin, FKreitzer, G. KIF17 stabilizes microtubules and contributes to epithelial morphogenesis by acting at MT plus ends with EB1 and APC. *J Cell Biol,* 2010 190, 443-460.

[108] Dikovskaya, D;Li, Z;Newton, I P;Davidson, I;Hutchins, J R;Kalab, P;Clarke, P RNathke, I S. Microtubule assembly by the Apc protein is regulated by importin-beta--RanGTP. *J Cell Sci*, 2010 123, 736-746.

[109] 1Barth, A I;Pollack, A L;Altschuler, Y;Mostov, K ENelson, W J. NH2-terminal deletion of beta-catenin results in stable colocalization of mutant beta-catenin with adenomatous polyposis coli protein and altered MDCK cell adhesion. *J Cell Biol,* 1997 136, 693-706.

[110] Etienne-Manneville, SHall, A. Cdc42 regulates GSK-3beta and adenomatous polyposis coli to control cell polarity. *Nature*, 2003 421, 753-756.

[111] Kroboth, K;Newton, I P;Kita, K;Dikovskaya, D;Zumbrunn, J;Waterman-Storer, C MNathke, I S. Lack of adenomatous polyposis coli protein correlates with a decrease in cell migration and overall changes in microtubule stability. *Mol Biol Cell,* 2007 18, 910-918.

[112] Yokota, Y;Kim, W Y;Chen, Y;Wang, X;Stanco, A;Komuro, Y;Snider, WAnton, E S. The adenomatous polyposis coli protein is an essential regulator of radial glial polarity and construction of the cerebral cortex. *Neuron*, 2009 61, 42-56.

[113] Votin, V;Nelson, W JBarth, A I. Neurite outgrowth involves adenomatous polyposis coli protein and beta-catenin. *J Cell Sci,* 2005 118, 5699-5708.

[114] Zhou, F Q;Zhou, J;Dedhar, S;Wu, Y HSnider, W D. NGF-induced axon growth is mediated by localized inactivation of GSK-3beta and functions of the microtubule plus end binding protein APC. *Neuron*, 2004 42, 897-912.

[115] Gartner, A;Huang, XHall, A. Neuronal polarity is regulated by glycogen synthase kinase-3 (GSK-3beta) independently of Akt/PKB serine phosphorylation. *J Cell Sci,* 2006 119, 3927-3934.

[116] Asada, NSanada, K. LKB1-mediated spatial control of GSK3beta and adenomatous polyposis coli contributes to centrosomal forward movement and neuronal migration in the developing neocortex. *J Neurosci,* 2010 30, 8852-8865.

[117] Baas, A F;Smit, LClevers, H. LKB1 tumor suppressor protein: PARtaker in cell polarity. *Trends Cell Biol*, 2004 14, 312-319.

[118] Rusan, N M;Akong, KPeifer, M. Putting the model to the test: are APC proteins essential for neuronal polarity, axon outgrowth, and axon targeting? *J Cell Biol*, 2008 183, 203-212.

[119] 1Matsumoto, S;Fumoto, K;Okamoto, T;Kaibuchi, KKikuchi, A. Binding of APC and dishevelled mediates Wnt5a-regulated focal adhesion dynamics in migrating cells. *Embo J,* 2010 29, 1192-1204.

[120] Ashton, G H;Morton, J P;Myant, K;Phesse, T J;Ridgway, R A;Marsh, V;Wilkins, J A;Athineos, D;Muncan, V;Kemp, R;Neufeld, K;Clevers, H;Brunton, V;Winton, D J;Wang, X;Sears, R C;Clarke, A R;Frame, M CSansom, O J. Focal adhesion kinase is required for intestinal regeneration and tumorigenesis downstream of Wnt/c-Myc signaling. *Dev Cell,* 2010 19, 259-269.

[121] Mili, S;Moissoglu, KMacara, I G. Genome-wide screen reveals APC-associated RNAs enriched in cell protrusions. *Nature*, 2008 453, 115-119.

[122] Collin, L;Schlessinger, KHall, A. APC nuclear membrane association and microtubule polarity. Biol Cell, 2008 100, 243-252.

[123] Murawala, P;Tripathi, M M;Vyas, P;Salunke, AJoseph, J. Nup358 interacts with APC and plays a role in cell polarization. *J Cell Sci,* 2009 122, 3113-3122.

[124] Olmeda, D;Castel, S;Vilaro, SCano, A. Beta-catenin regulation during the cell cycle: implications in G2/M and apoptosis. *Mol Biol Cell,* 2003 14, 2844-2860.

[125] Bhattacharjee, R N;Hamada, F;Toyoshima, KAkiyama, T. The tumor suppressor gene product APC is hyperphosphorylated during the M phase. *Biochem Biophys Res Commun*, 1996 220, 192-195.

[126] Trzepacz, C;Lowy, A M;Kordich, J JGroden, J. Phosphorylation of the tumor suppressor adenomatous polyposis coli (APC) by the cyclin-dependent kinase p34. *J Biol Chem*, 1997 272, 21681-21684.

[127] Beamish, H;de Boer, L;Giles, N;Stevens, F;Oakes, VGabrielli, B. Cyclin A/cdk2 regulates adenomatous polyposis coli-dependent mitotic spindle anchoring. *J Biol Chem,* 2009 284, 29015-29023.

[128] Green, R A;Wollman, RKaplan, K B. APC and EB1 function together in mitosis to regulate spindle dynamics and chromosome alignment. Mol Biol Cell, 2005 16, 4609-4622.

[129] Zhang, J;Ahmad, SMao, Y. BubR1 and APC/EB1 cooperate to maintain metaphase chromosome alignment. *J Cell Biol*, 2007 178, 773-784.

[130] Kaplan, K B;Burds, A A;Swedlow, J R;Bekir, S S;Sorger, P KNathke, I S. A role for the Adenomatous Polyposis Coli protein in chromosome segregation. *Nat Cell Biol*, 2001 3, 429-432.

[131] Fodde, R;Kuipers, J;Rosenberg, C;Smits, R;Kielman, M;Gaspar, C;van Es, J H;Breukel, C;Wiegant, J;Giles, R HClevers, H. Mutations in the APC tumour suppressor gene cause chromosomal instability. *Nat Cell Biol*, 2001 3, 433-438.

[132] Draviam, V M;Shapiro, I;Aldridge, BSorger, P K. Misorientation and reduced stretching of aligned sister kinetochores promote chromosome missegregation in EB1- or APC-depleted cells. *Embo J,* 2006 25, 2814-2827.

[133] Dikovskaya, D;Schiffmann, D;Newton, I P;Oakley, A;Kroboth, K;Sansom, O;Jamieson, T J;Meniel, V;Clarke, ANathke, I S. Loss of APC induces polyploidy as a result of a combination of defects in mitosis and apoptosis. *J Cell Biol,* 2007 176, 183-195.

[134] Caldwell, C M;Green, R AKaplan, K B. APC mutations lead to cytokinetic failures in vitro and tetraploid genotypes in Min mice. *J Cell Biol*, 2007 178, 1109-1120.

[135] Fleming, E S;Temchin, M;Wu, Q;Maggio-Price, LTirnauer, J S. Spindle misorientation in tumors from APC(min/+) mice. *Mol Carcinog,* 2009 48, 592-598.

[136] Green, R AKaplan, K B. Chromosome instability in colorectal tumor cells is associated with defects in microtubule plus-end attachments caused by a dominant mutation in APC. J Cell Biol, 2003 163, 949-961.

[137] Dikovskaya, D;Newton, I PNathke, I S. The adenomatous polyposis coli protein is required for the formation of robust spindles formed in CSF Xenopus extracts. *Mol Biol Cell,* 2004 15, 2978-2991.

[138] Banks, J DHeald, R. Adenomatous polyposis coli associates with the microtubule-destabilizing protein XMCAK. *Curr Biol,* 2004 14, 2033-2038.

[139] Tighe, A;Johnson, V LTaylor, S S. Truncating APC mutations have dominant effects on proliferation, spindle checkpoint control, survival and chromosome stability. *J Cell Sci,* 2004 117, 6339-6353.

[140] Aoki, K;Aoki, M;Sugai, M;Harada, N;Miyoshi, H;Tsukamoto, T;Mizoshita, T;Tatematsu, M;Seno, H;Chiba, T;Oshima, M;Hsieh, C LTaketo, M M. Chromosomal instability by beta-catenin/TCF transcription in APC or beta-catenin mutant cells. *Oncogene*, 2007 26, 3511-3520.

[141] Radulescu, S;Ridgway, R A;Appleton, P;Kroboth, K;Patel, S;Woodgett, J;Taylor, S;Nathke, I SSansom, O J. Defining the role of APC in the mitotic spindle checkpoint in vivo: APC-deficient cells are resistant to Taxol. *Oncogene*, 2010

[142] Henderson, B R. Nuclear-cytoplasmic shuttling of APC regulates beta-catenin subcellular localization and turnover. *Nat Cell Biol*, 2000 2, 653-660.

[143] Neufeld, K LWhite, R L. Nuclear and cytoplasmic localizations of the adenomatous polyposis coli protein. *Proc Natl Acad Sci U S A,* 1997 94, 3034-3039.

[144] 1Zhang, F;White, R LNeufeld, K L. Phosphorylation near nuclear localization signal regulates nuclear import of adenomatous polyposis coli protein. *Proc Natl Acad Sci U S* A, 2000 97, 12577-12582.

[145] Zhang, F;White, R LNeufeld, K L. Cell density and phosphorylation control the subcellular localization of adenomatous polyposis coli protein. *Mol Cell Biol*, 2001 21, 8143-8156.

[146] Fagman, H;Larsson, F;Arvidsson, Y;Meuller, J;Nordling, M;Martinsson, T;Helmbrecht, K;Brabant, GNilsson, M. Nuclear accumulation of full-length and truncated adenomatous polyposis coli protein in tumor cells depends on proliferation. *Oncogene*, 2003 22, 6013-6022.

[147] Schneikert, J;Grohmann, ABehrens, J. Truncated APC regulates the transcriptional activity of beta-catenin in a cell cycle dependent manner. *Hum Mol Genet,* 2007 16, 199-209.

[148] Henderson, B R;Galea, M;Schuechner, SLeung, L. Lymphoid enhancer factor-1 blocks adenomatous polyposis coli-mediated nuclear export and degradation of beta-catenin. Regulation by histone deacetylase 1. *J Biol Chem,* 2002 277, 24258-24264.

[149] Brocardo, M;Nathke, I SHenderson, B R. Redefining the subcellular location and transport of APC: new insights using a panel of antibodies. *EMBO Rep,* 2005 6, 184-190.

[150] Sierra, J;Yoshida, T;Joazeiro, C AJones, K A. The APC tumor suppressor counteracts beta-catenin activation and H3K4 methylation at Wnt target genes. *Genes Dev,* 2006 20, 586-600.

[151] Kouzmenko, A P;Takeyama, K;Kawasaki, Y;Akiyama, TKato, S. Truncation mutations abolish chromatin-associated activities of adenomatous polyposis coli. *Oncogene*, 2008 27, 4888-4899.

[152] Baeg, G H;Matsumine, A;Kuroda, T;Bhattacharjee, R N;Miyashiro, I;Toyoshima, KAkiyama, T. The tumour suppressor gene product APC blocks cell cycle progression from G0/G1 to S phase. *Embo J*, 1995 14, 5618-5625.

[153] Carson, D J;Santoro, I MGroden, J. Isoforms of the APC tumor suppressor and their ability to inhibit cell growth and tumorigenicity. *Oncogene*, 2004 23, 7144-7148.

[154] Qian, J;Sarnaik, A A;Bonney, T M;Keirsey, J;Combs, K A;Steigerwald, K;Acharya, S;Behbehani, G K;Barton, M C;Lowy, A MGroden, J. The APC tumor suppressor inhibits DNA replication by directly binding to DNA via its carboxyl terminus. *Gastroenterology*, 2008 135, 152-162.

[155] Narayan, S;Jaiswal, A SBalusu, R. Tumor suppressor APC blocks DNA polymerase beta-dependent strand displacement synthesis during long patch but not short patch base excision repair and increases sensitivity to methylmethane sulfonate. *J Biol Chem*, 2005 280, 6942-6949.

[156] Jaiswal, A SNarayan, S. A novel function of adenomatous polyposis coli (APC) in regulating DNA repair. *Cancer Lett,* 2008 271, 272-280.

[157] Wang, Y;Azuma, Y;Moore, D;Osheroff, NNeufeld, K L. Interaction between tumor suppressor adenomatous polyposis coli and topoisomerase IIalpha: implication for the G2/M transition. *Mol Biol Cell*, 2008 19, 4076-4085.

[158] Homma, M K;Li, D;Krebs, E G;Yuasa, YHomma, Y. Association and regulation of casein kinase 2 activity by adenomatous polyposis coli protein. *Proc Natl Acad Sci U S A*, 2002 99, 5959-5964.

[159] Balusu, R;Jaiswal, A S;Armas, M L;Kundu, C N;Bloom, L BNarayan, S. Structure/function analysis of the interaction of adenomatous polyposis coli with DNA polymerase beta and its implications for base excision repair. *Biochemistry*, 2007 46, 13961-13974.

[160] Jaiswal, A S;Balusu, R;Armas, M L;Kundu, C NNarayan, S. Mechanism of adenomatous polyposis coli (APC)-mediated blockage of long-patch base excision repair. *Biochemistry*, 2006 45, 15903-15914.

[161] Kinzler, K WVogelstein, B. Lessons from hereditary colorectal cancer. *Cell*, 1996 87, 159-170.

[162] Kundu, C N;Balusu, R;Jaiswal, A SNarayan, S. Adenomatous polyposis coli-mediated hypersensitivity of mouse embryonic fibroblast cell lines to methylmethane sulfonate treatment: implication of base excision repair pathways. Carcinogenesis, 2007 28, 2089-2095.

[163] Narayan, SJaiswal, A S. Activation of adenomatous polyposis coli (APC) gene expression by the DNA-alkylating agent N-methyl-N'-nitro-N-nitrosoguanidine requires p53. *J Biol Chem*, 1997 272, 30619-30622.

[164] Jaiswal, A S;Balusu, RNarayan, S. 7,12-Dimethylbenzanthracene-dependent transcriptional regulation of adenomatous polyposis coli (APC) gene expression in normal breast epithelial cells is mediated by GC-box binding protein Sp3. *Carcinogenesis*, 2006 27, 252-261.

[165] Jaiswal, A S;Multani, A S;Pathak, SNarayan, S. N-methyl-N'-nitro-N-nitrosoguanidine-induced senescence-like growth arrest in colon cancer cells is associated with loss of

adenomatous polyposis coli protein, microtubule organization, and telomeric DNA. Mol Cancer, 2004 3, 3.

[166] Jaiswal, A SNarayan, S. Protein synthesis and transcriptional inhibitors control N-methyl-N'-nitro-N-nitrosoguanidine-induced levels of APC mRNA in a p53-dependent manner. International Journal of Oncology, 1998 13, 733-740.

[167] Browne, S J;MacFarlane, M;Cohen, G MParaskeva, C. The adenomatous polyposis coli protein and retinoblastoma protein are cleaved early in apoptosis and are potential substrates for caspases. *Cell Death Differ,* 1998 5, 206-213.

[168] Qian, J;Steigerwald, K;Combs, K A;Barton, M CGroden, J. Caspase cleavage of the APC tumor suppressor and release of an amino-terminal domain is required for the transcription-independent function of APC in apoptosis. *Oncogene*, 2007 26, 4872-4876.

[169] Webb, S J;Nicholson, D;Bubb, V JWyllie, A H. Caspase-mediated cleavage of APC results in an amino-terminal fragment with an intact armadillo repeat domain. *Faseb J,* 1999 13, 339-346.

[170] Qian, J;Perchiniak, E M;Sun, KGroden, J. The Mitochondrial Protein hTID-1 Partners With the Caspase-Cleaved APC Tumor Suppressor to Facilitate Apoptosis. *Gastroenterology*, 2009

[171] Brocardo, M;Lei, Y;Tighe, A;Taylor, S S;Mok, M THenderson, B R. Mitochondrial targeting of adenomatous polyposis coli protein is stimulated by truncating cancer mutations: regulation of Bcl-2 and implications for cell survival. *J Biol Chem*, 2008 283, 5950-5959.

[172] Browne, S J;Williams, A C;Hague, A;Butt, A JParaskeva, C. Loss of APC protein expressed by human colonic epithelial cells and the appearance of a specific low-molecular-weight form is associated with apoptosis in vitro. *Int J Cancer*, 1994 59, 56-64.

[173] Venesio, T;Balsamo, A;Scordamaglia, A;Bertolaso, M;Arrigoni, A;Sprujevnik, T;Rossini, F PRisio, M. Germline APC mutation on the beta-catenin binding site is associated with a decreased apoptotic level in colorectal adenomas. *Mod Pathol,* 2003 16, 57-65.

[174] Morin, P J;Vogelstein, BKinzler, K W. Apoptosis and APC in colorectal tumorigenesis. *Proc Natl Acad Sci U S A*, 1996 93, 7950-7954.

[175] Huang, XGuo, B. Adenomatous polyposis coli determines sensitivity to histone deacetylase inhibitor-induced apoptosis in colon cancer cells. *Cancer Res*, 2006 66, 9245-9251.

[176] Zhang, T;Otevrel, T;Gao, Z;Ehrlich, S M;Fields, J ZBoman, B M. Evidence that APC regulates survivin expression: a possible mechanism contributing to the stem cell origin of colon cancer. *Cancer Res*, 2001 61, 8664-8667.

[177] Steigerwald, K;Behbehani, G K;Combs, K A;Barton, M CGroden, J. The APC tumor suppressor promotes transcription-independent apoptosis in vitro. *Mol Cancer Res,* 2005 3, 78-89.

[178] Clarke, A R. Studying the consequences of immediate loss of gene function in the intestine: *APC. Biochem Soc Trans,* 2005 33, 665-666.

[179] Ahmed, Y;Hayashi, S;Levine, AWieschaus, E. Regulation of armadillo by a Drosophila APC inhibits neuronal apoptosis during retinal development. *Cell*, 1998 93, 1171-1182.

[180] Zhang, L;Ren, X;Alt, E;Bai, X;Huang, S;Xu, Z;Lynch, P M;Moyer, M P;Wen, X FWu, X. Chemoprevention of colorectal cancer by targeting APC-deficient cells for apoptosis. *Nature*, 2010 464, 1058-1061.

In: Tumor Suppressors
Editor: Susan D. Nguyen

ISBN: 978-1-61761-986-1

Chapter 7

Emerging Roles of BRIT1/MCPH1 in Genome Maintenance and Tumor Suppression

Guang Peng and Shiaw-Yih Lin *

Department of Systems Biology, The University of Texas,
M. D. Anderson Cancer Center, Houston, Texas 77030, USA

Abstract

BRIT1 (BRCT-Repeat Inhibitor of hTERT expression) was originally identified from our laboratory as an inhibitor of human telomere reverse transcriptase (hTERT) by a genome-wide genetic screen[1]. The amino acid sequence of BRIT1 was later matched to a putative disease gene called microcephalin (MCPH1). Dysfunction of BRIT1/MCPH1 causes an autosomal recessive genetic disease known as primary microcephaly, which is characterized by reduced brain size of patients[2]. In addition to neuronal development disorder, aberrations of BRIT1 have been identified in various human cancers including breast, ovarian and prostate cancer. In order to gain the mechanistic insights into how BRIT1 deficiency leads to the pathogenesis of the human diseases, our studies and studies from other groups indicate BRIT1 functions as an early DNA damage responsive protein to coordinate cellular responses to genotoxic stresses and maintain genomic stability. In this chapter, we only focus on the function of BRIT1 as a tumor suppressor gene in tumorigenesis. We will discuss the emerging roles of BRIT1 in orchestrating cellular responses to DNA damage including DNA damage signaling, checkpoint activation, and DNA repair. As genomic instability is a hallmark of cancer cells, we will further discuss in the context of cancer development, how BRIT1 functions as a novel tumor suppressor by providing cells with a fundamental genome maintenance mechanism against tumorigenesis and how BRIT1 deficiency may provide a unique opportunity for targeted therapeutics in cancer treatment.

* Corresponding author: Dr. Shiaw-Yih Lin, Department of Systems Biology, Unit 950, The University of Texas M. D. Anderson Cancer Center, South Campus Research Building II, 7435 Fannin, Houston, TX 77054, USA, Phone: (713) 563-4217, Fax: (713) 563-4235, email: sylin@mdanderson.org

BRIT1 Functions as a Tumor Suppressor Gene in Human Cancers

BRIT1 is located on chromosomal 8p23.1, where genetic alterations are frequently identified in multiple human cancers including breast, ovarian and prostate cancer. By analyzing human tumor samples and a variety of cancer cell lines, our studies reveal a novel link between BRIT1 deficiency and human cancer development. We found that BRIT DNA copy number substantially decreased in 40% of advanced epithelial ovarian cancer. In line with the aberrations of BRIT1 DNA, expression levels of BRIT1 mRNA significantly decreased in 63% of ovarian cancer specimens. More interestingly, by using immunohistochemical staining, we observed that BRIT1 protein expression was reduced in benign prostate hypertrophy with further decreases in prostate cancer cells. This finding shows that the loss of BRIT1 expression contributes to the transition of cells from normal to malignant, indicating a tumor suppression function of BRIT1 in early lesions and against tumor progression[3].

Next we analyzed 54 breast cancer cell lines. We found that 72% of the breast cancer cell lines analyzed showed reduced BRIT1 DNA copy number, mRNA and protein levels compared to nontransformed breast epithelial cells. In consistent with its tumor suppression function, BRIT1 expression inversely correlates with the likelihood of breast cancer metastasis and with the duration of relapse-free survival. Notably, in addition to the reduced expression level of BRIT1, we also identified a genetic aberration occurred in the BRIT1 coding region in a breast cancer specimen. A deletion in exon 10 of BRIT1 resulted in a premature stop codon in exon 11, which led to a C-terminal truncated nonfunctional BRIT1 protein[3].

In a very recent study, 77 primary mantle cell lymphoma (MCL) were analyzed by high-resolution RNA expression and genomic profiling. BRIT1 is identified as a novel gene that is deregulated in MCL tumors and implicated in the pathobiology of MCL[4].

Collectively, these data show that BRIT1 functions as a tumor suppressor gene in which aberrations of BRIT1 contribute to both cancer initiation and progression. Then the next question is to understand the underlying mechanisms how BRIT1 deficiency contributes to tumorigenesis.

By protein sequencing analysis, we noticed that BRIT1 contains three BRCT (breast cancer carboxyl-terminal) domains, one in its N-terminus and two in its C-terminus[5]. BRCT domains are well characterized peptide- and phosphopeptide-binding modules, which are present in a wide variety of proteins involved in DNA damage response and genome maintenance[6]. One of the fundamental driving mechanisms of cancer development is the loss of genomic integrity. In consistent with this notion, both *in vitro* and *in vivo* studies from our group and others showed that BRIT1 deficiency leads to genomic instability and tumor prone phenotypes.

For example, in human ovarian cancer specimens, the loss of gene copy number of BRIT1 significantly correlated with overall genomic instability. Then we sought to assess whether depletion of BRIT1 in cells would lead to an increase in chromosome aberrations and genomic instability, which might contribute to the cancer development. We depleted BRIT1 by siRNAs in normal human mammary epithelial cells (HMECs) and found a wide range of chromosome aberrations, including chromosomal breaks, dicentric chromosomes and chromosomal telomeric association. More sever chromosomal aberrations were identified in BRIT1-deficient cells after exposing cells to ionizing radiation (IR), a DNA damage stimulus causing DNA double strand breaks (DBSs). Similar results were also observed in a variety of cell lines including normal human fibroblast BJ cells, MCF-7 cells and HeLa cells[3].

In addition to *in vitro* studies, the importance of BRIT1 in maintaining genomic stability and preventing tumorigenesis is further strengthen and supported by an *in vivo* study using the BRIT1 knockout mouse model[7]. BRIT1-/- mice are found to be more sensitive to irradiation with a shorter survival compared to wild-type control mice. Increased sensitivity to radiation has also been observed in BRIT1-/- mouse embryonic fibroblast (MEFs) and T cells. In consistent with the increased genomic instability in BRIT1-/- mice, BRIT1 knockout mice in the p53 null background exhibited enhanced cancer susceptibility. Moreover, tissue specific knockout of BRIT1 in the mammary glands readily led to breast tumors after exposure to low dosage of irradiation[8].

In summary, these findings indicate that BRIT1 functions as a guardian of genomic integrity against the development of human cancers. As the "central store" of our genetic information, DNA within our cells is constantly being exposed to endogenous and exogenous DNA damaging factors such as reactive oxygen species, ionizing radiation and radiomimetic drugs. In order to maintain genomic integrity, cells have evolved a complex network to detect, signal the presence of and repair DNA damage, which is referred as DNA damage response pathway (DDR). To further provide the mechanistic insights into the function of BRIT1 as a tumor suppressor gene in maintaining genomic stability, studies from our groups and others have led to fruitful findings of the function of BRIT1 in regulating cellular responses to DNA damage and genome integrity.

DNA Damage Response, A Potent Anti-cancer Barrier

DDR consists of a complex network of proteins, which function in a dynamic, hierarchically ordered and mutually coordinated manner to detect, signal and repair DNA lesions. In this network (as shown in Figure 1), two phosphatidylinositol-3-related kinases, ATM (ataxia telangiectasia mutated) and ATR (ATM-Rad3-related) are located at the top of signal cascades; ATM is activated primarily by DSBs induced by ionizing radiation, whereas ATR also responds to UV or stalled replication forks. Once activated in response to DNA damage, ATM and ATR phosphorylate and activate a variety of molecules to execute the DNA damage response. One of their substrates is H2AX, a histone variant, which is phosphorylated at serine 139 (referred to as γ–H2AX) and decorates the DSBs lesions. Sensors and early mediators, such as the Mre11/Rad50/NBS1 complex, MDC1, 53BP1, BRAC1, RPA and Rad17, are promptly recruited to the damaged DNA sites. Recruitment of these DNA damage responsive proteins result in the formation of immunostainable nuclear foci, called IRIF (irradiation-induced foci). Accumulation of IRIF serves as a platform where checkpoint and DNA repair proteins assemble to facilitate the transduction of the damage signal to cellular response pathways, including cell cycle checkpoints, DNA repair, transcription and the apoptotic and senescent pathway. The two effector kinases Chk1 and Chk2 are phosphorylated by ATM and ATR and then phosphorylate the downstream checkpoint protein Cdc25s, which results in its degradation that ,in turn, leads to activation of the G1/S, intra-S, and G2/M checkpoints. Activation of checkpoints by DDR delays cell-cycle progression to provide more time for repair of the lesions. Failure to properly repair damaged DNA results in potentially deleterious mutations. If such genetically altered cells potentially escape from the cellular elimination mechanisms such as senescence and/or apoptosis, the accumulation of these unstable cells may very likely lead to the development of cancer[9; 10; 11; 12; 13].

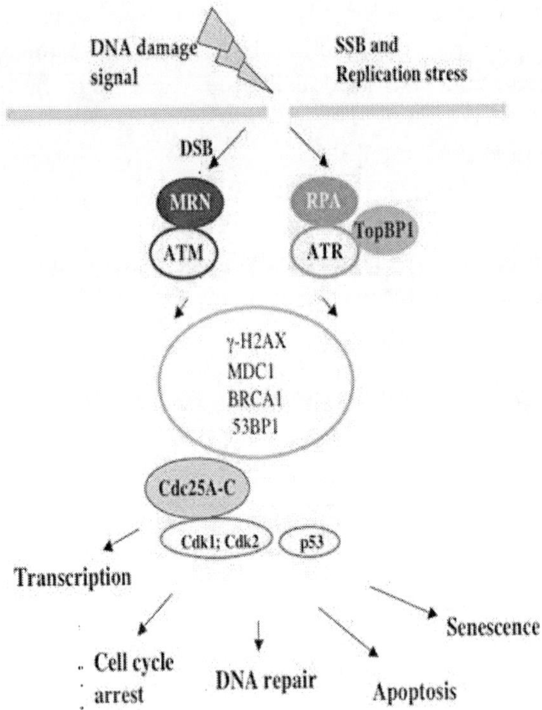

Figure 1. DNA damage Reponse Pathway.

The importance of such genome surveillance is best exemplified by numerous cancer-predisposing clinical syndromes, which are caused by aberrations in DDR components. For instance, mutations of tumor suppressor BRCA1 and BRCA2, two well-known DNA repair genes, result in elevated cancer incidence in both breast cancer and ovarian cancer. Moreover, the protein kinase ATM deficiency causes a human genetic disease with the cancer predisposition, particularly the development of lymphomas and leukemia. Another two human cancer predisposition disorders, Werner syndrome and Bloom syndrome, have also been implicated in impaired HR repair due to defective helicases, in which cancer susceptibility is seen in a wide range of human cancer types[11; 14].

Studies from our group and others have highlighted multiple roles of BRIT1 in DDR and in genome surveillance, which contribute to its function as a potent tumor suppressor.

BRIT1, An Early DNA Damage Responsive Protein

Several lines of evidence indicate that BRIT1 is a proximal factor in DDR. Following the DNA damage, BRIT1 is recruited to the DNA lesions to form IRIF as early as 2 min, which colocalized with multiple DNA damage sensor and mediator proteins such as NBS1, p-ATM, MDC1, and 53BP1[3; 5]. The functional significance of the recruitment of BRIT1 to DNA damage loci has been extensively studied in BRIT1 deficient-cells both by siRNA knockdown and by genetically gene knockout MEFs[15]. BRIT1 is required for transducing DNA damage signaling in both ATM and ATR pathways. BRIT1 depletion impairs the recruitment of 53BP1, NBS1, p-ATM, ATR, p-RAD17 and p-RPA34 to the DNA damage sites[3]. However, the formation of γ-H2AX foci is not altered in the absence of BRIT1[3]. To determine how BRIT1 is recruited to DNA damage loci, studies using chicken cells and MEFs showed that BRIT1 foci formation is independent of ATM, BRCA1 or MDC1, while it dependents on H2AX phosphorylation[15; 16]. Domain analysis indicates that C-terminal BRCT domains of BRIT1 are involved in self-oligomerization and are required for its foci formation. These data collectively support that BRIT1 is an early DNA damage responsive protein that regulates DDR signaling cascade.

BRIT1, A Cell Cycle Regulator

After exposure to IR, BRIT1-deficient cells failed to arrest with a G2/M DNA content compared to the control cells. By using phospho-histone H3 antibody, a marker for cells in M phase, we observed that BRIT1 knockdown cells had a significantly higher proportion of cells in mitosis phase compared to control cells after irradiation.These results indicate a defective G2-M checkpoint activation[5]. In addition, BRIT1 knockdown cells showed a remarkable resistance to the reduction of DNA synthesis after IR and significantly increased sensitivity to IR in contrast to the control cells[5]. These data support a critical role of BRIT1 in intra-S phase control.

BRIT1 functions in the control of checkpoint activation not only affecting DNA damage response signaling cascades and regulating the activity of the components inside this signaling network, but also through regulating the expression levels of key checkpoint regulators such as BRCA1 and Chk1[5; 17]. BRIT1 depletion significantly reduces BRCA1 and Chk1 expression, which potentially provide a second mechanism for the function of BRIT1 in regulating cell cycle checkpoint activation. Another study also showed that BRIT1 functions as a transcriptional regulator in controlling E2F1 pathway[18].

In the developmental perspective, BRIT1 is found to coordinate the S-M transition in fly embryos. Deficiency of BRIT1 in drosophila embryo results in premature chromosome condensation (PCC) and mitotic entry with unreplicated DNA and genomic instability[19; 20]. The function of BRIT1 in regulating mitotic entry is further supported by studies using cell lines derived from primary microcephaly patients with the characterized brain development defect[21; 22]. The function of BRIT1 in regulating PCC has also been shown in a genetic mouse model, which only disrupts the C-terminal BRCT-domain[23].

Besides its direct function in regulating the cell cycle entry into mitosis, BRIT1 has an additional role in centrosome regulation. BRIT has been found to play a significant role as a mitotic regulator. The function of BRIT1 is required for coordinating centrosomal and nuclear division cycles in multiple model systems including Drosophila and chicken[16; 24]. In the mammalian cells, BRIT1 is localized at the centrosomes and functions to maintain integrity and normal function of centrosomes[25]. A recent study reported that a lack of BRIT1 results in a loss of Chk1 from centrosomes with subsequently deregulated activation of centrosomal cyclin B-Cdk1[20], which provides additional support that dysfunction of BRIT1 in cell cycle regulation may contribute to the development of human diseases such as cancer and primary microcephaly.

BRIT1, A Linkage between Chromatin Remodeling and DDR

In order to gain mechanistic insights into a wide range effect of BRIT1 in genome maintenance, we undertook a proteomic approach to systematically identify BRIT1 interaction proteins. Among many binding partners of BRIT1, we discovered that BRIT1 interacts with ATP-dependent chromatin remodeling complex SWI/SNF and coordinates chromatin remodeling in DNA repair (Figure 2)[26].

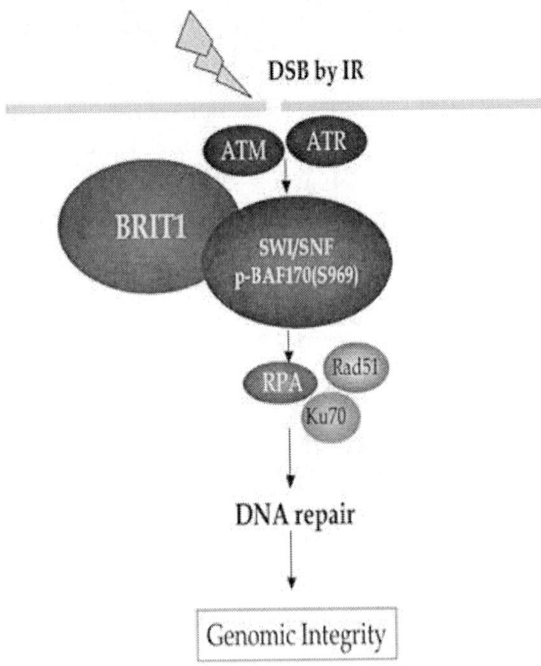

Figure 2. A Proposed Model of BRIT1-SWI/SNF in Regulating DNA Repair

Five subunits of human SWI/SNF complex were co-purified with BRIT1 including BRG1/BRM, BAF170, BAF155 and SNF5. Notably, these five subunits have been found to be the functional core of SWI/SNF as their *in vitro* remodeling activity was identical to the activity of whole complex. By depletion of individual subunits, we found that BRIT1 interacts with SWI/SNF complex via its core subunits BAF170 and BAF155 and the interaction is via the N-terminal domain of BRIT1. These interactions are enhanced in response to DNA damage signaling, and the enhanced binding affinity of BRIT1-SWI/SNF is mediated through an ATM/ATR-dependent phosphorylation of BAF170[26].

DSBs induced by numerous endogenous and environmental stimuli are the most dangerous DNA lesion of the many types of DNA damage existing within the cells. Inaccurate repair or lack of repair of DSBs can result in the introduction of gene mutations and amplifications, as well as chromosomal deletions and translocations. Such genome aberrations lead to genetic instability and consequently enhance the rate of cancer development[27; 28]. To elucidate the functional significance of BRIT1-SWI/SNF interaction, we systematically investigated how BRIT1-mediated DSB repair was impaired when BRIT1-SWI/SNF interaction was disrupted.

There are two conserved repairing pathways for DSBs, homologous recombination (HR) and nonhomologous end joining (NHEJ). The distinct difference between these two pathways is the requirement of homologous sequence for HR-mediated repair. Therefore, HR is generally error-free repair that uses a homologous information from a sister chromatid as template DNA to repair damaged lesions in the S/G2 phase. In contrast, NHEJ involves the direct linkage of broken ends, which is usually error-prone process and present throughout cell cycle. Different sets of proteins are required for these two distinct pathways. HR repair initially requires an MRN complex mediated 5'-3' resection followed by RAD51, RAD52 and RAD54 proteins to promote strand invasion and subsequent recombination. NHEJ repair involves the DNA dependent protein kinase (DNA-PK), K70, K80 and the DNA ligase IV complex, which together facilitate re-joining of broken non-compatible DNA ends[27; 28].

To dissect the role of BRIT1 in regulating DSB repair, we utilized I-SceI-induced DSBs repairing system to determine the efficiency of DSB repair in BRIT1-deficient cells. Notably, we found that BRIT1 is required for both HR and NHEJ. Via interaction with BRIT1, SWI/SNF can be specifically recruited to and maintained at DNA lesions. Thereby, BRIT1 promotes chromatin relaxation at DNA damage sites that, in turn, facilitates the recruitment of key DNA repair proteins such as RAD51, RPA, and Ku70 to DNA damage sites for efficient repair[26]. As a consequence, depletion of BRIT1 leads to impaired chromatin relaxation and DNA DSB repair, which may contribute to the development of cancer.

Highly condensed chromatin structure forms a significant barrier for the accesses of proteins to DNA. ATP-dependent chromatin remodeling is a fundamental mechanism utilized by cells to relax chromatin structure[29]. However, the remodeling complex, including SWI/SNF does not contain intrinsic specificity for particular nuclear process. In fact, how SWI/SNF complex is recruited to DNA lesions in response to DNA damage is still poorly understood. Our studies reveal a novel mechanism by which SWI/SNF complex is targeted to DNA lesions via an interaction with early DNA damage response protein BRIT1. DNA damage response proteins, such as BRIT1, may themselves directly regulate the function of chromatin remodeling complexes both spatially and temporally to facilitate the detection and repair of DNA lesions. It is tempting to suspect that multiple mechanisms may be involved regulating chromatin structure in order to cope with different stages of damage response and/or response to different types of DNA lesions and/or repair DNA lesions located in different regions of chromatin (euchromatin or heterochromatin)[30; 31].

Furthermore, our studies reveal that post-translational modifications such as phosphorylation may serve as critical mechanisms to regulate the functions of SWI/SNF. In response to DNA damage signaling, unique modifications, such as phosphorylation, can occur in various subunits of chromatin remodeling complexes. These modifications may provide remodeling complexes with the means of interacting with distinct cofactors in various cellular processes to maintain genomic integrity.

BRIT1, A Protein Repairing DNA DSBs

In consistent with our findings that BRIT1 is required for HR mediated DSBs repair, several studies from other groups also showed the extensive role of BRIT1 in HR repair.

BRIT1 is found to interact with the Condensin II complex, which is implicated in chromosome condensation. Biochemical analysis indicated that BRIT1 interacts with Condensin II via its central domain. Disruption of this interaction impairs HR repair[32]. Moreover, a recent study indicates that BRIT1 binds to DNA repair proteins BRCA2 through its C-terminal BRCT domain. The interaction between BRCA2 and BRIT1 is not essential for BRCA2 to form a complex with RAD51 but is required for their presence at DNA damage sites to perform their DNA repair function[33].

In addition to *in vitro* studies, the function of BRIT1 in HR repair has also been shown in a BRIT1 knockout mouse model[7]. BRIT1 knockout mice exhibited severe defects in meiotic recombination to produce sperm for reproduction. BRIT1 knockout spermatocytes exhibited a failure of chromosomal synapsis, and meiosis was arrested at late zygotene of prophase I accompanied by apoptosis. The meiotic phenotypes in BRIT1 knockout mice are attributed to the impaired recruitment of BRCA2/RAD51 to repair DSBs generated during meiotic recombination. In the absence of BRIT1, recruitment of BRCA2/RAD51 to chromatin is remarkably reduced while their protein levels are not altered. The interaction of BRIT1-BRCA2/RAD51 is also implicated in this study. As a consequence, male BRIT1 knockout mice are infertile with smaller testes and very few spermatids. This phenotype is consistent with previous studies in mice deficient with BRCA2 or RAD51.

The identification of BRIT1 as a repair protein in HR provides a molecular basis to use PARP inhibitors as therapeutic drugs in BRIT1-deficient tumors. PARP is an enzyme that facilitates repair of single-strand breaks. In normal cells, DNA damage generated by PARP inhibitors is well tolerated because of compensation from HR repair. In contrast, HR-repair-defective cancer cells, such as BRCA1/BRCA2-deficient cells, are unable to cope with this increased DNA damage and thereby exhibit hypersensitivity to PARP inhibitors[34; 35; 36]. This synthetic lethality interaction between HR repair-defective cancer cells and PARP inhibitors brings the most exciting therapeutic strategy to achieve cancer-specific targeting. Elucidating the role of BRIT1 in HR repair and tumorigenesis will expand the use of PARP inhibitors against tumors beyond BRCA1/BRCA2-deficient tumors. It will be of future research interests to investigate the potential effects of PARP inhibitors in BRIT1-deficient cancer cells and develop a rationale combination of therapeutic drugs in treating BRIT1-deficient tumors.

Perspective of BRIT1 Functions in Genome Maintenance

Having determined the function of BRIT1 in regulating DNA damage signaling, checkpoint activation, transcription and DNA repair in response to DNA damage, the next question is what the potential roles of BRIT1 in other aspects of genome maintenance.

BRIT1 in Telomere Maintenance

Telomeres are another crucial components required for genomic stability. As shown in Figure 3A, telomeres are highly specialized nucleoprotein structures that maintain genomic stability by stabilizing and protecting the chromosomes. In mammalian cells, the formation and stabilization of telomeres requires a minimal length of telomeric repeats as well as the direct binding of a number of specific telomeric repeat binding factors. These proteins form a complex known as shelterin (telosome), which includes six core proteins: TRF1, TRF2, RAP1, TIN2, TPP1, and POT1. This shelterin protein complex protects telomeres from being recognized as DSBs and prevents inappropriate engagement of the DNA repair apparatus[37; 38; 39; 40]. TRF2, an essential component of the shelterin complex, directly binds to double-stranded DNA and is involved in processes required for maintenance of telomere integrity, such as shelterin assembly; telomere-length regulation; DNA replication, repair, and endjoining; and cell-cycle control. Thus, TRF2 is postulated to serve as a protein hub in telomere maintenance[40].

When the protective function of telomeres is disrupted as a result of either physiological loss of telomeric sequences or genetic abnormalities affecting the shelterin complex, telomeres become dysfunctional[41]. Cells respond to the resulting unprotected chromosome ends as if they were DSBs and activate DNA damage response (Figure 3B), which induces the formation of telomere dysfunction-induced foci (TIFs), and the activation of downstream checkpoint regulators, such as Chk2, p53, and p21, leading to cell cycle arrest[42]. In addition, the DNA repair machinery recognizes unprotected chromosome ends as DSBs, resulting in inappropriate chromosomal end-to-end fusions, mainly through the nonhomologous end-joining (NHEJ) pathway. Telomere dysfunction contributes to tumorigenesis by promoting genome instability. Loss of functional telomere protection of chromosome ends leads to chromosomal end-to-end fusions, followed by random breakage and then subsequent fusions to generate aneuploidy, loss of heterozygosity, or amplification of certain chromosomal loci, which are the basis of tumorigenesis caused by dysfunctional telomeres. When telomeres become dysfunctional, cells activate an intrinsic defense mechanism by eliciting DNA damage responses to engage apoptosis and/or senescence pathways and suppress the process of tumorigenesis (Figure 3C).

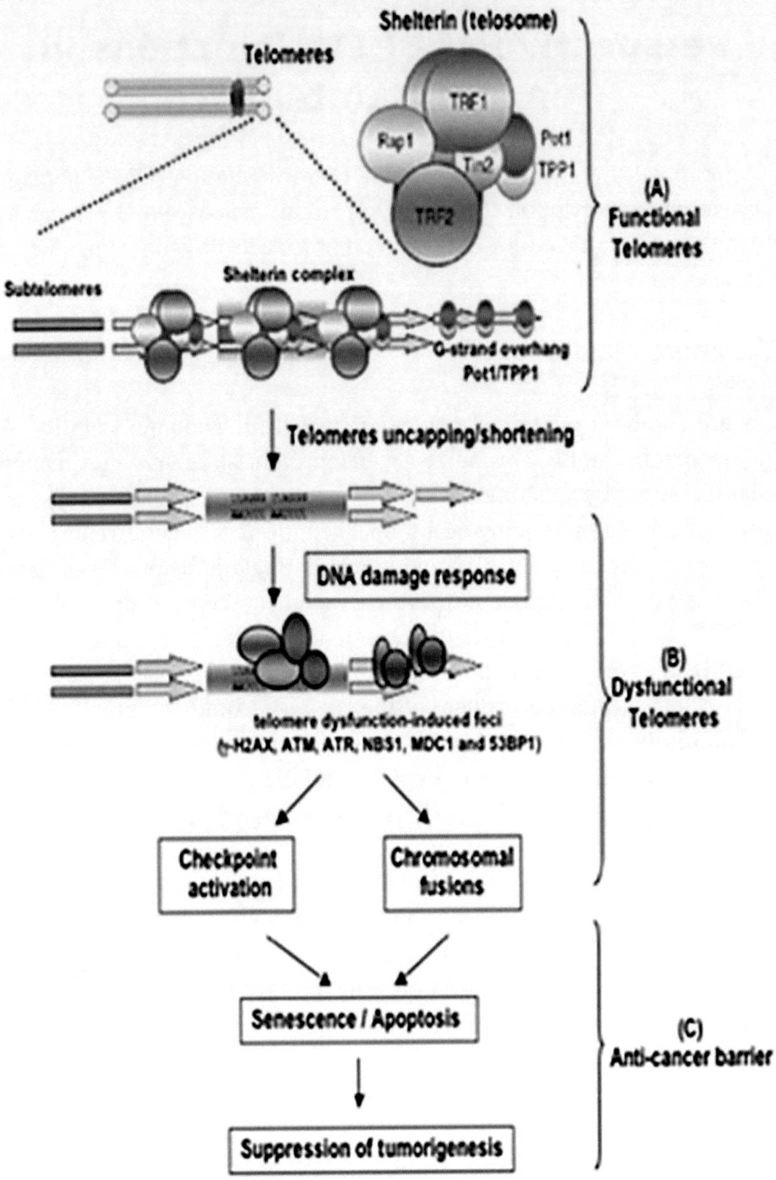

Figure 3. Implication of Telomere Stability in Preventing Tumorigenesis. (A) Schematic of telomeres with functional end protection by shelterin complex. (B) Dysfunctional Telomeres activate the canonical DNA damage responses. (C) DNA damage responses elicited by dysfunctional telmoeres can engage cellular senescence and/or apoptosis pathways to inhibit tumorigenesis.

Inactivated DNA damage response to dysfunctional telomeres has been found to provide a permissive environment that favors proliferation and survival of cells with dysfunctional telomeres and eventual progression to cancer. Therefore, both maintenance of functional telomeres and maintenance of intact DNA damage responses at dysfunctional telomeres are essential for telomere stability, which forms a potent anticancer barrier[42; 43]

Our proteomic assay identified TRF2 as a novel binding partner of BRIT1. Further experiments utilizing immunofluorescent staining clearly showed that BRIT1 foci co-localized with TRF2 foci at telomeres[40]. TRF2 is a core subunit of the shelterin complex, which exerts an essential function in maintaining telomere integrity. Thus, BRIT1 most likely has an additional biological function in regulating telomere stability.

Recent studies have indicated that TRF2 functions to organize telomeric chromatin structure and recruit other regulatory proteins to the telomeres. As a binding partner of TRF2 at telomeres, BRIT1 may facilitate the assembly of shelterin complex at telomere ends and contribute to establishing normal telomerestructure. Our previous studies demonstrated that BRIT1 is functionally implicated in various DNA damage responses to DSBs. Notably, when telomeres lose their end protection and become dysfunctional, both the DNA damage signaling pathway and the DNA damage repair reactions elicited by these unprotected chromosomal ends resemble the canonical response to DSBs. Activation of the canonical DNA damage response pathway can, in turn, initiate apoptosis and/or senescence, which serves as a potent barrier against tumorigenesis.

Based on the function of BRIT1 as a DNA damage responsive protein involved in the early response to DSB, we hypothesize that BRIT1 may also regulate cellular responses to dysfunctional telomeres, including DNA damage signaling, DNA repair, and checkpoint activation. A better understanding of BRIT1 in DNA damage response induced by dysfunctional telomeres may provide additional insights into BRIT1's role in tumor suppression.

Telomeres are specialized higher-order structures, which form constitutive heterochromatin regions and remain condensed through the cell cycle. These highly condensed structures protect telomeres and limit telomere length. However, they may also form a barrier against recruiting and tethering proteins at both functional and dysfunctional telomeres[44; 45]. As described above, BRIT1 may recruit SWI/SNF to the heterochromatin to enhance the access of the functional proteins to the regions. We, therefore, speculate that BRIT1 targets SWI/SNF complex to telomeres and helps to maintain telomere stability via altering the accessibility of proteins to telomeres.

BRIT1 in DNA replication

S phase represents the most valuable time for cells to faithfully replicate their DNA and ensure a high fidelity transmission of genetic information[46]. From our proteomic study, we also identified that BRIT1 interacts with multiple proteins involved in DNA replication such as PCNA. It is of our research interest to understand whether BRIT1 functions in the formation of replication complex and the initiation of replication process.

It is also possible that BRIT1 is involved in the response to replication stress. When cells are challenged with replication stress-inducing agents, the progression of the replication fork is stalled, which activates intra-S checkpoint and recruits repair proteins to remove DNA lesions. If DNA lesions are successfully resolved, the replication will resume. Otherwise, replication folks lose stability and collapse, which results in accumulation of DNA damage[46]. The biological functions of BRIT1 in DNA replication stress response may occur at multiple steps including the stabilization of stalled replication fork, recruiting intra-S checkpoint activation factors, resolving DNA lesions via facilitating DNA repair or resuming of replication after the removal of replication stress.

Regulatory Mechanisms of BRIT1 via Post-translational Modifications

Post-translational modifications have been highlighted to coordinate cellular responses to detect, signaling and repair DNA damage. Multiple protein modifications are implicated in DDR including phosphorylation, ubiquitination, acetylation and sumoylation[13; 47; 48]. The combined effects of these modifications not only allow temporal and spatial control of the initiation, amplification and propagation of DNA damage signaling, but also provide regulatory specificity for DDR components to response certain DNA damage stimuli at particular DDR stage. For example, recent studies show phosphorylation of H2AX recruits MDC1, which in turn facilitates the recruitment of RNF8 and RNF168[49; 50; 51; 52]. The ubiquitination cascade mediated by RNF8 and RNF168 at DNA damage sites coordinate to recruit RAP80 and BRCA1. It will be worthwhile to determine the potential posttranscriptional modification on BRIT1 in response to DNA damage, which may provide a fine-tuned regulatory mechanism to bridge BRIT1 in various processes of genome maintenance.

Post-translational modifications on BRIT1 such as phosphorylation, ubiquitination, acetylation and sumoylation may provide an important means of recruiting of BRIT1 to DNA damage sites. It is tempting to suspect that DNA damage-induced modifications of BRIT1 may change its binding affinity for its interaction partners, which serve as a regulatory mechanism to modulate its functions in various processes to maintain genomic integrity such as DNA repair, DNA replication, transcription regulation and telomere maintenance. In summary, to identify post-transcriptional modifications on BRIT1 may better our understandings on its distinct functions in genome maintenance.

References

[1] S.Y. Lin, and S.J. Elledge, Multiple tumor suppressor pathways negatively regulate telomerase. *Cell* 113 (2003) 881-9.

[2] A.P. Jackson, H. Eastwood, S.M. Bell, J. Adu, C. Toomes, I.M. Carr, E. Roberts, D.J. Hampshire, Y.J. Crow, A.J. Mighell, G. Karbani, H. Jafri, Y. Rashid, R.F. Mueller, A.F. Markham, and C.G. Woods, Identification of microcephalin, a protein implicated in determining the size of the human brain. *Am J Hum Genet* 71 (2002) 136-42.

[3] R. Rai, H. Dai, A.S. Multani, K. Li, K. Chin, J. Gray, J.P. Lahad, J. Liang, G.B. Mills, F. Meric-Bernstam, and S.Y. Lin, BRIT1 regulates early DNA damage response, chromosomal integrity, and cancer. *Cancer Cell* 10 (2006) 145-57.

[4] E.M. Hartmann, E. Campo, G. Wright, G. Lenz, I. Salaverria, P. Jares, W. Xiao, R.M. Braziel, L.M. Rimsza, W.C. Chan, D.D. Weisenburger, J. Delabie, E.S. Jaffe, R.D. Gascoyne, S.S. Dave, H.K. Mueller-Hermelink, L.M. Staudt, G. Ott, S. Bea, and A. Rosenwald, Pathway discovery in mantle cell lymphoma by integrated analysis of high resolution gene expression and copy number profiling. *Blood* (2010) Epub ahead of print.

[5] S.Y. Lin, R. Rai, K. Li, Z.X. Xu, and S.J. Elledge, BRIT1/MCPH1 is a DNA damage responsive protein that regulates the Brca1-Chk1 pathway, implicating checkpoint dysfunction in microcephaly. *Proc Natl Acad Sci USA* 102 (2005) 15105-9.

[6] X. Yu, C.C. Chini, M. He, G. Mer, and J. Chen, The BRCT domain is a phosphoprotein binding domain. *Science* 302 (2003) 639-42.

[7] Y. Liang, H. Gao, S.Y. Lin, G. Peng, X. Huang, P. Zhang, J.A. Goss, F.C. Brunicardi, A.S. Multani, S. Chang, and K. Li, BRIT1/MCPH1 is essential for mitotic and meiotic recombination DNA repair and maintaining genomic stability in mice. *PLoS Genet* 6 e1000826.

[8] S.Y. Lin, Y. Liang, and K. Li, Multiple roles of BRIT1/MCPH1 in DNA damage response, DNA repair, and cancer suppression. *Yonsei Med J* 51 (2010) 295-301.

[9] B.B. Zhou, and S.J. Elledge, The DNA damage response: putting checkpoints in perspective. *Nature* 408 (2000) 433-9.

[10] S.P. Jackson, Detecting, signalling and repairing DNA double-strand breaks. *Biochem Soc Trans* 29 (2001) 655-61.

[11] K.K. Khanna, and S.P. Jackson, DNA double-strand breaks: signaling, repair and the cancer connection. *Nat Genet* 27 (2001) 247-54.

[12] S.P. Jackson, Sensing and repairing DNA double-strand breaks. *Carcinogenesis* 23 (2002) 687-96.

[13] J.W. Harper, and S.J. Elledge, The DNA damage response: ten years after. *Mol Cell* 28 (2007) 739-45.

[14] S.P. Jackson, and J. Bartek, The DNA-damage response in human biology and disease. *Nature* 461 (2009) 1071-8.

[15] J.L. Wood, N. Singh, G. Mer, and J. Chen, MCPH1 functions in an H2AX-dependent but MDC1-independent pathway in response to DNA damage. *J Biol Chem* 282 (2007) 35416-23.

[16] L.J. Jeffers, B.J. Coull, S.J. Stack, and C.G. Morrison, Distinct BRCT domains in Mcph1/Brit1 mediate ionizing radiation-induced focus formation and centrosomal localization. *Oncogene* 27 (2008) 139-44.

[17] X. Xu, J. Lee, and D.F. Stern, Microcephalin is a DNA damage response protein involved in regulation of CHK1 and BRCA1. *J Biol Chem* 279 (2004) 34091-4.

[18] S.Z. Yang, F.T. Lin, and W.C. Lin, MCPH1/BRIT1 cooperates with E2F1 in the activation of checkpoint, DNA repair and apoptosis. *EMBO Rep* 9 (2008) 907-15.

[19] K. Brunk, B. Vernay, E. Griffith, N.L. Reynolds, D. Strutt, P.W. Ingham, and A.P. Jackson, Microcephalin coordinates mitosis in the syncytial Drosophila embryo. *J Cell Sci* 120 (2007) 3578-88.

[20] A. Tibelius, J. Marhold, H. Zentgraf, C.E. Heilig, H. Neitzel, B. Ducommun, A. Rauch, A.D. Ho, J. Bartek, and A. Kramer, Microcephalin and pericentrin regulate mitotic entry via centrosome-associated Chk1. *J Cell Biol* 185 (2009) 1149-57.

[21] G.K. Alderton, L. Galbiati, E. Griffith, K.H. Surinya, H. Neitzel, A.P. Jackson, P.A. Jeggo, and M. O'Driscoll, Regulation of mitotic entry by microcephalin and its overlap with ATR signalling. *Nat Cell Biol* 8 (2006) 725-33.

[22] M.W. Richards, J.W. Leung, S.M. Roe, K. Li, J. Chen, and R. Bayliss, A pocket on the surface of the N-terminal BRCT domain of Mcph1 is required to prevent abnormal chromosome condensation. *J Mol Biol* 395 (2010) 908-15.

[23] M. Trimborn, M. Ghani, D.J. Walther, M. Dopatka, V. Dutrannoy, A. Busche, F. Meyer, S. Nowak, J. Nowak, C. Zabel, J. Klose, V. Esquitino, M. Garshasbi, A.W. Kuss, H.H. Ropers, S. Mueller, C. Poehlmann, I. Gavvovidis, D. Schindler, K. Sperling,

and H. Neitzel, Establishment of a mouse model with misregulated chromosome condensation due to defective Mcph1 function. *PLoS One* 5 e9242.

[24] J.L. Rickmyre, S. Dasgupta, D.L. Ooi, J. Keel, E. Lee, M.W. Kirschner, S. Waddell, and L.A. Lee, The Drosophila homolog of MCPH1, a human microcephaly gene, is required for genomic stability in the early embryo. J *Cell Sci* 120 (2007) 3565-77.

[25] X. Zhong, G.P. Pfeifer, and X. Xu, Microcephalin encodes a centrosomal protein. *Cell Cycle* 5 (2006) 457-8.

[26] G. Peng, E.K. Yim, H. Dai, A.P. Jackson, I. Burgt, M.R. Pan, R. Hu, K. Li, and S.Y. Lin, BRIT1/MCPH1 links chromatin remodelling to DNA damage response. *Nat Cell Biol* 11 (2009) 865-72.

[27] C.L. Peterson, and J. Cote, Cellular machineries for chromosomal DNA repair. *Genes Dev* 18 (2004) 602-16.

[28] A. Sancar, L.A. Lindsey-Boltz, K. Unsal-Kacmaz, and S. Linn, Molecular mechanisms of mammalian DNA repair and the DNA damage checkpoints. *Annu Rev Biochem* 73 (2004) 39-85.

[29] M.A. Osley, T. Tsukuda, and J.A. Nickoloff, ATP-dependent chromatin remodeling factors and DNA damage repair. *Mutat Res* 618 (2007) 65-80.

[30] G. Peng, and S.Y. Lin, The linkage of chromatin remodeling to genome maintenance: contribution from a human disease gene BRIT1/MCPH1. *Epigenetics* 4 (2009) 457-61.

[31] G. Peng, and S.Y. Lin, BRIT1/MCPH1 is a multifunctional DNA damage responsive protein mediating DNA repair-associated chromatin remodeling. *Cell Cycle* 8 (2009) 3071-2.

[32] J.L. Wood, Y. Liang, K. Li, and J. Chen, Microcephalin/MCPH1 associates with the Condensin II complex to function in homologous recombination repair. *J Biol Chem* 283 (2008) 29586-92.

[33] X. Wu, G. Mondal, X. Wang, J. Wu, L. Yang, V.S. Pankratz, M. Rowley, and F.J. Couch, Microcephalin regulates BRCA2 and Rad51-associated DNA double-strand break repair. *Cancer Res* 69 (2009) 5531-6.

[34] H.E. Bryant, N. Schultz, H.D. Thomas, K.M. Parker, D. Flower, E. Lopez, S. Kyle, M. Meuth, N.J. Curtin, and T. Helleday, Specific killing of BRCA2-deficient tumours with inhibitors of poly(ADP-ribose) polymerase. *Nature* 434 (2005) 913-7.

[35] H. Farmer, N. McCabe, C.J. Lord, A.N. Tutt, D.A. Johnson, T.B. Richardson, M. Santarosa, K.J. Dillon, I. Hickson, C. Knights, N.M. Martin, S.P. Jackson, G.C. Smith, and A. Ashworth, Targeting the DNA repair defect in BRCA mutant cells as a therapeutic strategy. *Nature* 434 (2005) 917-21.

[36] A. Ashworth, A synthetic lethal therapeutic approach: poly(ADP) ribose polymerase inhibitors for the treatment of cancers deficient in DNA double-strand break repair. *J Clin Oncol* 26 (2008) 3785-90.

[37] T. de Lange, Shelterin: the protein complex that shapes and safeguards human telomeres. *Genes Dev* 19 (2005) 2100-10.

[38] P. Slijepcevic, and S. Al-Wahiby, Telomere biology: integrating chromosomal end protection with DNA damage response. *Chromosoma* 114 (2005) 275-85.

[39] R.E. Verdun, and J. Karlseder, Replication and protection of telomeres. *Nature* 447 (2007) 924-31.

[40] H. Kim, O.H. Lee, H. Xin, L.Y. Chen, J. Qin, H.K. Chae, S.Y. Lin, A. Safari, D. Liu, and Z. Songyang, TRF2 functions as a protein hub and regulates telomere maintenance by recognizing specific peptide motifs. *Nat Struct Mol Biol* 16 (2009) 372-9.

[41] M.P. Longhese, DNA damage response at functional and dysfunctional telomeres. *Genes Dev* 22 (2008) 125-40.

[42] A.L. Cheung, and W. Deng, Telomere dysfunction, genome instability and cancer. *Front Biosci* 13 (2008) 2075-90.

[43] Y. Deng, S.S. Chan, and S. Chang, Telomere dysfunction and tumour suppression: the senescence connection. *Nat Rev Cancer* 8 (2008) 450-8.

[44] E.Y. Yu, O. Steinberg-Neifach, A.T. Dandjinou, F. Kang, A.J. Morrison, X. Shen, and N.F. Lue, Regulation of telomere structure and functions by subunits of the INO80 chromatin remodeling complex. *Mol Cell Biol* 27 (2007) 5639-49.

[45] A.J. Morrison, and X. Shen, Chromatin remodelling beyond transcription: the INO80 and SWR1 complexes. *Nat Rev Mol Cell Biol* 10 (2009) 373-84.

[46] J. Bartek, C. Lukas, and J. Lukas, Checking on DNA damage in S phase. *Nat Rev Mol Cell Biol* 5 (2004) 792-804.

[47] M.S. Huen, and J. Chen, The DNA damage response pathways: at the crossroad of protein modifications. *Cell Res* 18 (2008) 8-16.

[48] S. Bergink, and S. Jentsch, Principles of ubiquitin and SUMO modifications in DNA repair. *Nature* 458 (2009) 461-7.

[49] M.S. Huen, R. Grant, I. Manke, K. Minn, X. Yu, M.B. Yaffe, and J. Chen, RNF8 transduces the DNA-damage signal via histone ubiquitylation and checkpoint protein assembly. *Cell* 131 (2007) 901-14.

[50] N.K. Kolas, J.R. Chapman, S. Nakada, J. Ylanko, R. Chahwan, F.D. Sweeney, S. Panier, M. Mendez, J. Wildenhain, T.M. Thomson, L. Pelletier, S.P. Jackson, and D. Durocher, Orchestration of the DNA-damage response by the RNF8 ubiquitin ligase. *Science* 318 (2007) 1637-40.

[51] N. Mailand, S. Bekker-Jensen, H. Faustrup, F. Melander, J. Bartek, C. Lukas, and J. Lukas, RNF8 ubiquitylates histones at DNA double-strand breaks and promotes assembly of repair proteins. *Cell* 131 (2007) 887-900.

[52] C. Doil, N. Mailand, S. Bekker-Jensen, P. Menard, D.H. Larsen, R. Pepperkok, J. Ellenberg, S. Panier, D. Durocher, J. Bartek, J. Lukas, and C. Lukas, RNF168 binds and amplifies ubiquitin conjugates on damaged chromosomes to allow accumulation of repair proteins. *Cell* 136 (2009) 435-46

In: Tumor Suppressors
Editor: Susan D. Nguyen

ISBN: 978-1-61761-986-1

Chapter 8

The Role of Histone Deacetylase (HDAC) and EZH2 in Oncogenesis: Epigenetic Silencing of Tumor Suppressors

Junpei Yamaguchi, Motoko Sasaki and Yasuni Nakanuma *

Department of Human Pathology,
Kanazawa University Graduate School of Medicine, Kanazawa, Japan

Abstract

Epigenetic mechanisms result in the silencing of genes without a change in their coding sequence. The most well-characterized alteration is DNA hypermethylation, and a modification of histones also contributes to tumor suppressor loss through epigenetic silencing.

Acetylation and deacetylation of histones play an important role in transcription regulation. The acetylation status of histones is determined by histone deacetylase (HDAC), and HDAC are strongly expressed in cancerous tissue. HDAC inhibitors are known to alter gene expression and to induce different phenotypes in various transformed cells, including growth arrest, apoptotic pathways and mitotic cell death. For example, the CDK inhibitor p21WAF1/CIP1 is one of most common genes induced by HDAC inhibitor.

Polycomb group proteins are epigenetic chromatin modifiers involved in cancer development. EZH2, one component of polycomb repressive complex, contain the signature domain providing the methylation active site, and its expression levels are abnormally elevated in malignant tissues. EZH2 mediates tumor suppressor genes such as p16INK4A and E-cadherin, affecting and controlling cell proliferation, differentiation

* Correspondence Address: Yasuni Nakanuma, M.D, Department of Human Pathology. Kanazawa University Graduate School of Medicine, Kanazawa 920-8640, Japan, Tel: +81-76-265-2197 (Japan), Fax: +81-76-234-4229 (Japan), E-mail: pbcpsc@kenroku.kanazawa-u.ac.jp

and invasiveness in cancer cells. As a consequence, a down-regulation of EZH2 induces significant growth inhibitory effects and represses its invasiveness in carcinoma cells.

HDAC and EZH2 are strongly expressed in cancer cells and they seem to interact each other and contribute to oncogenesis. HDAC inhibitor (SAHA) decreases EZH2 expression itself in carcinoma cells, in addition to HDAC repression. This double-repression effect might be an important mechanism in the anticancer effect of SAHA. Furthermore, HDAC inhibitor and/or EZH2-repression using siRNA affect trimethylated and acetylated levels at p16INK4A and E-cadherin promoter, and the combined treatment increases the expression level of p16INK4A and E-cadherin synergistically. Consequently, functional links between EZH2 and HDAC contribute to an emerging view that all these types of epigenetic silencing machinery play an important role in abnormal control of gene expression in malignant cells. Therefore, EZH2 and HDAC may be promising targets for treatment strategy.

Introduction

Deregulation of gene expression is a hallmark of cancer. Although genetic lesions have been the focus of cancer research for many years, it has been increasingly recognized that aberrant epigenetic modifications also play major roles in the tumorigenic process [1-3]. Epigenetic mechanisms, which involve DNA and histone modifications, result in the heritable silencing of genes without a change in their coding sequence. Chromatin alterations are causally related to the development and progression of malignant tumors. The most well-characterized alteration is CpG DNA hypermethylation, which contributes to tumor suppressor loss through epigenetic silencing, and epigenetic modification of histone is also implicated in oncogenesis. Both epigenetic changes and genetic alterations to DNA sequence in the malignant cell genome might contribute to disease progression. However, once the DNA sequence is changed by mutation, it is difficult to restore the gene. On the other hand, epigenetic changes can potentially be reserved with inhibitors that block the relevant chromatin-modifying enzymes. Thus, epigenetic silencing of the tumor suppressor gene in carcinoma has inspired potentially therapeutic strategies because of their dynamic nature and potential reversibility.

Epigenetic Modifications

DNA methylation and histone acetylation are major epigenetic modifications that are most intensively studied in the context of gene transcription and abnormal events that lead to oncogenic process. Evidence suggests that these marks are dynamically liked in the epigenetic control of gene expression and that their deregulation plays an important role in tumorigenesis [4]. Disruption of one of these two epigenetic marks inevitably affects the other. For example, hypermethylation of CpG island in gene promoters triggers deacetylation of local histone, whereas lower levels of histone acetylation seem to sensitize to targeted DNA methylation. Therefore, there is an intimate communication between histone acetylation and DNA methylation [1].

The methylation of DNA is the covalent addition of a methyl group to the five-carbon positions of cytosine basis in CpG dinucleotides. Cytosine methylation plays an important role in a number of central cellular functions. DNA methylation has gained wide importance, owing to implication of aberrant DNA methylation in human diseases, notably cancer [5, 6]. The methylation of CpG sites within the human genomes is maintained by a number of DNA methyltransferases (DNMTs) and has multifaceted roles for the silencing of transposable elements, for defense of viral sequences and for the transcriptional repression of certain genes. CpG islands, which are regions of more than 500 base pairs in size and with a GC content greater than 55 %, have been conserved during evolution because they are normally kept free of methylation. These stretches of DNA are located within the promoter regions of about 40 % of mammalian genes and, when methylated, cause stable heritable transcriptional silencing. Aberrant de novo methylation of CpG islands is a hallmark of human cancers and is found early during carcinogenesis [6].

Eukaryotic genomes are packaged into a highly compacted chromatin, which imposes constraints on gene transcription and other chromatin-based processes. To deal with this impediment, histone acetylation has evolved to open chromatin structure and facilitate accessibility of transcriptional machinery to DNA templates in chromatin. Histone acetylation is a reversible modification of specific residues in histone tails and is controlled by histone acetylases (HATs) and histone deacetylases (HDACs) that typically act as transcriptional co-activators and co-repressors, respectively. In addition to the acetylation of histone, methylation of conserved lysine residues on the amino-terminal tail domains have also defined as epigenetic modifiers and have been studied closely over the past few years. Generally, the acetylation of histones marks active, transcriptionally competent regions, whereas hypo-acetylated histones are found in transcriptionally inactive euchromatic or heterochromatic regions. Methylation of lysine 9 or 27 on the N terminus of histone H3 (H3-K9, H3-K27) is a hallmark of silent DNA and is globally distributed throughout heterochromatic regions such as centromeres and telomeres [7, 8]. In contrast, methylation of lysine 4 of histone H3 (H3-K4) denotes activity and is found predominantly at promoters of active genes [9, 10].

DNA methylation and histone modifications function in close interplay with nucleosome remodeling an positioning complex that bind specific histone modifications, such as tri-methylated H3K4 and methyl CpG binding proteins. The functional link between DNA methylation and histone modifications was initially established by studies showing that histone deacetylases (HDACs) are recruited to methylated DNA by methyl-CpG binding proteins [11, 12]. In general, regions silenced by DNA methylation also show hypoacethylation and hypermethylation of specific histone lysine residues, such as lysine 9 or 27 in histone H3 [8]. In addition, histone acetylation is thought to be able to prevent DNA methylation. This is supported by studies showing that the administration of HDAC inhibitors (HDACi), which restores the ability for the cell to acetylate histones, was able to increase the demethylation of promoters which were previously hypermethylated [13]. The use of HDACi like valporate (VPA) and Trichostatin (TSA) which influence DNA methylation was reported elsewhere, and strengthen the idea that histone acetylation may influence DNA methylation [14, 15].

Cancer and Epigenetics

When a general role for DNA methylation in gene silencing was established, it was proposed that aberrant patterns of DNA methylation might play a role in tumorigenesis. Initial studies found the occurrence of global hypomethylation in cancer, and this hypomethylation occurs mainly at DNA repetitive elements and might contribute to the genomic instability frequently seen in cancer [5]. Aberrant hypermethylation at normally unmethylated CpG islands occurs parallel to global hypomethylation. The CpG island promoter of the Rb (Retinoblastoma) gene, found to be hypermethylated in retinoblastoma, was the first tumor suppressor shown to harbor such a modification [16]. This discovery was soon followed by studies showing promoter hypermethylation and silencing of other tumor suppressor genes such as VHL (von Hippel-Lindau) in renal cancer [17], the cell cycle regulator CDKN2A/p16 in bladder cancer [18], the mismatch repair gene hMLH1 in colon cancer [19], and many others. On the basis of these findings, it was proposed that epigenetic silencing of tumor suppressor genes by DNA methylation can serve as an alternative hit to mutation. It is now established that aberrant hypermethylation at CpG island promoters is a hallmark of cancer.

In addition to DNA hypermethylation, transcriptional repression has been linked with histone deacetylation and histone methylation in carcinogenesis. Methylation at lysine residues in histones has been known for many years, but this modification was only recently recognized as crucially important for normal gene regulation [20, 21]. For example, methylation of lysine 9 in histone H3 correlates with silencing of the *CDKN2A* tumor suppressor in cancer cells [22]. Histone methylation is a parsimonious explanation for the perpetuation of silent epigenetic states through cell divisions, and the silent state can be maintained by a cycle of histone methylation, such as SUV39H1 histone methyltransferases followed by recruitment of the biding protein heterochromatin protein-1 (HP1). And also, RB has been shown to function as a brake on the cell cycle at least in part by establishing and enforcing stable epigenetic silencing of its target genes. It does this by participating in a multiprotein complex that includes chromatin-remodeling enzymes, as well as histone deacetylases (HDACs) [23, 24] and epigenetic silencing protein of the polycomb class [25]. Polycomb group complexes (PcGs) are protein complexes responsible for maintenance of long-term silencing of genes, which is mediated by methylation of lysine 27 of histone H3 at the repressed regions. The enzyme that catalyzes this modification is EZH2, which is known to be upregulated in tumors and involved in tumor progression.

HDACs and HDAC Inhibitors

Histone deacetylases can be grouped into three classes based on their homology to yeast enzymes. The first class contains HDACs 1-3 and 8 shows homology to the yeast enzyme RPD3. HDACs 4-7, 9, and 10 are grouped in the second class with similarity to the yeast HDA1 enzyme, while the third class of HDACs displays NAD-dependent deacetylation and homology to the yeast enzyme Sir2. Recent studies have disclosed that HDACs have many protein substrates involved in the regulation of gene expressions, cell proliferation, and cell death. Acetylation and deacetylation of histones plays an important role in the transcriptional regulation of cells and the acetylation status of histones and non-histone proteins is determined by HDACs [26-28]. A direct involvement of HDACs in human cancers is well documented in the case of promyelocytic leukemia (PML) [29], and recently, several reports showed that HDACs are strongly expressed in cancerous tissue, and the expression of class I HDACs is an independent prognostic marker in various cancers, such as ovarian, colorectal and cervical cancer [30-32].

Many inhibitors target either DNA methyltransferases or HDACs [26]. Inhibition of HDACs cause the accumulation of acetylated forms of histones with alteration of their function, and the CDK inhibitor $p21^{WAF1/CIP1}$ is one of the most common genes induced by HDAC inhibitor [33]. HDAC inhibitors are a group of recently discovered targeted anticancer agents. HDAC inhibitors induce different phenotypes in various transformed cells, including growth arrest, activation of extrinsic and/or intrinsic apoptotic pathways, autophagic cell death, mitotic cell death, and senescence [34]. In comparison, normal cells are relatively more resistant to HDAC inhibitor-induced cell death [35-37]. This selectivity of the effect can be beneficial when HDAC inhibitors are applied to clinical trials, but the mechanism underlying this difference is not well understood.

HDAC inhibitors have been found to have profound anticancer effects in clinical trials [38, 39]. Among HDAC inhibitors, suberoylanilide hydroxamic acid (SAHA) is one of the most advanced in clinical fields as an anticancer agent, which interacts directly with the catalytic site of HDAC-like protein and inhibits its enzymatic activity [28]. SAHA inhibits all 11 members of the class I and II HDAC family, and causes specific modifications in the pattern of acetylation and methylation of lysines in histones H3 and H4 associated with the proximal promoter of the p21 gene [28]. Although considerable progress has been made in elucidating the role of HDACs and the effects of HDAC inhibitors, these areas are still in the early stages of discovery.

Polycomb Group Protein

The polycomb group (PcG) proteins are transcriptional repressors that regulate lineage choices during development and differentiation [40]. Recent studies have advanced our understandings of how the PcG proteins regulate cell fate decisions and how their deregulation potentially contributes to cancer, and understanding this might facilitate the design of more effective cancer therapies.

The PcG proteins form multiprotein repressive complexes, called Polycomb Repressive Complexes (PRC), which repress transcription by a mechanism that probably involves the modification of chromatin [41, 42]. Two major PRCs have been described. The PRC2 complex contains the histone methyltransferase enhancer of zeste homologue 2 (EZH2), which together with embryonic ectoderm development (EED) and suppressor of zeste 12 homolog (SUZ12) catalyses the trimethylation of histone H3 at lysine K27 (H3K27me3). The EZH2 SET domain confers this activity. Multiple forms of the PRC1 complex exist and these contain combinations of at least four PC proteins (CBX2, CBX4, CBX7 and CBX8), six PSC proteins (BMI1, MEL18, MBLR, NSPC1, RNF159 and RNF3), two RING proteins (RNF1 and RNF2), three PH proteins (HPH1, HPH2 and HPH3) and two SCML proteins (SCML11 and SCML12).

Several genetic studies in different organisms have firmly established the vital and conserved role for PcG proteins in embryonic development and adult somatic cell differentiation [43]. Moreover, recent studies have demonstrated that the PcG proteins are required for maintaining correct identities of stem, progenitor and differentiated cells [44]. The PcG proteins have been found to bind and repress the promoters of genes that encode proteins with key roles in cell fate determination in many different cellular lineages. The examples of genes to which PcG proteins bind and repress are the *CDKN2B* and *CDKN2A*, which encode the tumor suppressors INK4B, INK4A and ARF [45, 46]. In addition to frequent genetic alterations, this locus is often epigenetically silenced by DNA methylation in cancer, and the PcG proteins have been proposed to contribute to this. The reports that EZH2 [47] and CBX7 [48] can physically associate with DNA methyltransferases (DNMTs) suggest a mechanism whereby the PcG proteins directly contribute to the altered DNA methylation profiles that are observed in multiple cancer types. These results suggest possibility that PcG proteins and DNA methylation enzymes cooperate to aberrantly silence pro-differentiation and anti-proliferative genes, which leads to the accumulation of a population of cells unable to respond to differentiation signals.

Among the histone modifications associated with gene silencing and cancer, much has been learned recently about the enzymes responsible for methylation of histone lysine residues [43, 49]. PRC2 contain a conserved catalytic subunit, EZH2, which contains the signature SET domain that provides the methyltransferase active site. Since the basic discovery that EZH2 functions as a chromatin-modifying enzyme, many reports have appeared that link EZH2 to the altered properties of cancer cells. The common findings is that EZH2 levels are abnormally elevated in cancer tissue versus corresponding normal tissues, with the highest EZH2 levels correlating with advanced stages of disease and poor prognosis. Among them, altered EZH2 levels have been most extensively documented in prostate and breast cancer [50, 51].

Interaction of HDAC and EZH2

In human cells, PRC2 interacts with class I HDAC [28], and recent data suggest that transient interactions likely provide functional synergy between the silencing enzymes for tumor suppressor genes *in vivo*. The precise mechanisms of this synergy are not yet clear. Functional links between EZH2 and HDACs contribute to an emerging view that all of these types of epigenetic silencing machinery contribute to abnormal control of gene expression in malignant cells.

We studied the expression pattern of HDCA1 and 2 in normal gallbladder epithelial cells and gallbladder carcinoma cells [37]. Unlike other organs such as ovary and colon [30-32], HDAC expression is not specific to carcinoma cells in gallbladder. HDAC 1 and 2 are expressed in the nuclei of non-neoplastic epithelial cells and carcinoma cells, however, expression levels are slightly weaker in the former than in the latter. Therefore, it is compatible to make a hypothesis that HDAC play a role in gallbladder carcinogenesis. To evaluate the effect of HDAC inhibitor, carcinoma cells and normal epithelial cells were treated with SAHA. This treatment reduced the number of carcinoma cells , but had no effect on the number of normal epithelial cells in spite of their HDAC expression. These differences in sensitivity to SAHA-induced cell reduction of carcinoma cells compared with normal cells appeared not to be caused by a difference in the expression levels of HDACs, because normal cells has relatively weak but significant expression level of HDACs, and moreover, it was found that the expression level of HDACs was significantly repressed in normal cells and carcinoma cells by SAHA treatment.

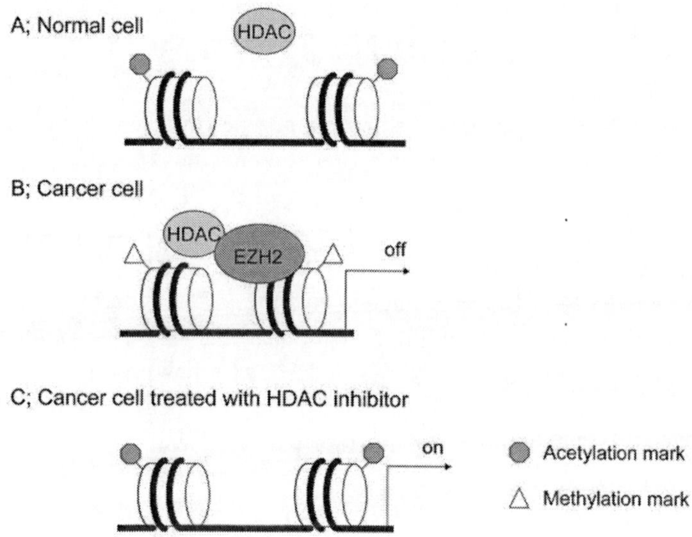

Figure 1. Hypothesis; collaboration of HDAC and EZH2.

In normal cells, HDAC are not recruited to histones and not responsible for repression of target genes (A). In cancer cells, target genes are silenced through histone deacetylation and methylation, which is caused by HDAC in collaboration with EZH2 (B). Treated with HDAC inhibitor (SAHA), HDAC and EZH2 is repressed. Histones are re-acetylated, resulting in the re-activation of silenced genes, such as p21$^{WAF1/CIP1}$, p16^{INK4A} and E-cadherin (C).

HDAC inhibitors are known to alter gene expression followed by the expression of the proteins responsible for composing the transcription factor complex to which HDACs are recruited [52]. We therefore examined whether tumor suppressor genes are activated by SAHA treatment. It was found that p21$^{WAF1/CIP1}$ was expressed in carcinoma cells but not in normal cells, indicating that HDACs forcibly repress the p21$^{WAF1/CIP1}$ gene in carcinoma cells, that inhibition of HDACs by SAHA treatment re-activated the p21$^{WAF1/CIP1}$ gene, and that HDACs are not responsible for p21$^{WAF1/CIP1}$ gene expression in normal cells.

Almost all carcinomas have multiple alterations in the expression and/or structure of proteins that regulate cell proliferation and death. The multiple alterations of tumor suppressor genes in cancer cells might explain why transformed cells are more sensitive than normal cells to the HDAC inhibitor. EZH2 are reported to mediate tumor suppressor genes, such as p16^{INK4A} and E-cadherin [45, 53]. In this context, the effect of HDAC inhibitor might be linked to EZH2 expression (Fig. 1). In the link between EZH2 and HDACs it has been reported to that PRC2-mediated transcriptional silencing is impeded by the HDAC inhibitor, trichostatin A (TSA) [51, 54]. Moreover, SAHA decreased EZH2 itself in carcinoma cells, in addition to HDAC repression [37]. Whether the mechanism by which HDAC inhibitors such as SAHA deplete EZH2 level is transcriptional, post-transcriptional, or increased protein degradation remains to be addressed in future study. From this point of view, the effect of SAHA on carcinoma cells might be associated with EZH2 expression, rather than HDACs expression.

Epigenetic Therapy

The epigenetic silencing of tumor suppressor genes in cancer has inspired potential therapeutic strategies that use inhibitors of epigenetic enzymes [55, 56]. A goal of epigenetic therapy is to achieve pharmacological reactivation of abnormally silenced genes in cancer patients, which could arrest or even reverse processes contributing to tumorigenesis. There are many inhibitors available that target either DNMTs or HDACs and clinical trials are underway to assess them [56]. Since epigenetic enzymes often synergize in vivo, there is also great interest in testing combined inhibitor treatments that target more than one epigenetic enzyme. Simultaneous disruption of DNMTs and HDACs has produced encouraging results on gene reactivation [3]. Some early clinical trials are beginning to test efficacies of combined DNMT/HDAC inhibitors in leukemia patients, with at least one study reporting reveral of DNA methylation and hematological improvement [57].

We found that the combination of SAHA treatment and EZH2 repression decreased cell numbers more than either single treatment [37]. It was disclosed that cell cycle arrest, not apoptosis, might be related to the synergistic effect of the combined treatment. Furthermore, this study showed that SAHA and/or EZH2 repression affect trimethylated and acetylated levels at the $p16^{INK4A}$ and E-cadherin promoter and the combined treatment increased the expression levels of $p16^{INK4A}$ and E-cadherin. Although the mechanism how the addition of EZH2 repression enhanced antitumor activity of SAHA remains to be clarified, EZH2 downregulation might affect other members of PRC2 and HDAC activity, which result in the enhanced antitumor effect of SAHA.

Similar to DNMTs and HDACs, EZH2 histone methyltransferase has emerged as a key target in potential epigenetic strategies. However, specific inhibitors of EZH2 histone methyltransferase have not yet been described. A high-resolution structure for the EZH2 SET domain, which houses the methyltransferase active site, would profoundly influence design of small molecule inhibitors specific for PRC2. The availability of these histone methyltransferase inhibitors should expand the repertoire of new possibilities in combined epigenetic therapy.

Conclusion

Epigenetic mechanisms, which involve DNA and histone modifications, result in the heritable silencing of genes without a change in their coding sequence. The study of human disease has shown that disruption of the balance of epigenetic networks can cause several major pathogenesis including cancer. Several inhibitors of enzymes controlling epigenetic modifications have anti-tumorigenic effects for some malignancies, and EZH2 and HDAC may be promising targets for treatment strategy.

References

[1] Vaissiere T, Sawan C, Herceg Z. Epigenetic interplay between histone modifications and DNA methylation in gene silencing. *Mutation Research-Reviews in Mutation Research* 2008; 659:40-48.

[2] Gal-Yam EN, Saito Y, Egger G, Jones PA. Cancer epigenetics: Modifications, screening, and therapy. *Annual Review of Medicine* 2008; 59:267-280.

[3] Egger G, Liang GN, Aparicio A, Jones PA. Epigenetics in human disease and prospects for epigenetic therapy. *Nature* 2004; 429:457-463.

[4] Fischle W, Wang YM, Allis CD. Binary switches and modification cassettes in histone biology and beyond. *Nature* 2003; 425:475-479.

[5] Feinberg AP, Tycko B. Timeline - The history of cancer epigenetics. *Nature Reviews Cancer* 2004; 4:143-153.

[6] Jones PA, Baylin SB. The fundamental role of epigenetic events in cancer. *Nature Reviews Genetics* 2002; 3:415-428.

[7] Lachner M, Jenuwein T. The many faces of histone lysine methylation. *Current Opinion in Cell Biology* 2002; 14:286-298.

[8] Kouzarides T. Chromatin modifications and their function. *Cell* 2007; 128:693-705.

[9] Heintzman ND, Stuart RK, Hon G, Fu YT, Ching CW, Hawkins RD, Barrera LO, et al. Distinct and predictive chromatin signatures of transcriptional promoters and enhancers in the human genome. *Nature Genetics* 2007; 39:311-318.

[10] Liang GN, Lin JCY, Wei VV, Yoo C, Cheng JC, Nguyen CT, Weisenberger DJ, et al. Distinct localization of histone H3 acetylation and H3-K4 methylation to the transcription start sites in the human genome. *Proceedings of the National Academy of Sciences of the United States of America* 2004; 101:7357-7362.

[11] Jones PL, Veenstra GJC, Wade PA, Vermaak D, Kass SU, Landsberger N, Strouboulis J, et al. Methylated DNA and MeCP2 recruit histone deacetylase to repress transcription. *Nature Genetics* 1998; 19:187-191.

[12] Nan XS, Ng HH, Johnson CA, Laherty CD, Turner BM, Eisenman RN, Bird A. Transcriptional repression by the methyl-CpG-binding protein MeCP2 involves a histone deacetylase complex. *Nature* 1998; 393:386-389.

[13] Dong E, Guidotti A, Grayson DR, Costa E. Histone hyperacetylation induces demethylation of reelin and 67-kDa glutamic acid decarboxylase promoters. *Proceedings of the National Academy of Sciences of the United States of America* 2007; 104:4676-4681.

[14] Milutinovic S, D'Alessio AC, Detich N, Szyf M. Valproate induces widespread epigenetic reprogramming which involves demethylation of specific genes. *Carcinogenesis* 2007; 28:560-571.

[15] Ou JN, Torrisani J, Unterberger A, Provencal N, Shikimi K, Karimi M, Ekstrom TJ, et al. Histone deacetylase inhibitor Trichostatin A induces global and gene-specific DNA demethylation in human cancer cell lines. *Biochemical Pharmacology* 2007; 73:1297-

1307.

[16] Greger V, Passarge E, Hopping W, Messmer E, Horsthemke B. Epigenetic changes may contribute to the formation and spontaneous regression of retinoblastoma. *Human Genetics* 1989; 83:155-158.

[17] Herman JG, Latif F, Weng YK, Lerman MI, Zbar B, Liu S, Samid D, et al. Silencing of the VHL tumor-suppressor gene by DNA methylation in renal-carcinoma. *Proceedings of the National Academy of Sciences of the United States of America* 1994; 91:9700-9704.

[18] Gonzalezzulueta M, Bender CM, Yang AS, Nguyen TD, Beart RW, Vantornout JM, Jones PA. Methylation of the 5'-CpG island of the p16/CDKN2 tumor-suppressor gene in normal and transformed human tissues correlates with gene silencing. *Cancer Research* 1995; 55:4531-4535.

[19] Kane MF, Loda M, Gaida GM, Lipman J, Mishra R, Goldman H, Jessup JM, et al. Methylation of the hMLH1 promoter correlates with lack of expression of hMLH1 in sporadic colon tumors and mismatch repair-defective human tumor cell lines. Cancer Research 1997;57:808-811.

[20] Rea S, Eisenhaber F, O'Carroll N, Strahl BD, Sun ZW, Schmid M, Opravil S, et al. Regulation of chromatin structure by site-specific histone H3 methyltransferases. Nature 2000; 406:593-599.

[21] Strahl BD, Ohba R, Cook RG, Allis CD. Methylation of histone H3 at lysine 4 is highly conserved and correlates with transcriptionally active nuclei in Tetrahymena. *Proceedings of the National Academy of Sciences of the United States of America* 1999; 96:14967-14972.

[22] Nguyen CT, Weisenberger DJ, Velicescu M, Gonzales FA, Lin JCY, Liang GN, Jones PA. Histone H3-lysine 9 methylation is associated with aberrant gene silencing in cancer cells and is rapidly reversed by 5-Aza-2 '-deoxycytidine. *Cancer Research* 2002; 62:6456-6461.

[23] Luo RX, Postigo AA, Dean DC. Rb interacts with histone deacetylase to repress transcription. *Cell* 1998; 92:463-473.

[24] Magnaghi-Jaulin L, Groisman R, Naguibneva I, Robin P, Lorain S, Le Villain JP, Troalen F, et al. Retinoblastoma protein represses transcription by recruiting a histone deacetylase. *Nature* 1998; 391:601-605.

[25] Dahiya A, Wong S, Gonzalo S, Gavin M, Dean DC. Linking the Rb and polycomb pathways. *Molecular Cell* 2001; 8:557-568.

[26] Lehrmann H, Pritchard LL, Harel-Bellan A. Histone acetyltransferases and deacetylases in the control of cell proliferation and differentiation. *Advances in Cancer Research*, Vol 86 2002; 86:41-65.

[27] Mai A, Massa S, Rotili D, Cerbara I, Valente S, Pezzi R, Simeoni S, et al. Histone deacetylation in epigenetics: An attractive target for anticancer therapy. *Medicinal Research Reviews* 2005; 25:261-309.

[28] Bhalla KN. Epigenetic and chromatin modifiers as targeted therapy of hematologic malignancies. *Journal of Clinical Oncology* 2005; 23:3971-3993.

[29] Melnick A, Licht JD. Deconstructing a disease: RAR alpha, its fusion partners, and their roles in the pathogenesis of acute promyelocytic leukemia. *Blood* 1999; 93:3167-3215.

[30] Weichert W, Denkert C, Noske A, Darb-Esfahani S, Dietel M, Kalloger SE, Huntsman

DG, et al. Expression of class I histone deacetylases indicates poor prognosis in endometrioid subtypes of ovarian and endometrial carcinomas. *Neoplasia* 2008; 10:1021-1027.

[31] Weichert W, Roske A, Niesporek S, Noske A, Buckendahl AC, Dietel M, Gekeler V, et al. Class I histone deacetylase expression has independent prognostic impact in human colorectal cancer: Specific role of class I histone deacetylases in vitro and in vivo. *Clinical Cancer Research* 2008; 14:1669-1677.

[32] Lin ZH, Bazzaro M, Wang MC, Chan KC, Peng SW, Roden RBS. Combination of Proteasome and HDAC Inhibitors for Uterine Cervical Cancer Treatment. *Clinical Cancer Research* 2009; 15:570-577.

[33] Gui CY, Ngo L, Xu WS, Richon VM, Marks PA. Histone deacetylase (HDAC) inhibitor activation of p21(WAF1) involves changes in promoter-associated proteins, including HDAC1. *Proceedings of the National Academy of Sciences of the United States of America* 2004; 1 01:1241-1246.

[34] Xu WS, Parmigiani RB, Marks PA. Histone deacetylase inhibitors: molecular mechanisms of action. *Oncogene* 2007; 26:5541-5552.

[35] Burgess A, Ruefli A, Beamish H, Warrener R, Saunders N, Johnstone R, Gabrielli B. Histone deacetylase inhibitors specifically kill nonproliferating tumour cells. *Oncogene* 2004; 23:6693-6701.

[36] Ungerstedt JS, Sowa Y, Xu WS, Shao Y, Dokmanovic M, Perez G, Ngo L, et al. Role of thioredoxin in the response of normal and transformed cells to histone deacetylase inhibitors. *Proceedings of the National Academy of Sciences of the United States of America* 2005; 102:673-678.

[37] Yamaguchi J, Sasaki M, Sato Y, Itatsu K, Harada K, Zen Y, Ikeda H, et al. Histone deacetylase inhibitor (SAHA) and repression of EZH2 synergistically inhibit proliferation of gallbladder carcinoma. *Cancer Science* 2010; 101:355-362.

[38] Marks PA, Breslow R. Dimethyl sulfoxide to vorinostat: Development of this histone deacetylase inhibitor as an anticancer drug. *Nature Biotechnology* 2007; 25:84-90.

[39] Tan JH, Cang SD, Ma YH, Petrillo RL, Liu DL. Novel histone deacetylase inhibitors in clinical trials as anti-cancer agents. Journal of *Hematology & Oncology* 2010; 3.

[40] Bracken AP, Helin K. Polycomb group proteins: navigators of lineage pathways led astray in cancer. *Nature Reviews Cancer* 2009; 9:773-784.

[41] Ohm JE, Baylin SB. Stem cell chromatin patterns - An instructive mechanism for DNA hypermethylation? *Cell Cycle* 2007; 6:1040-1043.

[42] Schlesinger Y, Straussman R, Keshet I, Farkash S, Hecht M, Zimmerman J, Eden E, et al. Polycomb-mediated methylation on Lys27 of histone H3 pre-marks genes for de novo methylation in cancer. *Nature Genetics* 2007; 39:232-236.

[43] Sparmann A, van Lohuizen M. Polycomb silencers control cell fate, development and cancer. *Nature Reviews Cancer* 2006; 6:846-856.

[44] Pietersen AM, van Lohuizen M. Stem cell regulation by polycomb repressors: postponing commitment. *Current Opinion in Cell Biology* 2008; 20:201-207.

[45] Bracken AP, Kleine-Kohlbrecher D, Dietrich N, Pasini D, Gargiulo G, Beekman C, Theilgaard-Monch K, et al. The Polycomb group proteins bind throughout the INK4A-ARF locus and are disassociated in senescent cells. *Genes & Development* 2007; 21:525-530.

[46] Dietrich N, Bracken AP, Trinh E, Schjerling CK, Koseki H, Rappsilber J, Helin K, et al.

Bypass of senescence by the polycomb group protein CBX8 through direct binding to the INK4A-ARF locus. *Embo Journal 2007*; 26:1637-1648.

[47] Vire E, Brenner C, Deplus R, Blanchon L, Fraga M, Didelot C, Morey L, et al. The Polycomb group protein EZH2 directly controls DNA methylation. *Nature* 2006; 439:871-874.

[48] Mohammad HP, Cai Y, McGarvey KM, Easwaran H, Van Neste L, Ohm JE, O'Hagan HM, et al. Polycomb CBX7 Promotes Initiation of Heritable Repression of Genes Frequently Silenced with Cancer-Specific DNA Hypermethylation. *Cancer Research* 2009; 69:6322-6330.

[49] Simon JA, Lange CA. Roles of the EZH2 histone methyltransferase in cancer epigenetics. *Mutation Research-Fundamental and Molecular Mechanisms of Mutagenesis* 2008; 647:21-29.

[50] Yu J, Rhodes DR, Tomlins SA, Cao X, Chen G, Mehra R, Wang X, et al. A polycomb repression signature in metastatic prostate cancer predicts cancer outcome. *Cancer Research* 2007; 67:10657-10663.

[51] Kleer CG, Cao Q, Varambally S, Shen RL, Ota L, Tomlins SA, Ghosh D, et al. EZH2 is a marker of aggressive breast cancer and promotes neoplastic transformation of breast epithelial cells. *Proceedings of the National Academy of Sciences of the United States of America* 2003; 100:11606-11611.

[52] Kuzmichev A, Nishioka K, Erdjument-Bromage H, Tempst P, Reinberg D. Histone methyltransferase activity associated with a human multiprotein complex containing the Enhancer of Zeste protein. *Genes & Development* 2002; 16:2893-2905.

[53] Cao Q, Yu J, Dhanasekaran SM, Kim JH, Mani RS, Tomlins SA, Mehra R, et al. Repression of E-cadherin by the polycomb group protein EZH2 in cancer. *Oncogene* 2008; 27:7274-7284.

[54] Varambally S, Dhanasekaran SM, Zhou M, Barrette TR, Kumar-Sinha C, Sanda MG, Ghosh D, et al. The polycomb group protein EZH2 is involved in progression of prostate cancer. *Nature* 2002; 419:624-629.

[55] Lyko F, Brown R. DNA methyltransferase inhibitors and the development of epigenetic cancer therapies. *Journal of the National Cancer Institute* 2005; 97:1498-1506.

[56] Yoo CB, Jones PA. Epigenetic therapy of cancer: past, present and future. Nature Reviews Drug Discovery 2006; 5:37-50.

[57] Gore SD, Jiemjit A, Silverman LB, Aucott T, Baylin S, Carraway H, Douses T, et al. Combined Methyltransferase/Histone deacetylase inhibition with 5Azacitidine and MS-275 in patients with MDS, CMMoL and AML: Clinical response, Histone Acetylation and DNA damage. *Blood* 2006; 108:517.

In: Tumor Suppressors
Editor: Susan D. Nguyen

ISBN: 978-1-61761-986-1

Chapter 9

Functions of Kank1 and Carcinogenesis

Naoto Kakinuma[1], Yun Zhu[2], Takunori Ogaeri[2], Jun-ichiro Suzuki[2] and Ryoiti Kiyama[2,*]

[1] Department of Anatomy and Cell Biology, Interdisciplinary Graduate School of Medicine & Engineering, University of Yamanashi, Japan

[2] Biomedical Research Institute, National Institute of Advanced Industrial Science and Technology (AIST), Japan

Abstract

The *Kank1* gene was found at 9p24 in a human chromosome showing loss of function through allelic loss/mutation/epigenetic modification in renal cell carcinoma cells. Loss or mutation of the gene has been found in cases of other diseases including cancers. The functions of the Kank1 protein, such as inhibition of cell migration, intracellular transport and cytokinesis, are discussed here in association with carcinogenesis/metastasis.

Introduction

More than 340,000 people die of cancer in Japan annually and the number is still increasing [1]. Owing to extensive search for the genes responsible for cancer, we now know a number of oncogenes and tumor suppressor genes. However, knowledge about cancer is not enough to cure or even properly diagnose it, as is evident in the statistics. Meanwhile, when the knowledge is applied for cancer therapy or diagnosis, it needs good techniques for good outcomes, and the demand for mechanism- and molecular-based techniques is increasing because we now know that proper targeting is crucial for the effective therapy and the

* Corresponding author, AIST Central 6, 1-1-1 Higashi, Tsukuba, Ibaraki 305-8566, Japan, E-mail address: kiyama.r@aist.go.jp

reduction of the side effect caused by drugs. Since bio-molecules mostly mediate signal from molecules at the cell membrane to those at various functional sites within the cell via specific pathways, the study about the signaling pathways will give important information about the targets. Here, we discuss potential targets in the signaling pathways related to the *Kank1* gene by focusing on several cellular functions.

1. *Kank1* as a Tumor Suppressor Gene

Genome subtraction combined with a comprehensive analysis of human chromosomes for loss of heterozygosity revealed a new gene, *Kank1* (or *KANK1* for the human gene), encoding a potential tumor suppressor for renal cell carcinoma (RCC) at 9p24 [2, 3]. The *Kank1* gene encodes an ankyrin-repeat domain-containing protein, and belongs to a family of genes that includes *Kank1*, *Kank2*, *Kank3*, and *Kank4* [2-4]. Deletions of the *KANK1* locus have been reported not only in RCC [2, 5] but also in other carcinomas, such as cervical carcinoma, bladder cancer, and lung cancer [6-8]. In addition, DNA microarray-based expression profiling of human lung cancer cell lines showed that *KANK1* is inactivated by epigenetic alterations [9]. Therefore, the loss of *Kank1* may be related to carcinogenesis. Moreover, the overexpression of *Kank1* suppressed cell growth and arrested the cell cycle at G_0/G_1 in HEK293 cells [2]. In addition, tumor growth was inhibited in nude mice, when *Kank1* was expressed in the tumor cells injected [2]. Furthermore, overexpression of Kank-family proteins decreased the formation of actin stress fibers [2, 4, 10]. These results suggest that *Kank1* and the other family members function as tumor suppressors.

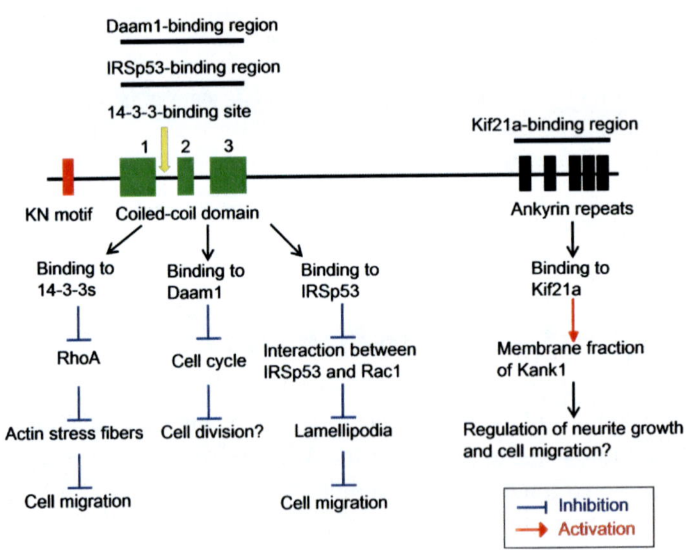

Figure 1. A schematic diagram showing the multiple domains of full-length Kank1 (Kank1-L; [3, 18]) and their potential functions. Kank1 inhibits the formation of actin stress fibers and lamellipodia through interaction with 14-3-3 and IRSp53, respectively, which results in negative regulation of cell migration. The membraneous fraction of Kank1 is increased when it binds to Kif21a, and this interaction may contribute to the regulation of neurite growth or cell migration. Kank1 is also involved in regulating cytokinesis possibly through binding to Daam1, which may inhibit cell division.

Kank1 may function in regulatory activities, relating to the actin cytoskeleton, cell migration, and the cell cycle [2, 10, 11; summarized in Figure 1). Kank1 protein has a motif at the N-terminus (the KN motif), five ankyrin-repeats at the C-terminus, and three coiled-coil motifs, and all these domains are conserved among the Kank-family [4]. According to yeast-two hybrid or mass-spectrometrical studies, Kank1 can directly bind to 14-3-3 proteins, the insulin receptor substrate (IRS) p53, KIF21A, and Disheveled-associated activator of morphogenesis 1 (Daam1) ([10-12], Suzuki et al., unpublished data). KIF21A is a member of the Kif4-class of kinesin motors and acts as a plus-end kinesin motor [13]. Heterozygous mutations in KIF21A cause congenital fibrosis of the extraocular muscles type 1 (CFEOM1), a disorder of eye movement accompanying bilateral ptosis and ophthalmoplegia [14]. Kank1 interacts with the third and fourth coiled-coil domains of KIF21A at its ankyrin-repeat domain. A major mutant of KIF21A found in patients with CFEOM1 (R954W) enhances the interaction with Kank1 and the translocation of Kank1 to the membrane [12]. Although the mechanisms involved need further study, the interaction of these two proteins may affect neurite outgrowth or cell migration.

14-3-3 is a family of acidic regulatory proteins found in all eukaryotes. 14-3-3 proteins act as molecular scaffolds by altering the conformation of their binding partners [15]. Among the seven isoforms of 14-3-3, 14-3-3θ, 14-3-3γ, 14-3-3η, and 14-3-3ε bind to Kank1 at its Akt-phosphorylation motif. This interaction regulates the activation of RhoA through the phoshoinositide 3-kinase (PI3K)/Akt signaling pathway, resulting in a decrease in actin stress fibers and the inhibition of cell migration [10]. IRSp53 was identified as another binding partner of Kank1, with Kank1 negatively regulating the formation of lamellipodia by inhibiting the interaction between Rac1 and IRSp53 [11]. The coiled-coil domain of Kank1 binds to another protein, Daam1. Daam1 belongs to a novel protein family containing formin homology domains and has been implicated in the regulation of cell polarity in association with the Wnt/Frizzled/Rho signaling pathway [16, 17]. Although how is not clear, the interaction results in the blocking of cytokinesis in some cancer cells (Suzuki et al., unpublished data). Below, we discuss advances in the study of Kank1 in association with the cytoskeleton, cell migration, and the cell cycle.

2. Function of Kank1 in Cell Migration

Cell migration is an essential process in all multicellular organisms and important not only during development but throughout life, for example, in wound repair and during immune surveillance. Cell migration is controlled by soluble factors, or local signals received from neighboring cells or the extracellular matrix. However, this control is lost when it comes to cancer cells. The mechanisms of cell migration have been studied extensively in tissue cultures, where the environment can be controlled and easily manipulated. In addition, genetic analyses of whole organisms have made significant contributions [19]. More recently, the dream of visualizing cell migration in live animals has become a reality through the direct imaging of fluorescently tagged cells [20]. It is now widely accepted that a major driving force of cell migration is the extension of the leading edge of cells, where a lamellipodial protrusion with filopodia is formed, establishment of new adhesion sites at the front, and detachment of adhesion sites at the rear (Figure 2) (reviewed in Raftopoulou and Hall, 2004, and Narumiya et al., 2009; [21, 22]). All these steps involve the assembly and disassembly of the actin cytoskeleton, and each must be coordinated both in space and in time to generate a productive, net forward movement. A huge variety of intracellular signaling molecules have been implicated in cell migration, such as MAPK-cascade mediators and PI3K-signaling molecules [23, 24]. However, one particular family of proteins seem to play a pivotal role in regulating the biochemical pathways most relevant to cell migration, the Rho-family GTPases, such as Rac1, Cdc42, and RhoA [21, 22, 25, 26]. Activated Rac1 and Cdc42 promote the formation of lamellipodia and filopodia, respectively, at the leading edge of migrating cells. The lamellipodium is composed of broad actin networks. The filopodium is a spike-like structure forming dendrites. Active RhoA promotes the formation of actin stress fibers in the cell body. Moreover, RhoA is activated at both the front and the rear of migrating cells, where it may function in the retraction of the cell tail, the turnover of focal adhesion sites, and the initiation of cell protrusion [22, 27]. Thus, the regulation of Rho-family GTPases is important for the control of cell migration. Kank1 regulates the Rac1-dependent formation of lamellipodia and the activity of RhoA, resulting in the inhibition of cell migration. This function is mediated through at least two signaling pathways: the regulation of Rac1 signaling through inhibition of Rac1's interaction with IRSp53, and the regulation of RhoA activity through PI3K/Akt signaling.

IRSp53 is a 'missing link' between Rac1 and WAVE2. Activated Rac1 binds to the N-terminal region of IRSp53, and the C-terminal Src-homology-3 (SH3) domain of IRSp53 binds to WAVE2, forming a trimolecular complex [28]. From studies of ectopic expression, Miki *et al.* found that IRSp53 is essential for Rac1 to induce membrane ruffling, probably because it recruits WAVE2 and stimulates actin polymerization mediated by the Arp2/3 complex [28]. The coiled-coil domain of Kank1 binds to the coiled-coil domain of IRSp53, which is also the site of interaction with active Rac1, with which Kank1 interferes. Indeed, overexpression of Kank1 inhibits the formation of lamellipodia induced by active Rac1 in NIH3T3 cells, while knockdown of Kank1 enhances it. Furthermore, endogenous Kank1 and IRSp53 are co-localized at sites of membrane protrusions such as lamellipodia. Thus, Kank1 may regulate the active-Rac1-dependent formation of lamellipodia at the leading edge of cells. Membrane protrusions form when cells are stimulated with growth factors such as insulin or when an integrin is stimulated with fibronectin [29, 30]. Kank1 inhibits their formation in both cases. Thus, Kank1 regulates membrane protrusions at the leading edge of cells, which is needed for cell migration, by preventing active Rac1 from interacting with IRSp53 [11].

PI3K/Akt signaling regulates multiple biological functions such as cell cycling, apoptosis, cell growth, and cell migration. This signaling is activated by insulin and various growth factors. Serine at position 167 of Kank1 is phosphorylated by Akt [10]. 14-3-3 binds to Kank1 through the 14-3-3 binding motif including this phosphorylated serine. The interaction between Kank1 and 14-3-3 is enhanced by growth factors such as insulin and epidermal growth factor (EGF).

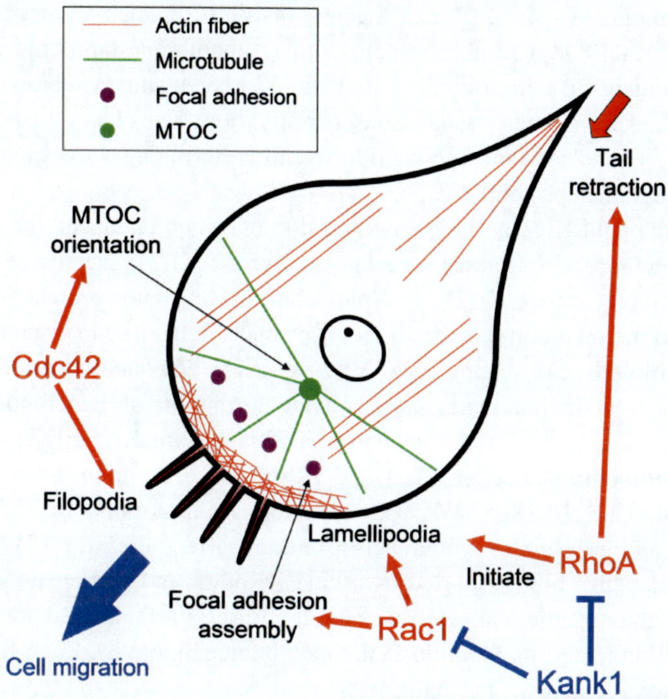

Figure 2. A scheme of cell migration. Cells perform a series of coordinated steps as follows: Cdc42 induces filopodia at the leading edge of cells and regulates the orientation of the microtubule-organizing center (MTOC) to control direction. Rac1 induces membrane protrusions and the integrin-mediated formation of adhesion complexes at the front of cells by activating actin polymerization. RhoA promotes the initiation of cell protrusion and tail retraction at the rear. Kank1 is involved by regulating RhoA and Rac1 activities.

Furthermore, this interaction regulates the formation of actin stress fibers. RhoA stimulates actin stress fibers [25], and the active form of RhoA enhances the formation of actin stress fibers and vinculin-containing focal adhesion sites [30]. Growth factors activate RhoA through PI3K/Akt signaling. Conversely, Kank1 inactivates active RhoA by retreaving 14-3 3 when the 14-3-3 binding motif of Kank1 is phosphorylated by Akt. RhoA also controls cell motility and invasion [31-33]. Cell migration is regulated by the interaction between Kank1 and 14-3-3 through inhibition of RhoA [10]. Thus, PI3K/Akt signaling is activated by stimulating cells with growth factors, which accelerates cell migration through activation of RhoA. At the same time, Kank1 may act as a negative regulator in this feedback system.

Taken together, Kank1 regulates cell migration through inhibition of IRSp53 in Rac1 signaling and inactivation of RhoA through PI3K/Akt signaling. As the *Kank1* locus shows loss of heterozygosity and the expression of the *Kank1* gene is suppressed in RCC cells as described above, Kank1 may contribute to the malignant transformation of cells and metastasis.

3. Kank1 and Intracellular Transport

Kank1 regulates cell migration by inhibiting Rac1 signaling and RhoA activity (Section 2; 10, 11]. To do this, it needs to be located at the leading edge of cells and affect the neighboring membrane. In fact, Kank1 occurs at sites of membrane ruffling such as lamellipodia [11]. Kank1 is a soluble protein with no membrane-targeting motif, such as a transmembrane domain or a lipid-binding domain. Moreover, no membrane-related protein associated with Kank1 has been found. Consequently, how Kank1 is transported to sites of membrane ruffling is unclear. One explanation would be through its association with Kif21a (or KIF21A for the human protein) [12].

Kank1 interacts with Kif21a, the overexpression of which enhanced the translocation of Kank1 to the membrane. In contrast, the knockdown of Kif21a decreased the amount of Kank1 at the membrane. Since Kif21a is a plus-end kinesin motor protein [13], it may help transport Kank1 to the membrane. Kinesin motor proteins deliver actin-organizing proteins to the leading edge of cells. For example, WAVE2, which is activated by active Rac1 through IRSp53 and induces actin polymerazation and the formation of lamellipodia [28, 34], is transported to the membrane through a kinesin motor protein, Kif5B [35], resulting in the formation of lamellipodia. As active Rac1 and IRSp53 also occur in lamellipodia [28], the distribution of the Rac1/IRSp53/WAVE2 complex is important to the formation of lamellipodia, and a kinesin motor protein acts as a transporter, at least, for WAVE2 [35]. Like WAVE2, Kank1 may also be transported by a kinesin motor and participate in the regulation of actin polymerization at the leading edge of cells. Based on this, we made a model of the transportation of Kank1 and its function at the membrane (Figure 3). First, Kank1 associates with Kif21a via some unknown mechanism. Second, Kank1 is transported to the membrane through microtubules with the help of Kif21a. Third, Kank1 is located in areas of membrane ruffling, such as lamellipodia, where there is a high level of actin polymerization mediated by active Rac1 and RhoA. Fourth, the inhibition of Rac1 signaling suppresses the activity of IRSp53 and RhoA at membrane ruffles. While Kank1 may regulate cell migration as a tumor suppressor, its translocation mediated by Kif21a may also be an important anti-metastatic step.

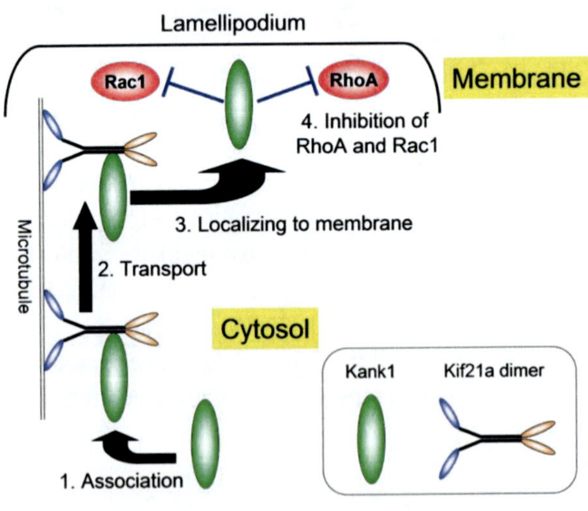

Figure 3. A model of the transportation of Kank1 and its function at the membrane. Kank1 associates with Kif21a via unknown mechanisms (step 1). The Kank/Kif21a complex is transported toward the membrane through microtubules (step 2). When the complex reaches the membrane, Kank1 is set free at lamellipodia (step 3). The Kank1 in lamellipodia stops Rac1-signaling by inhibiting IRSp53 and RhoA activity (step 4), which prevents lamellipodia from forming and results in the regulation of cell migration.

Kif21a is associated with CFEOM1. Kif21a mutations have been found in patients with CFEOM1 [14, 36], and one of the mutations (R954W) enhances the association of Kif21a with Kank1 and the translocation of Kank1 to the membrane compared with wild-type Kif21a [12]. Kif21a may be important to the develpment of the oculomoter nerve in embryogenesis [14, 37]. In addition, the activation of Rac1 is essential for the extension of axons in neuronal cells [reviewed in Luo, 2000; 38]. As Kank1 inhibits neurite outgrowth [11], we hypothesized that the Kif21a mutation enhances its association with Kank1, resulting in too much Kank1 being transported to the top of axons in the oculomotor nerve, where it inhibits Rac1 activity. As a result, axons of the oculomotor nerve may not be able to extend toward oculomotor muscles including the levator palpebrae superioris.

4. Function of Kank1 in Cell Division

Overexpression of Kank1 suppresses cell cycling and cell growth [2]. However, the mechanism involved has not been elucidated. We observed that the overexpression of Kank1 blocked cytokinesis and generated binucleate cells (Suzuki et al., unpublished results). Cytokinesis is a step in the separation of the cytoplasm after nuclear division at the final stage of mitosis [39, 40]. Its failure results in the generation of polyploid cells [41]. In these cells, the cell cycle is arrested through activation of a tumor suppressor, p53 protein. This p53 protein and several other tumor suppressors, BRCA1, LATS1 and LAPSER1, also regulate cytokinesis [42-45]. Moreover, drugs that target cytokinesis, such as an inhibitor of Aurora kinase, have been developed for treating cancer [46, 47]. Thus, cytokinesis is also a key process for tumor suppression.

During cytokinesis, a single cell divides into two daughter cells through four steps: the formation of a cleavage furrow (step 1); the assembly of a contractile ring (step 2); the constriction of the cleavage furrow (step 3); and the abscission of daughter cells (step 4). The contractile ring, important for the constriction of the cytoplasm, is assembled from actin and myosin. RhoA is a key regulator of its formation and of the cleavage furrow's ingression [48-50]. In RhoA inhibited or depleted cells, cytokinesis is impaired [51, 52]. RhoA activates downstream effectors to induce ingression of the cleavage furrow by activating myosin. Downstream effectors of RhoA involved in cytokinesis include a Rho-dependent kinase, Rock [53], and Citron kinase [54, 55], both implicated in myosin activity. Myosin consists of two heavy chains, two essential light chains, and two regulatory myosin light chains (MLCs). The activity of myosin depends on the phosphorylation of MLCs, which is regulated by Rock [53, 56], Citron kinase [57] and MLC kinase [58]. Activated myosin binds to actin in the contractile ring and induces the constriction of the cytoplasm. Thus, RhoA is required in cytokinesis to regulate the constriction of the contractile ring.

We observed the colocalization of endogenous Kank1 with Rho at the contractile ring during the cytokinesis of NIH3T3 cells (Figure 4A). Kank1 inhibits the activation of RhoA by binding to upstream signaling molecules such as Daam1, which is activated through a non-canonical Wnt signaling pathway [16, 17]. Kank1 may block cytokinesis by regulating Rho activity through interaction with Daam1 (Figure 4B). This may reveal a new way of regulating cytokinesis and tumor suppression.

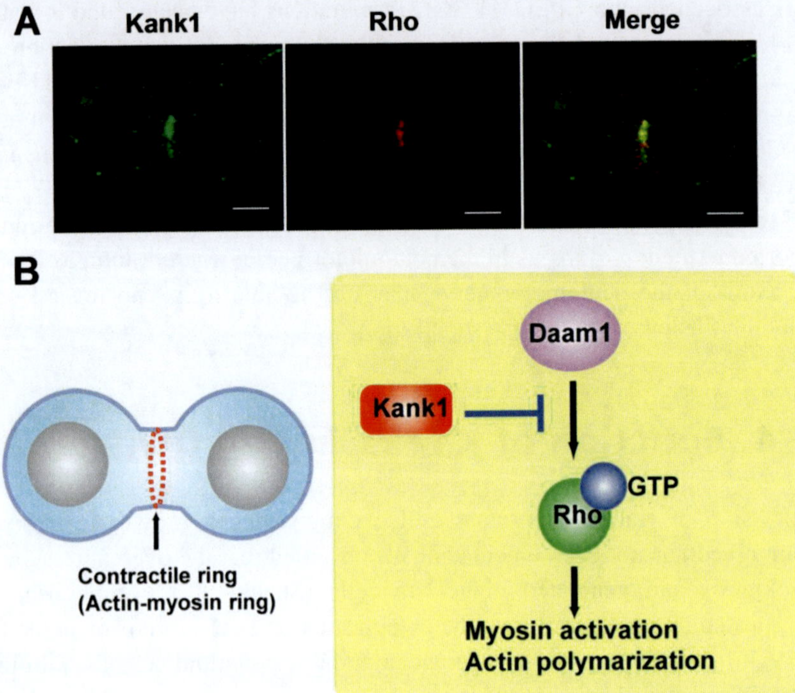

Figure 4. (**A**) Kank1 is co-localized with Rho in a contractile ring. NIH3T3 cells in anaphase were stained with an anti-Kank1 polyclonal antibody (green) and an anti-Rho monoclonal antibody (red). Bar: 10 μm. (**B**) A hypothetical model of the regulation of cytokinesis by Kank1. Kank1 inhibits Rho's activation by binding to Rho-regulating proteins, and activation of myosin and actin polymerization are not induced when Rho activity is inhibited. Therefore, Kank1 may play a role in the negative regulation of cytokinesis.

Conclusion

The *Kank1* gene was obtained by positional cloning from the region potentially responsible for sporadic RCC [2]. Some characteristics of the gene, loss of functions in RCC and growth suppression of tumor cells at G_0/G_1, suggest it to be a tumor suppressor gene. However, its relationship with tumorigenesis is still not clear despite an extensive search for tumor suppressors or related proteins interacting with Kank1. We have found several proteins interacting with Kank1, including IRSp53, 14-3-3, Kif21a, and Daam1. These proteins are related to cell migration (Section 2), intracellular transport (Section 3), and cell division (Section 4). Although they are not tumor suppressors or directly related to tumorigenesis, their roles in cells are important for understanding the role of Kank1 in tumorigenesis.

There are two cellular functions that could be related to the role of Kank1 as a tumor suppressor. One is the inhibition of cell migration, and the other is the inhibition of the cell cycle. Changes in cell migration are important to tumorigenesis. When tumor cells become malignant (as in the case of metastasis), cell migration can be enhanced significantly. A number of reports described the involvement of signal mediators related to cell migration, or more specifically, cell adhesion, such as Rho-family proteins (reviewed in Evers et al., 2000; [59]). Some regulators of cell migration are also known as tumor suppressors, including

DLC1, gelsolin and DCC (reviewed in Stafford et al., 2008; [60]). Meanwhile, oncogenes generally enhance cell growth, and classic tumor suppressors, such as pRB and p16 [61-63], are also cell-cycle regulators. While *Kank1* was found as a tumor suppressor gene, how its function is related to tumor suppression is not yet known. However, knowledge about the regulatory mechanism of cell migration and cell cycle would provide clues to understanding the function of Kank1 as a tumor suppressor.

References

[1] Cancer statistics in Japan 2008. *Foundation of cancer research* (2008).

[2] Sarkar, S; Roy, BC; Hatano, N; Aoyagi, T; Gohji, K; Kiyama, R. A novel ankyrin repeat-containing gene *(Kank)* located at 9p24 is a growth suppressor of renal cell carcinoma. *J Biol Chem*. (2002) 277(39): 36585-36591.

[3] Kakinuma, N; Zhu, Y; Wang, Y; Roy, BC; Kiyama, R. Kank proteins: structure, functions and diseases. *Cell Mol Life Sci*. (2009) 66(16): 2651-2659.

[4] Zhu, Y; Kakinuma, N; Wang, Y; Kiyama, R. Kank proteins: a new family of ankyrin-repeat domain-containing proteins. *Biochim Biophys Acta.* (2008) 1780 (2): 128-133.

[5] Roy, BC; Aoyagi, T; Sarkar, S; Nomura, K; Kanda, H; Iwaya, K; Tachibana, M; Kiyama, R. Pathological characterization of Kank in renal cell carcinoma. *Exp Mol Pathol*. (2005) 78(1): 41-48.

[6] Zimonjic, DB; Simpson, S; Popescu, NC; DiPaolo, JA. Molecular cytogenetics of human papillomavirus-negative cervical carcinoma cell lines. *Cancer Genet Cytogenet*. (1995) 82(1): 1-8.

[7] Simon, R; Burger, H; Semjonow, A; Hertle, L; Terpe, HJ; Bocker, W. Patterns of chromosomal imbalances in muscle invasive bladder cancer. *Int J Oncol.* (2000) 17(5): 1025-1029.

[8] Lo, KC; Stein, LC; Panzarella, JA; Cowell, JK; Hawthorn, L. Identification of genes involved in squamous cell carcinoma of the lung using synchronized data from DNA copy number and transcript expression profiling analysis. *Lung Cancer*. (2008) 59(3): 315-331.

[9] Kohno, T; Otsuka, A; Girard, L; Sato, M; Iwakawa, R; Ogiwara, H; Sanchez-Cespedes, M; Minna, JD; Yokota, J. A catalog of genes homozygously deleted in human lung cancer and the candidacy of PTPRD as a tumor suppressor gene. *Genes Chromosomes Cancer*. (2010) 49(4): 342-352.

[10] Kakinuma, N; Roy, BC; Zhu, Y; Wang, Y; Kiyama, R. Kank regulates RhoA-dependent formation of actin stress fibers and cell migration via 14-3-3 in PI3K-Akt signaling. *J Cell Biol*. (2008) 181(3): 537-549.

[11] Roy, BC; Kakinuma, N; Kiyama, R. Kank attenuates actin remodeling by preventing interaction between IRSp53 and Rac1. *J Cell Biol*. (2009) 184(2): 253-267.

[12] Kakinuma, N; Kiyama, R. A major mutation of KIF21A associated with congenital fibrosis of the extraocular muscles type 1 (CFEOM1) enhances translocation of Kank1 to the membrane. *Biochem Biophys Res Commun*. (2009) 386(4): 639-644.

[13] Marszalek, JR; Weiner, JA; Farlow, SJ; Chun, J; Goldstein, LS. Novel dendritic kinesin sorting identified by different process targeting of two related kinesins: KIF21A and KIF21B. *J Cell Biol.* (1999) 145(3): 469-479.
[14] Yamada, K; Andrews, C; Chan, WM; McKeown, CA; Magli, A; de Berardinis, T; Loewenstein, A; Lazar, M; O'Keefe, M; Letson, R; London, A; Ruttum, M; Matsumoto, N; Saito, N; Morris, L; Del Monte, M; Johnson, RH; Uyama, E; Houtman, WA; de Vries, B; Carlow, TJ; Hart, BL; Krawiecki, N; Shoffner, J; Vogel, MC; Katowitz, J; Goldstein, SM; Levin, AV; Sener, EC; Ozturk, BT; Akarsu, AN; Brodsky, MC; Hanisch, F; Cruse, RP; Zubcov, AA; Robb, RM; Roggenkäemper, P; Gottlob, I; Kowal, L; Battu, R; Traboulsi, EI; Franceschini, P; Newlin, A; Demer, JL; Engle, EC. Heterozygous mutations of the kinesin KIF21A in congenital fibrosis of the extraocular muscles type 1 (CFEOM1). *Nat Genet.* (2003) 35(4): 318-321.
[15] Mhawech, P. 14-3-3 proteins--an update. *Cell Res.* (2005) 15(4): 228-236.
[16] Habas, R; Kato, Y; He, X. Wnt/Frizzled activation of Rho regulates vertebrate gastrulation and requires a novel Formin homology protein Daam1. *Cell.* (2001) 107 (7): 843–854.
[17] Liu, W; Sato, A; Khadka, D; Bharti, R; Diaz, H; Runnels, LW; Habas, R. Mechanism of activation of the Formin protein Daam1. *Proc Natl Acad Sci USA.* (2008)105 (1): 210–215.
[18] Wang, Y; Onishi, Y; Kakinuma, N; Roy, BC; Aoyagi, T; Kiyama, R. Alternative splicing of the human Kank gene produces two types of Kank protein. *Biochem Biophys Res Commun.* (2005) 330(4): 1247-1253.
[19] Lehmann, R. Cell migration in invertebrates: clues from border and distal tip cells. *Curr Opin Genet Dev.* (2001) 11(4): 457-463.
[20] Ahmed, F; Wyckoff, J; Lin, EY; Wang, W; Wang, Y; Hennighausen, L; Miyazaki, J; Jones, J; Pollard, JW; Condeelis, JS; Segall, JE. GFP expression in the mammary gland for imaging of mammary tumor cells in transgenic mice. *Cancer Res.* (2002) 62(24): 7166-7169.
[21] Raftopoulou, M; Hall, A. Cell migration: Rho GTPases lead the way. *Dev Biol.* (2004) 265(1): 23-32.
[22] Narumiya, S; Tanji, M; Ishizaki, T. Rho signaling, ROCK and mDia1, in transformation, metastasis and invasion. *Cancer Metastasis Rev.* (2009) 28(1-2): 65-76.
[23] Huang, C; Jacobson, K; Schaller, MD. MAP kinases and cell migration. *J Cell Sci.* (2004) 117(Pt 20): 4619-4628.
[24] Cain, RJ; Ridley, AJ. Phosphoinositide 3-kinases in cell migration. (2009) 101(1): 13-29.
[25] Ridley, A.J. and Hall, A. The small GTP-binding protein rho regulates the assembly of focal adhesions and actin stress fibers in response to growth factors. *Cell.* (1992) 70(3): 389-399.
[26] Ridley, AJ. The small GTP-binding protein rac regulates growth factor-induced membrane ruffling. *Cell.* (1992) 70(3): 401-410.
[27] Machacek, M; Hodgson, L; Welch, C; Elliott, H; Pertz, O; Nalbant, P; Abell, A; Johnson, GL; Hahn, KM; Danuser, G. Coordination of Rho GTPase activities during cell protrusion. *Nature.* (2009) 461(7260): 99-103.

[28] Miki, H; Yamaguchi, H; Suetsugu, S; Takenawa, T. IRSp53 is an essential intermediate between Rac and WAVE in the regulation of membrane ruffling. *Nature*. (2000) 408(6813): 732-735.

[29] Price, LS; Leng, J; Schwartz, MA; Bokoch, GM. Activation of Rac and Cdc42 by integrins mediates cell spreading. *Mol Biol Cell*. (1998) 9(7); 1863-1871.

[30] Nobes, CD; Hall, A. Rho, rac, and cdc42 GTPases regulate the assembly of multimolecular focal complexes associated with actin stress fibers, lamellipodia, and filopodia. *Cell*. (1995) 81(1): 53-62.

[31] Takaishi, K; Kikuchi, A; Kuroda, S; Kotani, K; Sasaki, T; Takai, Y. Involvement of rho p21 and its inhibitory GDP/GTP exchange protein (rho GDI) in cell motility. *Mol Cell Biol*. (1993) 13(1): 72-79.

[32] Yoshioka, K; Nakamori, S; Itoh, K. Overexpression of small GTP-binding protein RhoA promotes invasion of tumor cells. *Cancer Res*. (1999) 59(8): 2004-2010.

[33] Kurokawa, K; Matsuda, M. Localized RhoA activation as a requirement for the induction of membrane ruffling. *Mol Biol Cell*. (2005) 16(9): 4294-4303.

[34] Suetsugu, S; Kurisu, S; Oikawa, T; Yamazaki, D; Oda, A and Takenawa, T. Optimization of WAVE2 complex-induced actin polymerization by membrane-bound IRSp53, PIP(3), and Rac. *J Cell Biol*. (2006) 173(4): 571-585.

[35] Takahashi, K and Suzuki, K. Requirement of kinesin-mediated membrane transport of WAVE2 along microtubules for lamellipodia formation promoted by hepatocyte growth factor. *Exp Cell Res*. (2008) 314(11-12): 2313-2322.

[36] Yamada, K; Hunter, DG; Andrews, C and Engle, EC. A novel KIF21A mutation in a patient with congenital fibrosis of the extraocular muscles and Marcus Gunn jaw-winking phenomenon. *Arch Ophthalmol*. (2005) 123(9): 1254-1259.

[37] Engle, EC; Goumnerov, BC; Mckeown, CA; Schatz, M; Johns, DR; Porter, JD and Beggs, AH. Oculomotor nerve and muscle abnormalities in congenital fibrosis of the extraocular muscles. *Ann Neurol*. (1997) 41(3): 314-325.

[38] Luo, L. Rho GTPases in neuronal morphogenesis. *Nat Rev Neurosci*. (2000) 1(3): 173-180.

[39] Robinson, DN; Spudich, JA. Mechanics and regulation of cytokinesis. *Curr Opin Cell Biol*. (2004) 16(2): 182-188.

[40] Wolf, WA; Chew, TL; Chisholm, RL. Regulation of cytokinesis. *Cell Mol Life Sci*. (1999) 55(1): 108-120.

[41] Ganem, NJ; Pellman, D. Limiting the proliferation of polyploid cells. *Cell*. (2007) 131(3): 437-40.

[42] Tarapore, P; Fukasawa, K. Loss of p53 and centrosome hyperamplification. *Oncogene*. (2002) 21(40): 6234-6240.

[43] Xu, X; Weaver, Z; Linke, SP; Li, C; Gotay, J; Wang, XW; Harris, CC; Ried, T; Deng, CX. Centrosome amplification and a defective G2-M cell cycle checkpoint induce genetic instability in BRCA1 exon 11 isoform-deficient cells. *Mol Cell*. (1999) 3(3): 389-395.

[44] Yang, X; Yu, K; Hao, Y; Li, DM; Stewart, R; Insogna, KL; Xu, T. LATS1 tumour suppressor affects cytokinesis by inhibiting LIMK1. *Nat Cell Biol*. (2004) 6(7): 609-617.

[45] Sudo, H; Maru, Y. LAPSER1 is a putative cytokinetic tumor suppressor that shows the same centrosome and midbody subcellular localization pattern as p80 katanin. *FASEB J*. (2007) 21(9): 2086-2100.

[46] Harrington, EA; Bebbington, D; Moore, J; Rasmussen, RK; Ajose-Adeogun, AO; Nakayama, T; Graham, JA; Demur, C; Hercend, T; Diu-Hercend, A; Su, M; Golec, JM; Miller, KM. VX-680, a potent and selective small-molecule inhibitor of the Aurora kinases, suppresses tumor growth in vivo. *Nat Med*. (2004) 10(3): 262-267.

[47] Atilla-Gokcumen, GE; Castoreno, AB; Sasse, S; Eggert, US. Making the cut: the chemical biology of cytokinesis. *ACS Chem Biol*. (2010) 5(1): 79-90.

[48] Kamijo, K; Ohara, N; Abe, M; Uchimura, T; Hosoya, H; Lee, JS; Miki, T. Dissecting the role of Rho-mediated signaling in contractile ring formation. *Mol Biol Cell*. (2006) 17(1): 43-55.

[49] Li, J; Wang, J; Jiao, H; Liao, J; Xu, X. Cytokinesis and cancer: Polo loves ROCK'n' Rho(A). *J Genet Genomics*. (2010) 37(3): 159-172.

[50] Piekny, A; Werner, M; Glotzer, M. Cytokinesis: welcome to the Rho zone. *Trends Cell Biol*. (2005) 15(12): 651-658.

[51] Kishi K; Sasaki T; Kuroda S; Itoh T; Takai Y. Regulation of cytoplasmic division of Xenopus embryo by rho p21 and its inhibitory GDP/GTP exchange protein (rho GDI). *J Cell Biol*. (1993) 120(5): 1187-1195.

[52] Jantsch-Plunger, V; Gönczy, P; Romano, A; Schnabel, H; Hamill, D; Schnabel, R; Hyman, AA; Glotzer, M. CYK-4: A Rho family gtpase activating protein (GAP) required for central spindle formation and cytokinesis. *J Cell Biol*. (2000) 149(7): 1391-1404.

[53] Kosako, H; Yoshida, T; Matsumura, F; Ishizaki, T; Narumiya, S; Inagaki, M. Rho-kinase/ROCK is involved in cytokinesis through the phosphorylation of myosin light chain and not ezrin/radixin/moesin proteins at the cleavage furrow. *Oncogene*. (2000) 19(52): 6059-6064.

[54] Eda, M; Yonemura, S; Kato, T; Watanabe, N; Ishizaki, T; Madaule, P; Narumiya, S. Rho-dependent transfer of Citron-kinase to the cleavage furrow of dividing cells. *J Cell Sci*. (2001) 114(Pt 18): 3273-3284.

[55] Madaule, P; Eda, M; Watanabe, N; Fujisawa, K; Matsuoka, T; Bito, H; Ishizaki, T; Narumiya, S. Role of citron kinase as a target of the small GTPase Rho in cytokinesis. *Nature*. (1998) 394(6692): 491-494.

[56] Amano, M; Ito, M; Kimura, K; Fukata, Y; Chihara, K; Nakano, T; Matsuura, Y; Kaibuchi, K. Phosphorylation and activation of myosin by Rho-associated kinase (Rho-kinase). *J Biol Chem*. (1996) 271(34): 20246-20249.

[57] Yamashiro, S; Totsukawa, G; Yamakita, Y; Sasaki, Y; Madaule, P; Ishizaki, T; Narumiya, S; Matsumura, F. Citron kinase, a Rho-dependent kinase, induces di-phosphorylation of regulatory light chain of myosin II. *Mol Biol Cell*. (2003) 14(5): 1745-1756.

[58] Matsumura, F; Totsukawa, G; Yamakita, Y; Yamashiro, S. Role of myosin light chain phosphorylation in the regulation of cytokinesis. *Cell Struct Funct*. (2001) 26(6): 639-644.

[59] Evers, EE; Zondag, GC; Malliri, A; Price, LS; ten Klooster, JP; van der Kammen, RA; Collard, JG. Rho family proteins in cell adhesion and cell migration. *Eur J Cancer*. (2000) 36(10): 1269-1274.

[60] Stafford, LJ; Vaidya, KS; Welch, DR. Metastasis suppressors genes in cancer. *Int J Biochem Cell Biol*. (2008) 40(5): 874-891.

[61] Chellappan, SP; Hiebert, S; Mudryj, M; Horowitz, JM; Nevins, JR. The E2F transcription factor is a cellular target for the RB protein. *Cell*. (1991) 65(6): 1053-1061.

[62] Kamb, A; Gruis, NA; Weaver-Feldhaus, J; Liu, Q; Harshman, K; Tavtigian, SV; Stockert, E; Day, RS 3rd; Johnson, BE; Skolnick, MH. A cell cycle regulator potentially involved in genesis of many tumor types. *Science*. (1994) 264(5157): 436-440.

[63] Nobori, T; Miura, K; Wu, DJ; Lois, A; Takabayashi, K; Carson, DA. Deletions of the cyclin-dependent kinase-4 inhibitor gene in multiple human cancers. *Nature*. (1994) 368(6473): 753-756.

In: Tumor Suppressors
Editor: Susan D. Nguyen

ISBN: 978-1-61761-986-1

Chapter 10

The Relationship Between MicroRNA and Tumor Suppressors

Douglus Wu and Mary Waye*

School of Biomedical Sciences, The Chinese University of Hong Kong, Shatin, N.T. Hong Kong

Abstract

This review attempts to examine some of evidence that support the role of microRNA in tumor suppression, and to review those reports that shown promise of alteration of microRNAs as a strategy for cancer therapy. There are several ways that microRNA can affect tumor suppressors. Some reports have demonstrated that MicroRNA can act as tumor suppressors themselves (e.g. let-7, mir-125a), while others have shown that they act by affecting the up-stream regulators of tumor suppressors or downstream targets of oncogenes. The picture is also complicated by the fact that some microRNAs are regulated by other microRNAs (e.g. miR 16-1 precursor abolishes the expression of the mature miR-16), and some microRNAs can be regulated by oncogenes (e.g. miR-17-92 is regulated by c-Myc).

Introduction

There is an increasing body of evidence that shows microRNAs are implicated in carcinogenesis (as reviewed by Chen 2005), this is not surprising because of the following reasons:

* Corresponding author: Mary Waye, Ph.D., Professor, School of Biomedical Sciences, The Chinese University of Hong Kong, Shatin, N.T. Hong Kong, Tel: (852)26096874, Fax: (852)26037732, Email: mary-waye@cuhk.edu.hk

1. In lower organisms, microRNAs have been shown to play an important role in genetic programs including apoptosis, proliferation, differentiation, development and metabolism- which are the same programs central to tumor formation.
2. Target proteins of microRNAs have been shown to include various signaling molecules, cytokines, growth factors, transcription factors, proteins related to apoptosis and angiogenesis, etc which are molecules known to be important in tumor formation.
3. According to recent computational predictions, as many as 200 target genes can be regulated by a single microRNA, which implies that over one third of protein-coding genes in humans are regulated by microRNAs, and therefore even by random chance one third of oncogenes and tumor suppressors would be expected to be targets of microRNAs.
4. It was shown that microRNA microarrays are more effective in cancer classification than mRNA microarrays (Lu et al, 2005).

MicroRNA and Cancer Cells

The role of microRNAs is evidenced in many different steps of tumorigenesis: including the enhancement of the cancer cells' self-sufficiency in replication or growth, their independence of extrinsic signals to proliferate, or their insensitivity to antigrowth signals such as contact inhibition, their abnormal apoptosis pattern (Garofalo et al, 2010), abnormal angiogenesis, and tissue invasion or metastasis (Santarpia et al, 2010; Zhang et al, 2010). Negrini and Calin 2008 have summerized the findings of microRNA dysregulation in breast cancer, including 3 major studies: miR-10b indirectly activates the pro-metastatic gene RHOC by suppressing HOXD10, miR-373 and miR-520c function by regulating the gene CD44 and the loss of miR-335 leads to the activation of SOX4 and TNC (encoding tenascin C) (Negrini and Calin, 2008). The dysregulation is not limited to female breast cancer but also male breast cancer, as miR-21, miR519d, miR-183, miR-197, and miR-493-5p were identified as most prominently up-regulated, miR-145 and miR-497 as most prominently down-regulated in male breast cancer (Lehmann et al., 2010).

According to Yu, miR-96 directly targets the KRAS oncogene and functions as a tumor-suppressing miRNA in pancreatic cancer cells. Ectopic expression of miR-96 through a synthetic miRNA precursor inhibited KRAS, dampened Akt signaling, and triggered apoptosis in cells. In human clinical specimens, miR-96 was downregulated or deleted where an association with KRAS elevations was observed. The same group identified miR-96 as a potent regulator of KRAS (Yu et al., 2010).

A. MicroRNA as Tumor Suppressors

Using different breast carcinoma cells and correlation of gene expression level of HuR and the microRNA mir-125a, Guo et al, have concluded that miR-125a may function as a tumor suppressor for breast cancer, with HuR as a direct and functional target. This confirms earlier observation that microRNA such as let-7 is reduced in human lung cancers.

microRNA	Protein Target	Tumor	Reference:
miR-125a	HuR	Human Breast Cancer, difference carcinoma cell lines, e.g. MCF-7 breast cancer cells	Guo et al., 2009
Reduced let-7	mlin 41	Human Lung Cancers	Takamizawa et al., 2004
miR-335, miR-206, and miR-126	SOX4 and TNC (encoding tenascin C)	Breast cancer	Reviewed by Negrini and Calin 2008

B. MicroRNA Acting as Regulators of Tumor Suppressors Either by Positive Regulation (i.e. activation of tumor suppressors) or by negative regulation (i.e. inhibition/repression of tumor suppressors)

By conducting miRNA microarray expression profiling on normal lung versus adjacent lung cancers from transgenic mice, it was shown that miR-31 acts as an oncogenic miRNA (oncomir) in lung cancer by targeting specific tumor suppressors for repression. The targets included the tumor-suppressive genes- large tumor suppressor 2 (LATS2) and PP2A regulatory subunit B alpha isoform (PPP2R2A) (Liu et al, 2010).

Similar experiment of Cimmino, A. et al. have shown the negative regulation of Bcl2 at a posttranscriptional level by miRNA 15 and miRNA 16. It is known that the overexpression antiapoptotic B cell lym- phoma 2 (Bcl2) protein is a major cause of Chronic lymphocytic leukemia (CLL) which is a popular leukemia in human. The Levels of miR-15a and miR-16-1 are inversely correlated with BCL2 Protein Expression in Chronic lymphocytic leukemia (CLL) Cells (Cimmino, A. et al, 2005).

Reported by Minh et al, miRNA125b was tested on the binding site for p53. The experiment used human cells such as neural and lung cells which are known to express p53 in the experiment. The experiment was tested on the relationship between the amount of miR-125b and that of p53 in the cells. According to the result, the amount of p53 is inversely proportional to the amount of miRNA125b in the cells. Conversely, the decrease in amount of miRNA125b resulted in increasing amount of p53 in the cells. The same procedures were processed on zebrafish embryos and the same result was obtained. This confirmed that the p53 pathway is a major target of miRNA125b. Cells would undergo apoptosis under the influence of p53 protein, As cancer is formed by uncontrolled proliferation, p53 protein has especially significantly effect in the tumor cell. Therefore, p53 is a tumor suppressor protein. As a result, the decrease in miRNA125b, would suppress the formation of tumor.

In addition, miRNA-221 and miRNA-222 are hypothesized to be a regulator of p27Kip1 expression while p27Kip1 gene is a member of the Cip/Kip family of cyclin-dependent kinase (CDK) inhibitors that function to negatively control cell cycle progression (Koff 2006). It also acts as a tumor suppressor and its expression is often disrupted in human cancers. Announced by Sage, in a condition with high miRNA-221 & 222 levels, it shows a decrease in the level of p27Kip1. Therefore, miRNA -221 & 222 are also indicated as regulators of tumor suppressor (Sage, et al 2007).

microRNA	Protein Target	Tumor	Reference:
miR-31	LATS2 & PP2A regulatory subunit B alpha isoform (PPP2R2A)	Lung Cancer (mice)	Liu et al, 2010
miR-125b	tumor protein p53		Minh et al., 2009
mir-15/ mir-16	Bcl2 protein	Chronic lymphocytic leukemia	Cimmino, A. et al, 2005
miR-222/ miR-221	$p27^{Kip1}$		Sage, et al, 2007

C. MicroRNA Acting as Regulators of Transcription Proteins (TF) of Tumor Suppressors Either by Positive Regulation (i.e. activate TF of tumor suppressors) or by Negative Regulation (i.e. inhibit TF of tumor suppressors)

A microRNA miR-21 posttranscriptionally regulates Pdcd4, which is a novel tumor suppressor that inhibits neoplastic transformation, tumor progression and translation of colon cancer and Pdcd4 was thought to function at least partly by suppressing expression of the invasion-related urokinase receptor (u-PAR) gene via the transcription factors Spl/Sp3 (Allgayer, 2010).

Furthermore, Imam et al. suggested that miRNA-185 translationally represses Six1 by binding to its 3'-untranslated region. In their analyses of ovarian cancers, pediatric renal tumors and multiple breast cancer cell lines showed decreased miR-185 expression, paralleling an increase in Six1 levels. They pointed out that miR-185 mediates its tumor suppressor function by regulating cell-cycle proteins and Six1 transcriptional targets c-myc and cyclin A1 (Imam, 2010).

MicroRNA	Target protein	Tumor	Reference
miR-21	Pdcd4, which function by by suppression of u-PAR via Sp1/Sp3	colon cancer	Allgayer, 2010
miRNA-185	Six1, which targets c-myc and cyclin A1	ovarian cancers, pediatric renal tumors and multiple breast cancer cell lines	Imam, 2010
miRNA 34a	E2F3 protein	neuroblastoma tumors	Welch, C. et al, 2007

On the other hand, miRNA 34a expresses at a low level in unfavorable primary neuroblastoma tumors and cell lines relative to normal adrenal tissue and that reintroduction of this miRNA into three different NB cell lines causes a dramatic reduction in cell proliferation through the induction of a caspase-dependent apoptotic pathway. A potential explanation for the effect of miRNA 34a in neuroblastoma tumor is that miRNA 34a influences the mRNA, which encodes E2F3, directly and reduces the levels of E2F3 protein, a potent transcriptional inducer of cell-cycle progression (Welch, C. et al, 2007).

D. MicroRNA Regulated by other MicroRNAs

While microRNA serves as regulators of many genes via 3' UTR region or translational repression, it is also possible that the promoters of microRNAs are regulated by other microRNAs directly or indirectly. It has been shown that some microRNAs are regulated by other microRNAs (e.g. miR-16-1 precursor abolishes the expression of the mature miR-16). Currently known regulatory pathways of miRNA processing have been reviewed by Slezak-Prochazka et al, 2010. Zhou et al have examined the core promoters of microRNA in four model species (Caenorhabditis elegans, Homo sapiens, Arabidopsis thaliana, and Oryza sativa) and shown that most known microRNA genes in these four species have the same type of promoters as protein-coding genes have. So far, several miRNA-TF mediated regulatory modules have been verified. Furthermore, it has been hypothesized that miRNAs and TFs might play combinatory regulatory roles for tumor suppression.

E. MicroRNA Regulated by Oncognes:

E1. Positive regulation

Androgen Receptor (AR) is a nuclear hormone receptor and transcription factor which plays a paramount role in prostate cancer (PCa) pathobiology, and activates AR directly interacts with miR-21 regulatory regions which can in turn lead to induction of transcription and androgen-independent proliferation (Ribas and Lupold, 2010).

E2. Negative regulation

microRNA	Protein Target	Tumor	Reference:
miR-17-92 cluster highly expressed in amplified 13q31–32 chromosomal fragments	E2F1- downstream target of c-Myc	malignant lymphoma	O'Donnell et al, 2005
miR-21	Androgen receptor	Prostate cancer	Ribas & Lupold, 2010

F. MicroRNA Regulated by Tumor Suppressors by Positive and Negative Regulation

Induction by the tumor suppressor p53 was observed for the microRNAs miR-34a and miR-34b/c, which turned out to be direct p53 target genes, (Hermeking, H. 2010) MiR-34a expression was markedly reduced in p53-mutant cells U251 compared with A172 and SHG-44 cells expressing wild-type p53 and normal brains (Luan et al, 2010). The mechanism of such regulation is not clear but Boominathan have used comparative and computational miRNA analyses to show that curated p53-dependent miRNA expression data can be used to identify p53-miRs that target the components of the miRNA-processing complex. From such bioinformatics analyses, it was predicted that p53/p73/p63 regulate the major components of the miRNA processing, such as Drosha-DGCR8, Dicer-TRBP2, and Argonaute proteins so that the processing of let-7, miR-200c, miR-143, miR-107, miR-16, miR-145, miR-134, miR-449a, miR-503, and miR-21 can be affected as a result (Boominathan, L., 2010). PRDM5 belongs to PR domain-containing family of tumor suppressors. It has 16 zinc fingers and acts as a sequence-specific, DNA binding transcription factor that targets hematopoiesis-associated protein-coding and microRNA genes, including many that are also targets of Gfi1 (Duan et al, 2007).

Tumor suppressor that targets micro RNA	Targeted protein	MicroRNA	Tumor/method used	Reference:
p53		miR-34a and miR-34b/c	Tumor or cell line	Hermeking, H. 2010
mutant p53		miR-34a (reduction)	Glioma cell lines U251, A172 and SHG-44 cells	Luan et al., 2010
p53, p63, and p73	MicroRNA Processing Complex (as both positive and negative regulators) Drosha-DGCR8, Dicer-TRBP2, and Argonaute proteins	let-7, miR-200c, miR-143, miR-107, miR-16, miR-145, miR-134, miR-449a, miR-503, and miR-21	Comparative/ computationalmiRNA analysis	Boominathan, L., 2010
PRDM5	targets of Gfi1	microRNA	hematopoiesis tissues	Duan et al., 2007

G. MicroRNA Regulating Downstream Targets of Oncogenes by Positive Regulation or Negative Regulation

The tumor suppressor miR-34 may provide a novel molecular therapy for p53-mutant gastric cancer since miR-34-mediated suppression of self-renewal appears to be related to the direct modulation of downstream targets Bcl-2, Notch, and HMGA2 (Ji et al., 2008). As most microRNA affects multiple genes, miR-34 is no exception, and it was shown to affect multiple protein expression by proteomic studies of transfected hepatocelullar carcinoma HepG2 cells, in addition to its function as a key mediator of p53 tumor suppression (Cheng et al., 2010).

H. Possible Mechanisms of MicroRNA Dysregulation

1. Epigenetic events
2. Amplifications, deletion and insertions
3. Dysregulation of transcription factors that target specific miRNAs (as mentioned in section C)

The causes or microRNA dysregulation in cancer has been reviewed (Croce CM., 2009: Rossi et al., 2008).

1. Epigenetic events

The role of epigenetic mechanisms has been well documented in many different tumor types. Epigenetic events include DNA methylation (Veeck et al, 2010), post-translational histone and other protein modifications, and nucleosome positioning, all might act together influencing microRNA expression. Such changes in the cancer epigenome could lead to development of biomarkers and the prospects for epigenetic based pharmacologic treatments. It has been suggested that the analysis of DNA methylation has the advantage over other molecular methods (e.g. single gene mutation, microsatellite analysis) that it can be detected with a very high degree of specificity even in the presence of excess unmethylated DNA (Parrella 2010; Ferracin et al, 2010; Sharma et al, 2010)

2. Amplification or deletion

The genomic region encoding the miR-17-92 microRNA (miRNA) cluster is often amplified in lymphoma and other cancers. The miR-17-92 miRNA suppressed expression of the tumor suppressor PTEN and the proapoptotic protein Bim and thus lead to development of lymphoma (Xiao et al., 2008). Furthermore, amplification of the oncogenic mir-17-92 microRNA cluster and deletion of the tumor suppressor PTEN were recurrent can be used to distinguish two types of B-cell lymphoma (Lenz et al., 2008).

I. Possible Therapeutic/preventive Strategies

1. Overexpression of microRNA that are tumor suppressors
2. Elimination or knockdown of microRNA that are oncogenes (or Oncomirs)
3. Modulation of the protein complex that process microRNA
4. Use of drugs
5. Change of environmental factors in modulation of microRNA expression

1. Overexpression of MicroRNA that are Tumor Suppressors

One can overexpress microRNA that are thought to be tumor suppressors thereby regaining control of normal cell proliferation, e.g. Overexpression of let-7 in A549 lung adenocarcinoma cell line inhibited lung cancer cell growth in vitro (Takamizawa et al, 2004). Epigenetic therapy was used to activate tumor Suppressor miR-126, which is located within an intron of the EGFL7 gene. The mechanism of such activation was due to direct activation of the miRNAs' own promoter and also activation of its host gene-EGFL7 (Saito et al., 2009). Such strategy would apply for any tumors that have downregulated microRNA, e.g. reduction of miR-221 and miR-222 in Sporadic Ovarian Carcinoma which negatively regulate expression of CDKN1B (p27) and CDKN1C (p57) (Wurz et al., 2010).

2. Elimination or Knockdown of MicroRNA that are Oncogenes (or Oncomirs)

As a corollary to the above treatment strategy, elimination or knockdown should be successful in cancer that has increased microRNA, e.g. up-regulation of miR-21, miR-16 and miR-30a-5p in human head and neck (HNSCC) and esophagus (ESCC) (Kimura et al., 2010)

3. Modulation of the Protein Complex that Process MicroRNA

Alternatively, one strategy would be to modulate processing of microRNA by affecting the proteins that are involved in processing, such that it might lead to the overexpression of microRNA that are tumor suppressors, or elimination of microRNA that are oncogenes (or Oncomirs). One study that aims to address the question studied a mouse model of retinoblastoma with different Dicer1 gene dosage. They have found that monoallelic loss of Dicer1 does not affect normal retinal development, it dramatically accelerates tumor formation on a retinoblastoma-sensitized background; however, complete loss of Dicer1 function in mice did not accelerate retinoblastoma formation (Lambertz et al, 2010). Thus the study implicates that such therapeutic strategies need to consider the multiple effects of such type of manipulation of global expression of microRNA.

4. Use of Drugs

Use of drugs such as curcumin (Sharma et al, 2004; Sun et al, 2008), indole-3-carbinol (Melkamu et al, 2009), and epigallocatechin-3-gallate (Tsang and Kwok 2009), resveratrol (Whyte et al, 2007; Leong et al, 2007) etc. could alter miRNA expression profiles, leading to the inhibition of cancer cell growth,modulation of the chemopreventive agents or promotion of cell cycle arrest (Li et al, 2010) and induction of apoptosis which lead to the naming of some of these small molecules with a novel name as Apoptomirs, Vecchione and Croce, 2010)

5. Change of Environmental Factors in Modulation of MicroRNA Expression

Preventive medicine has taken a strong hold in public health and prevention of various types of diseases such as cancer is no exception. It have suggested using dietary changes to modulate of miRNA expression is a feasible preventive measure for prostate carcinogenesis. (Saini et al, 2010)

Conclusions

With more than 93% of the human genome occupied by non-coding genes and non-coding RNAs, it is increasingly thought that the understanding of the relationship between these non-coding RNAs and human diseases (including cancer) might lead to the development of new anticancer drugs (Fabbri eet al, 2010; Saunders and Lim 2009). Such prediction has led to an exponential increase in research studies aimed at studying microRNA in cancer cell lines, animal models and tumor tissues, and microRNA has been found to be dysregulated in many caners and it was also note-worthy that MicroRNA genes are frequently located near mouse cancer susceptibility loci (Sevignani et al., 2007). The three most well-documented signaling pathways that are dysregulated in tumors: the NF kappa B and Ras prosurvival signaling cascades, and the tumor suppressor p53 pathway naturally became the likely candidates of potential micoRNA targets (Kasinski and Slack, 2010; Hoshida et al, 2010). There are many different approaches that one could potentially use to change microRNA expression and thus reverse the fate of cancer cells. Many of such approaches are being actively investigated both clinically and in animal model systems (Negrini et al., 2007; Altomare et al., 2010; Boni et al., 2009). It is predicted that complementation with microRNA therapy will help to answer some of p53 as yet unfulfilled promise (Desilet et al, 2010). However the prediction of microRNA targets by informatics is still at its embryonic stage and much has to be learnt by studying the complicated pathways that involves microRNA. Learning from simpler organisms such as drosophila might provide some insight into the mechanisms of regulation of genes with microRNA as active participants of such pathways (Polesello et al., 2006).

References

Allgayer, H. (2010). Pdcd4, a colon cancer prognostic that is regulated by a microRNA. *Critical Reviews in Oncology Hematology,* 73: 185-191.

Altomare, DA., Rybak, SM., Pei, JM., et al. (2010). Onconase responsive genes in human mesothelioma cells: implications for an RNA damaging therapeutic agent. *BMC Cancer*, 10(34).

Boni, V., Bandres, E., Zarate, R., et al. MicroRNAs as a New Potential Therapeutic Opportunity in Gastrointestinal Cancer. *Oncology*, 2009. 77(1): 75-89.

Boominathan, L. The Tumor Suppressors p53, p63, and p73 Are Regulators of MicroRNA Processing Complex. *PLoS One*, 2010, 5(5): e10615.

Chen, Chang-Zheng. MicroRNAs as Oncogenes and Tumor Suppressors . *New Eng. J. Med.*, 2005; 353(17): 1768-1771. Available from: *http://content.nejm.org/cgi /content/full/353/17/1768 and http://www. euchromatin. om/ChenCZ01.htm.*

Cheng, J., Zhou, L., Xie, QF, et al. The impact of miR-34a on protein output in hepatocellular carcinoma HepG2 cells. Proteomics, APR 2010. 10(8): 1557-1572.

Cimmino, M. Amelia, Calin, George Adrian, Fabbri, Muller, Iorio, Marilena V., Ferracin, Manuela, Shimizu, Masayoshi, Wojcik Sylwia E., Aqeilan, Rami I. , Dono, Simona , Zupo, Mariella, Rassent, Laura, Hansjuerg, Alder, Stefano,Volinia, Liu, Chang-gong, Thomas, J. Kipps, Massimo, Negrini, and Carlo, M. Croce. miR-15 and miR-16 induce apoptosis by targeting BCL2. *PNAS*, 2005; 102(39): 13944-13949.

Croce, CM. Causes and consequences of microRNA dysregulation in cancer. *Nature Reviews Genetics*, Oct 2009; 10(10): 704-714.

Desilet, N., Campbell, TN., Choy, FYM. p53-based Anti-cancer Therapies: an Empty Promise? *Current Issues in Molecular Biology*, 2010, 12: 143-146.

Duan, Z., Person, RE., Lee, HH., et al. Epigenetic regulation of protein-coding and MicroRNA genes by the gfi 1-interacting tumor suppressor PRDM5. *Molecular and Celluar Biology*, Oct 2007; 27(19): 6889-6902.

Fabri, M., Calin, GA. Beyond genomics: Interpreting the 93% of the human genome that does not encode proteins. *Current Opinion in Drug Discovery and Development*, 2010; 13(3): 350-358.

Ferracin, M, Veronese, A., Negrini M. Micromarkers: miRNAs in cancer diagnosis and prognosis. *Expert Review of Molecular Diagnostics*, 2010; 10(3): 297-308.

Garofalo, M., Condorelli, GL., Croce, CM., Condorelli, G.. MicroRNAs as regulators of death receptors signaling. *Cell Death and Differentation*, 2010; 17: 200-208

Guo, X., Wu, YH., Hartley, RS. MicroRNA-125a represses cell growth by targeting HuR in breast cancer. *RNA Biology*, Nov-Dec 2009; 6(5): 575-583.

Hermeking, H. The miR-34 family in cancer and apoptosis. *Cell Death and Differentation*, 2010; 17(2): 193-199.

Hoshida, Y., Toffanin, S., Lachenmayer, A., Villanueva, A., Minguez, B., Llovet, J. M. (2010) Molecular Classification and Novel Targets in Hepatocellular Carcinoma: Recent Advancements. *Seminars in Liver Disease*, 30: 35-51.

Imam, JS, et al. MicroRNA-185 suppresses tumor growth and progression by targeting the Six1 oncogene in human cancers. *Oncogene*, 2010.

Ji, Q., Hao, XB., Meng, Y., et al. (2008). Restoration of tumor suppressor miR-34 inhibits human p53-mutant gastric cancer tumorspheres. *BMC Cancer*, 8(266).

Kasinski, AL., Slack, FJ. (2010). Potential microRNA therapies targeting Ras, NF kappa B and p53 signaling, *Current Opinion in Molecular Therapeutics*, 12:147-157.

Kimura, S., Naganuma, S., Susuki, D., et al. Expression of microRNAs in squamous cell carcinoma of human head and neck and the esophagus: miR-205 and miR-21 are specific markers for HNSCC and ESCC. *Oncology Reports*, Jun 2010; 23(6): 1625-1633.

Koff, A. How to decrease p27Kip1 levels during tumor development. *Cancer Cell*, 2006; 9(2): 75-6.

Lehmann, U., Streichert, T., Otto, B., et al (MAR 23 2010). Identification of differentially expressed microRNAs in human male breast cancer. *BMC Cancer*, 10(109).

Lenz, G., Wright, GW., Emre, NCT., et al. Molecular subtypes of diffuse large B-cell lymphoma arise by distinct genetic pathways. *Proceedings of the National Academy of Sciences of the United States of America*, 105(36): 13520-13525.

Leong, CW., Wong, CH., Lao, SC., Leong, EC., Lao, IF., Law, PT., Fung, KP., Tsang, KS., Waye, MM., Tsui, SK., Wang, YT., Lee, SM. Effect of resveratrol on proliferation and differentiation of embryonic cardiomyoblasts. *Biochem Biophys Res Commun*, 2007; 360(1):173-80.

Li, Yiwei, Dejuan Kong, Zhiwei Wang and Fazlul H. Sarkar (2010) Regulation of microRNAs by Natural Agents: An Emerging Field in Chemoprevention and Chemotherapy Research. *Pharmaceutical Research*, 2010; 27(6): 1027-1041.

Liu, D., Shen, BF, Guo N. (2010). Helpers of the cellular gatekeeper-miRNAs dance in P53 network. *Biochimica et Biophysica Acta-Reviews on Cancer*, 1805: 218-225.

Liu, X., Sempere, LF., Ouyang, HX., et al. MicroRNA-31 functions as an oncogenic microRNA in mouse and human lung cancer cells by repressing specific tumorsuppressors. Journal of Clinical Investigation, Apr 2010; 120(4): 1298-1309.

Lu, J., Getz, G., Miska, EA., Alvarez-Saavedra, E., Lamb, J., Peck, D., Sweet-Cordero, A., Ebert, BL., Mak, RH., Ferrando, AA., Downing, JR., Jacks, T., H. Robert Horvitz HR, and Golub TR MicroRNA expression profiles classify human cancers. *Nature*, 2005;435(7043):834-838 Available from: *http://www.nature.com/nature/journal/v435/n7043/abs/ nature03702.html.*

Luan, SH., Sun, LL., Huang, FP.. MicroRNA-34a: A Novel_Tumor_Suppressor in p53-mutant Glioma Cell Line U251. *Archives of Medical Research*, 2009; 41(2): 67-74.

Melkamu, T., Zhang, X., Tan, J., Zeng, Y., Kassie, F. Alteration of microRNA expression in vinyl-carbamate-induced mouse lung tumors and modulation by the chemopreventive agent indole-3-carbinol. *Carcinogenesis*, 2010; 31(2): 252-258.

Minh, T. N. Le, Cathleen, The, Ng, Shyh-Chang, Xie, Huangming , Zhou, Beiyan, Vladimir Korzh, Harvey F. Lodish, Bing Lim. MicroRNA-125b is a novel negative regulator of p53. *Genes & Development*, 2009; 23 (862-876).

Negrini, M., Calin, GA. Breast cancer metastasis: a microRNA story. *Breast Cancer Research*, 2008; 10(2): 303.

Negrini, M., Ferracin, M., Sabbioni, S., et al. MicroRNAs in human cancer: from research to therapy. *Journal of Cell Science*, 2007; 120(11): 1833-1840.

O'Donnell, KA., Wentzel, EA., Zeller, KI., Dang, CV., Mendell, JT. c-Myc-regulated microRNAs modulate E2F1 expression. *Nature*, 2005; 435(7043): 839-843 Available from: *http://www.nature.com/nature/ journal/v435/n7043/ abs/nature03677.html.*

Parrella, P (2010). Epigenetic Signatures in Breast Cancer: *Clinical Perspective Breast Care* 5: 66-7.

Polesello, C., Huelsmann, S., Brown, NH., et al. The Drosophila RASSF homolog antagonizes the hippo pathway. Current Biology, Dec 19 2006; 16(24): 2459-2465.

Ribas, J., Lupold, SE.. The transcriptional regulation of miR-21, its multiple transcripts, and their implication in prostate cancer. *Cell Cycle*, Mar 2010; 9(5): 923-929.

Rossi, S., Sevignani, C., Nnadi, SC., et al. Cancer-associated genomic regions (CAGRs) and noncoding RNAs: bioinformatics and therapeutic implications. *Mammalian Genome*, Aug 2008; 19(7-8): 526-540

Sage, Carlos, et al. Regulation of the p27Kip1 tumor suppressor by miR-221 and miR-222 promotes cancer cell proliferation. *The EMBO Journal*, 2007; 26(15): 3699–3708.

Saini, S., Majid, S., Dahiya, R. Diet, MicroRNAs and Prostate Cancer. *Pharmaceutical Research*, 2010;27(6): 1014-1026.

Saito, Y., Friedman, JM., Chihara, Y., et al. Epigenetic therapy upregulates the tumor suppressor microRNA-126 and its host gene EGFL7 in human cancer cells. *Biochemical and Biophysical Research Communications*, Feb 13 2009; 379(3): 726-731.

Santarpia, L., Nicoloso, M., Calin GA (2010). MicroRNAs: a complex regulatory network drives the acquisition of malignant cell phenotype. *Endocrine-Related Cancer*, 17 :F51-F75.

Saunders, MA., Lim, LP.. (micro)genomic medicine microRNAs as therapeutics and biomarkers. *RNA Biology*, 2009; 6(3):324-328.

Sevignani, C., Calin, GA., Nnadi, SC., et al. MicroRNA genes are frequently located near mouse cancer susceptibility loci. *Proceedings of the National Academy of Sciences of the United States of America,* MAY 8 2007. 104(19): 8017-8022.

Sharma, RA., Euden, SA., Platton, SL., Cooke, DN., Shafayat, A., Hewitt, HR., et al. Phase I clinical trial of oral curcumin: biomarkers of systemic activity and compliance. *Clin Cancer Res*., 2004; 10(20): 6847–6854.

Sharma, S., Kelly, TK., Jones, PA. Epigenetics in cancer. *Carcinogenesis*, Jan 2010; 31(1): 27-36.

Slezak-Prochazka, Izabella, Selvi, Durmus, Bart-Jan, Kroesen and van den Berg, Anke. MicroRNAs, macrocontrol: Regulation of miRNA processing RNA. *RNA*, 2010; 16: 1087-1095.

Sun, M., Estrov, Z., Ji, Y., Coombes, KR., Harris, DH., Kurzrock, R.. Curcumin (diferuloylmethane) alters the expression profiles of microRNAs in human pancreatic cancer cells. *Mol Cancer Ther*., 2008; 7(3): 464–73.

Takamizawa, J., Konishi, H,, Yanagisawa, K., Tomida, S., Osada, H., Endoh, H., Harano, T., Yatabe, Y., Nagino, M., Nimura, Y., Mitsudomi, T., and Takahashi. T. Reduced Expression of the let-7 MicroRNAs in Human Lung Cancers in Association with Shortened Postoperative Survival. *Cancer Res*., 2004; 64(11): 3753-3756.

Tsang, WP., Kwok, TT. Epigallocatechin gallate up-regulation of miR-16 and induction of apoptosis in human cancer cells. The Journal of Nutritional *Biochemistry*, Feb 2010;21(2): 140-146.

Vecchione ,A., Croce, CM. (2010). Apoptomirs: small molecules have gained the license to kill. *Endocrine-Related Cancer*, 17: F37-F50.

Veeck, J., Esteller, M. Breast Cancer Epigenetics: From DNA Methylation to microRNAs. *Journal of Mammary Gland Biology and Neoplasia*, Mar 2010;15(1): 5-17.

Welch, C., Chen, Y. and Stalling, R.L. MicroRNA-34a functions as a potential tumor suppressor by inducing apoptosis in neuroblastoma cellsMicroRNA-34a as a tumor suppressor in neuroblastoma. *Oncogen*, 2007; 26:5017-5022.

Whyte, L., Huang, YY., Torres, K., Mehta, RG. Molecular mechanisms of resveratrol action in lung cancer cells using dual protein and microarray analyses. *Cancer Res*. 2007; 67(24): 12007–12017.

Wurz, K., Garcia, RL., Goff, BA., et al. MiR-221 and MiR-222 Alterations in Sporadic Ovarian Carcinoma: Relationship to CDKN1B, CDKN1C and Overall Survival. *Genes Chromosomes and Cancer*, Jul 2010; 49(7): 577-584.

Xiao, CC., Srinivasan, L., Calado, DP., et al. Lymphoproliferative disease and autoimmunity in mice with increased miR-17-92 expression in lymphocytes. *Nature Immunology*, Apr 2008. 9(4):405-414.

Yu, S., Lu, Z., Liu, C., Meng, Y., Ma, Y., Zhao, W., Liu, J., Yu, J., Chen, J. miRNA-96 Suppresses KRAS and Functions as a Tumor Suppressor Gene in Pancreatic Cancer. *Cancer Res*. 2010 Jul 15;70(14):6015-6025.

Zhang, H., Li, Y., Lai, M. (2010). The microRNA network and tumor metastasis. *Oncogene*, 29: 937-948.

In: Tumor Suppressors
Editor: Susan D. Nguyen

ISBN: 978-1-61761-986-1

Chapter 11

Biomarkers for Radiosensitivity and Radiosensitization Targets in Prostate Cancer

***WeiWei Xiao*[1,2,3], *Peter Graham*[1,3], *Carl Power*[1,4] *and Yong Li*[*1,3]**

[1]Faculty of Medicine, University of New South Wales, Kensington NSW 2052, Australia
[2]Sun Yat-Sen Cancer Center, Dongfeng Road, Guangzhou, Guangdong, China
[3]Cancer Care Centre, St George Hospital, Kogarah, NSW, Australia
[4]Oncology Research Centre, Prince of Wales Hospital, Randwick, NSW, Australia

Abstract

Prostate cancer (CaP) is the main cause of cancer death in men in Western countries. Radiation has been serving as an indispensable component of therapy for CaP patients. Local CaP recurrence after radiotherapy is a pattern of treatment failure attributable to radioresistance of cancer cells. Identification of predictive biomarkers for radioresistance offers the potential to select appropriate patients for multi-modality anti-cancer treatment or selection of an alternative modality.

Numerous membranous, cytoplasmic and intranuclear oncoproteins involved in prominent cell signaling pathways, such as PI3K/AKT, MAPK/ERK and apoptosis pathways, have been proven to contribute to the radioresistance of CaP. Assessing expression of these proteins will help to predict the radiation responsiveness of CaP patients.

The discovery of the existence of cancer stem cells (CSCs) provides another explanation of tumor recurrence after radiation. This is an interesting research area providing promise for overcoming cancer radioresistance. CSCs have been identified in

* Correspondence to: Dr Yong Li, Cancer Care Centre, St George Hospital, Gray St Kogarah, NSW 2217, Australia. Tel: +61-2-9113 2514, Fax: +61-2-9113 2514, and email address: y.li@unsw.edu.au

CaP cells, which are more tumorigenic than the non-tumor initiating cells *in vitro* and *in vivo* studies. Understanding the mechanisms of radioresistance of the CSCs will help to overcome recurrence after radiotherapy in CaP patients.

In this chapter, we aim to discuss the biomarkers related to radioresistance in CaP from two aspects: the markers involved in major signaling pathways and those associated with CSCs. The potential beneficial effects associated with targeting these markers and overcoming the observed clinical radioresistance to current treatments and CaP recurrence are also discussed.

Key words: Prostate cancer; radioresistance; radiosensitization; biomarkers; signaling pathways; cancer stem cell

Introduction

Prostate cancer (CaP) is one of the commonest cancers and accounts for approximately 30% of all male malignancies in Western Countries. It is estimated that more than 192000 new CaP patients were diagnosed in 2009 in the United State (Jemal *et al*, 2009) and close to 27,300 and 3,300 men die of CaP, respectively each year in the United State and Australia. (www.cancer.gov; www.prostate.org.au).

For localized CaP, surgery and radiation therapy can be curative. Local treatment modalities such as surgery, external beam radiotherapy (EBRT) and brachytherapy combined with systemic treatments (chemotherapy and hormonal therapy) can decrease tumor recurrence and distant metastasis. Radiotherapy, including external beam irradiation and radioactive isotopes, is a relatively effective therapeutic modality for localized CaP. EBRT is commonly used in treating CaP (Stephenson *et al*, 2004; Torres-Roca, 2006; Koukourakis *et al*, 2006; Sandler *et al*, 2009) while radioactive isotopes are mainly used locally at the tumor site in lower risk CaP patients by seed brachytherapy (Kwok *et al*, 2002; Yoshioka, 2009; Nguyen *et al*, 2009).

However, radioresistance is a major problem in radiation therapy, which occurs in nearly 1/3 of CaP patients treated with curative doses. Understanding the biology and signaling pathways that determine radiosensitivity in CaP cells is vital for selecting appropriate treatment modalities for patients and developing novel molecular agents to enhance radiosensitivity of CaP. Various factors (markers) have been identified that influence radiation responsiveness of CaP cells. Skvortsova *et al* (2008) established three radioresistant CaP cell lines from PC-3, DU145 and LNCaP. Higher levels of androgen receptor (AR) and epidermal growth factor receptor (EGFR) were detected in the radioresistant cell lines compared with the parental cell lines, accompanied by the activation of their downstream pathways including Ras-mitogen-activated protein kinase (MAPK) and phosphatidyl inositol 3-kinase (PI3K)-Akt and Jak-STAT (Skvortsova *et al*, 2008). This finding implied that multiple mechanisms contribute to radioresistance, including activation of cell receptors and related downstream signal transduction pathways.

Cancer stem cells (CSCs) are a small proportion of cells in a malignant tumor, which have the ability of self-renewal, differentiation and maintaining tumor growth (Yang *et al*, 2008). Existence of CSCs has been proven in different tumors (Sengupta *et al*, 2010), including CaP (Li *et al*, 2008; Lang *et al*, 2009; Li *et al*, 2010). Biological function of CSCs is quite different from non-CSCs. Contribution of CSCs to radioresistance is one of the hot topics in cancer research in recent years. Investigation of the relationship between the radioresistance of cancer and CSCs is useful for predicting radioresistance of cancer and developing more effective and specific radiosensitizers.

Here, we focus on some potential biomarkers involved in major signaling pathways in CaP, which have been demonstrated to influence radiosensitivity. We also discuss the roles of the CSC markers in the treatment of cancers. These markers are very promising and may be useful targets to overcome radioresistance in the treatment of CaP in the future.

Biomarkers Related with Radiosensitivity and Radiosensitization Targets in Cap

The term biomarkers refer to measurable and quantifiable biological parameters that can serve as indicators for health and physiology-related assessments, such as pathogenic processes, environmental exposure, disease diagnosis and prognosis, or pharmacologic responses to a therapeutic intervention. In this section, we focus on the cytoplasmic and intranuclear oncogenic proteins and their roles in CaP radiosensitivity and radiosensitization. Other biomarkers related to diagnosis, pathogenic processes or prognosis will not be discussed in this chapter.

Cytoplasmic Factors

1. PI3K/PTEN/Akt Pathway in CaP

PI3K signaling is important for regulating cell growth and survival, particularly during tumor progression and metastases. PI3K activates a number of downstream targets including the serine/threonine kinase Akt, a downstream member of the PI3K cascade, which plays an important role in cell growth, death, adhesion and migration, and is frequently activated in cancer cells (Jiang *et al*, 1999; Lin *et al*, 2003) (**Figure 1**). Recent studies highlight the importance of the PI3K/Akt signaling pathway in CaP invasion, progression and angiogenesis (Pommery *et al*, 2005; Fang *et al*, 2007; Shukla *et al*, 2007). Clinical CaP specimens are reported to show upregulation of the PI3K/Akt pathway associated with phosphorylation of the AR during development of castration-resistant prostate cancer (CRPC) (McCall *et al*, 2008). PI3K activation can also lead to the development of chemoresistant CaP cells, through the up-regulation of multidrug resistance protein 1 (MRP-1) (Lee *et al*, 2004).

Teng reported that 42% of CaP tissues have abnormal phosphatase and tensin homolog (PTEN)/Akt expression (Teng *et al*, 1997). Using antibodies against Akt, PTEN, its downstream targets and the respective phosphorylated proteins, Jendrossek *et al* (2008) demonstrated that up-regulated expression and phosphorylation of Akt in the CaP tissues was found in 78% and 82% of patients, respectively, and in patients with Gleason scores of ≥6, the number were even higher (84% and 100%, respectively). PTEN expression levels of cancer cells relative to adjacent benign cells were diminished in only 20% of the CaP tissues compared with benign tissues, and the rate was 30% in those with Gleason scores of ≥6, while the expression level of p-Akt was elevated without obvious abrogation of PTEN-function in a proportion of the patients (Jendrossek *et al*, 2008). These results suggest both PTEN-dependent and PTEN-independent mechanisms of Akt-activation in localized CaP and demonstrate the important role of deregulation of PI3k/PTEN/Akt pathway in localized CaP.

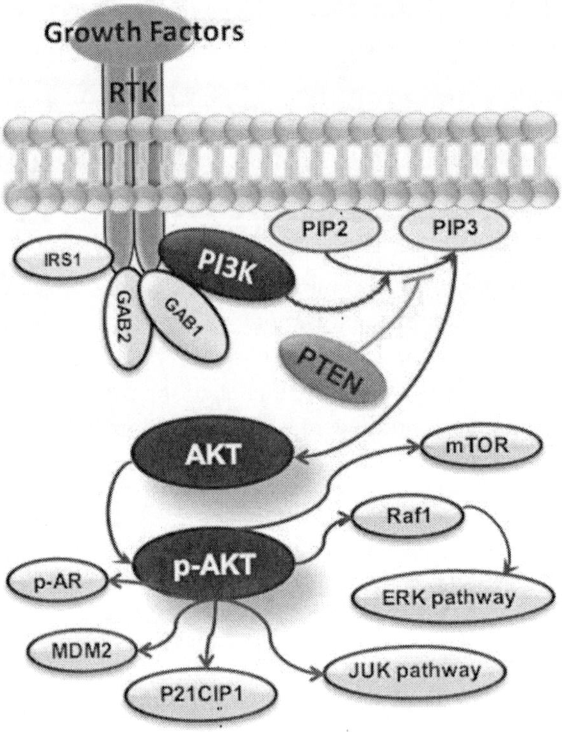

Figure 1. PI3K/PTEN/Akt pathway. This pathway plays a crucial role in regulating a broad range of cellular functions including cell growth, death, adhesion and migration among others. Phosphoinositide 3-kinase (PI3K) converts PIP2 into PIP3, while PTEN antagonizes PI3K function by converting PIP3 back to PIP2, and thus inhibiting downstream signaling. Akt, which is the downstream in the pathway, is activated and phosphorylated by PIP3 which subsequently causes alteration of numerous cell functions.

PI3K/Akt pathway also plays an important role in CaP radioresistance. It has been reported that the PI3K/Akt activity contributes to the resistance of human cancer cells to ionizing radiation via three major mechanisms: intrinsic radioresistance, tumor-cell proliferation and hypoxia (Bussink *et al*, 2008). Gottschalk *et al* (2005) tested the *in vitro* radiosensitization effect of LY294002, a broad inhibitor of PI3K, in the LNCaP human CaP cell line and found that clonogenic survival of LNCaP cells decreased after combined treatment with irradiation and LY294002 compared with each modality alone (Gottschalk *et al*, 2005). They further demonstrated that the PI3K inhibition by LY294002 increased radiosensitivity of CaP cells through inactivation of Akt, supporting the hypothesis that PI3K/Akt pathway is a target for enhancing radiosensitivity in CaP patients (Gottschalk *et al*, 2005). Although LY294002 is promising in preclinical studies, it has not progressed through clinical trials because it also inhibits a number of other proteins and is toxic to patients. Other more specific PI3K inhibitors are under development, such as IC486068 (Geng *et al*, 2004) and IC87114 (Soond *et al*, 2010) and potentially could be useful radiosensitization agents.

As a major regulator of the PI3K pathway (see **Figure 1**), Akt is a target for radiosensitization. Palomid 529 (P529) (an inhibitor for Akt) has been shown to target Akt without *in vivo* toxicity (Xue *et al*, 2008). Diaz *et al* (2009) recently reported that P529 combined with radiotherapy could increase radiosensitivity in PC-3 CaP cells *in vitro* compared with radiation alone, and retard tumor growth in a xenograft animal model (Diaz *et al*, 2009). The mechanisms of the action were shown to be decreased expression of p-Akt, vascular endothelial growth factor (VEGF), matrix metalloproteinase-2 (MMP-2), MMP-9, and inhibitors of DNA binding/differentiation protein 1 (Id-1) levels and Bcl-2/Bax ratio in CaP cells after radiation treatment.

PTEN, the gene for which is localized on chromosome 10q23, is a PI(3,4,5)P3 phosphatase which antagonizes the PI3K/Akt signaling pathway by dephoshorylation of PI(3,4,5)P3 to PI(3,4)P2 (see Figure 1) (Steelman *et al*, 2004). Functional studies demonstrate that PTEN is a highly effective tumor suppressor, but it is frequently mutated, deleted, or epigenetically silenced in various human cancers (Birck *et al*, 2000; Harima *et al*, 2001; Byun *et al*, 2003; Pedrero *et al*, 2005) including CaP (Sircar *et al*, 2009; de Muga *et al*, 2010; Reid *et al*, 2010). Inactivation or deletions of PTEN, which occur frequently in metastatic CaP, lead to Akt activation (Wang *et al,* 2003). At least 70% of CaP patients show loss or alteration of at least one PTEN allele, which may result in activation of the PI3K/Akt pathway (Gray *et al*, 1998). Loss of PTEN activity plays a role in tumor resistance to treatment with chemoagent and molecular-targeted antineoplastic agents (Faratian *et al*, 2009; Sos *et al*, 2009; Loupakis *et al*, 2009; Negri *et al*, 2010; Mao *et al*, 2010). Since PTEN mutations and deletions can lead to abnormal Akt activation, it is thought to play an important role in the resistance of CaP to radiation therapy (Li *et al*, 2009; Jung *et al*, 2010; Pattje *et al*, 2010).

Using gene therapy, Rosser *et al* (2004) transfected four CaP cell lines - PC-3-Bcl-2 (Bcl-2 overexpression, deleted PTEN), PC-3-Neo (wild-type Bcl-2, deleted PTEN), LNCaP (Bcl-2 overexpression, deleted PTEN) and DU145 (wild-type Bcl-2 and PTEN) with a recombinant adenovirus-5 vector expressing the human wild-type PTEN cDNA under the control of a human cytomegalovirus promoter (Ad-MMAC), which led to changed morphology and reduced cellular proliferation (Rosser *et al,* 2004). By clonogenic assay, they showed that Ad-MMAC treatment could reduce the fraction of cells surviving after irradiation at 2 Gy: PC-3-Bcl-2, reduction from 60.5 to 3.6%; PC-3-Neo, no reduction; LNCaP, reduction from 29.6 to 16.3%; and DU145, from 32.7 to 25.7%, which shows that PTEN restoration sensitizes some CaP cells to radiation (Rosser *et al*, 2004). In a subsequent study, this group further confirmed the radiosensitization effect of PTEN gene therapy *in vivo* in a xenograft animal model using the human CaP cell line PC-3-Bcl-2, and found that median tumor size on day 48 post inoculation was 1030 mm^3 in untreated controls, compared to 656 mm^3 in mice treated with radiation (5 Gy) alone, 640 mm^3 in mice treated with adenoviral vector-expressed PTEN (AdPTEN) alone, and 253 mm^3 in mice treated with the a combination therapy (radiation and AdPTEN) (Anai *et al*, 2006). In addition, increased apoptosis, reduced cell proliferation and tumor-induced neovascularity have also been observed in the combination group (radiation and AdPTEN) (Anai *et al*, 2006). In another study, Tomioka *et al* (2008) generated a new type of gene transfer drug, GelaTen, which is a microsphere of cationized gelatin hydrogels incorporating PTEN plasmid DNA and designed for sustained release of PTEN plasmid DNA *in vitro* and *in vivo* (Tomioka *et al*, 2008). Clonogenic assay showed that after transfection of PTEN gene in PC-3 and LNCaP cell lines, which have a PTEN gene deletion, cell surviving fraction for both cell lines was decreased (Tomioka *et al,* 2008). They also demonstrated a synergistic effect of GelaTen with irradiation in a subcutaneous (s.c) PC-3-Bcl-2 xenograft tumor model. Tumor volume was 105±31 mm^3, 420±43 mm^3, and 221±25 mm^3 on day 54 after treated with GelaTen + radiation (5Gy), Control gelatin + radiation (5Gy), and pCA14/PTEN (a PTEN expression plasmid vector driven by the human cytomegalovirus promoter) + radiation (5Gy), respectively (Tomioka *et al*, 2008). The results from this study suggested that delivery of PTEN via the novel gene microcapsule, GelaTen, could sensitize the radioresistant Bcl-2-overexpressing CaP cell line to irradiation both *in vitro* and *in vivo*.

Although the PI3K/PTEN/Akt pathway is of vital importance to tumor genesis and treatment responses, there is limited information on the association between treatment outcome in CaP patients and expression of proteins in the pathway in clinical tumor tissue. Using tissue microarrays (TMAs), Ayala *et al* (2004) has reported the predictive value of p-Akt-1 expression in CaP and non-neoplastic prostate tissues in CaP patients and found that p-Akt-1 was expressed in 45.8% of CaP patients and 8.4% in non-neoplastic tissues. In a multivariate analysis, p-Akt-1 expression in both the CaP tissues and non-neoplastic tissues was an independent prognostic indicator for the biochemical recurrence-free survival in the whole patients' series. This finding suggests that abnormal expression of p-Akt-1 in benign tissue is also a clue to distinguish patients with favorable prognosis from patients with poor prognosis because the root of cancer may have already existed in some patients due to inherent predisposition. In a further study, this group reported that p-Akt-1 expression was inversely correlated with apoptotic index and was predictive of both biochemical recurrence and CaP-specific death in 840 radical prostatectomy (RP) CaP cases (Li *et al*, 2009). These results indicate that p-Akt-1 expression in CaP tissue is a potential indicator for CaP recurrence and could be useful for monitoring radiotherapy outcome.

To the best of our knowledge, no data have been published regarding PI3K/PTEN/Akt pathway conferring tumor recurrence after radiotherapy in CaP patients. Studies using CaP cell lines are underway in our laboratory to investigate the relationship of PI3K/Akt pathway and CaP radiosensitivity.

2. Other Biomarkers Upstream and Downstream Of PI3K/PTEN/Akt Pathway in CaP

In addition to PI3K and Akt, markers upstream and downstream in this pathway such as EGFR, mammalian target of rapamycin (mTOR), COX-2, and Bcl-2 and others have also been explored as targets for enhancing radiosensitivity in CaP.

1). EGFR in CaP

EGFR is one of the most important downstream signaling kinases in the PI3K/Akt pathway. AEE788, a dual inhibitor for EGFR/VEGF receptor (VEGFR), has been assessed in combination with radiation in CaP animal models with different levels of EGFR expression (Huamani *et al*, 2008). In this study, AEE788 could enhance the efficacy of radiation for DU145 cells, which have high expression of EGFR. Furthermore, concurrent AEE788 (25 mg/kg) + radiation (2-3 Gy per day x 7 consecutive fractions) led to significant tumor growth delay in an *in vivo* DU145 tumor model compared with either alone, while no added benefit of combined modality therapy was derived in PC-3 tumor xenograft models (Huamani *et al*, 2008). C225 (cetuximab), a chimeric (mouse/human) monoclonal antibody, is another EGFR inhibitor under investigation. Its radio-enhancing effect was first reported by Wagener *et al* (2008). Compared with radiation alone, the combination of C225 and radiation inhibited *in vitro* DU145 cell viability and proliferation and retarded *in vivo* DU145 tumor growth accompanied by increased necrotic cell death (Wagener *et al*, 2008). Another study which evaluated the impact of C225 on the radiosensitivity of human CaP cells showed similar results to those of Wagener, but they also demonstrated the mechanisms as antiproliferative effects, inhibition of clonogenic growth, G0/G1 phase arrest, and down-regulation of MAPK activation in addition to apoptosis induction (Liu *et al*, 2010).

Gefitinib is the first selective inhibitor of the EGFR tyrosine domain which has been approved by Food and Drug Administration (FDA), USA. Gefitinib is recommended as monotherapy for second line treatment of patients with locally advanced or metastatic non-small cell lung cancer after failure of platinum or taxol-based chemotherapies. Joensuu *et al* (2009) initiated a phase I/II clinical trial of gefinitib given concurrently with radiotherapy in nonmetastatic CaP patients. A total of 42 patients with T2-T3N0M0 CaP were enrolled in the study and given 250 mg of gefitinib concurrently with three-dimensional conformal radiotherapy. 50.4 Gy was prescribed to the tumor, prostate, and seminal vesicles, followed by a 22-Gy booster (2 Gy/day) for a total dose of 72.4 Gy. Maximum tolerated dose was not reached in the phase I trial. After a median follow-up of 38 months, no deaths were recorded because of CaP. The 4 years' prostate specific antigen (PSA) relapse-free survival rate, salvage therapy-free survival rate and overall survival rate was 97%, 91%, and 87%, respectively. Compared with matched historical data in which patients were treated with radiotherapy alone, the survival results in this study were more promising. Randomized controlled phase III clinical trial(s) are required to determine if EGFR inhibitor will give further benefit to CaP patients when combined with radiation.

2). mTOR in CaP

mTOR is another very important downstream signaling kinase in the PI3K/Akt pathway. Cao *et al* (2006) tested the ability of the mTOR inhibitor-RAD001 (everolimus) to enhance the cytotoxic effects of radiation on two CaP cell lines, PC-3 and DU145, and found that both cell lines became more vulnerable to irradiation after treatment with RAD001, with the PTEN-deficient PC-3 cell line showing greater sensitivity, as expected (Cao *et al*, 2006). They suggested that nonapoptotic modes of cell death may play a crucial role in improving tumor cell killing because the increased susceptibility to radiation is associated with induction of autophagy. Furthermore, Bax/Bak small interfering RNA (siRNA) in these cells enhanced radiation-induced mortality and also induced autophagy.

3) COX-2 In CaP

Cyclooxygenase-2 (COX-2) is an enzyme that specifically catalyzes prostaglandins, and is responsible for promoting inflammation (Rajakariar *et al*, 2006), and plays an important role in tumor genesis. It is expressed in various cancers including breast, colorectal, lung, ovarian, liver and prostate cancers and esophageal carcinoma, and its overexpression is correlated with poor prognosis in several cancers (Wolf *et al*, 1998; Sheehan *et al*, 1999;

Zimmerman *et al*, 1999; Khuri *et al*, 2001; Richardsen *et al*, 2010; Breinig *et al*, 2007; Zhang XH *et al*, 2008; Menczer *et al*, 2009). Exposure to irradiation increases the expression of COX-2 in both normal and tumor cells including CaP cells (Dubois *et al*, 1987; Michalowski, 1994; Steinauer *et al*, 2000; Petersen *et al*, 2000; Wen *et al*, 2003; Anai *et al*, 2007B), which may be protective from the lethal effect of irradiation.

Preclinical studies have demonstrated that COX-2 overexpression is associated with radioresistance in CaP cells and targeting COX-2 with COX-2 inhibitors may render cells susceptible to the killing effects of the radiation (Wen *et al*, 2003; Anai *et al*, 2007B; Handrick *et al*, 2009). LNCaP cells transfected with COX-2 (LNCaP-COX-2) produced more colonies than the control LNCaP-Neo cells after irradiation with identical doses (Anai *et al*, 2007B). After treating CaP cells with celecoxib (a highly selective COX-2 inhibitor) for 48 hours, down-regulation of COX-2 sensitized both LNCaP-Neo and LNCaP-COX-2 to radiation with associated reduction in p-Akt and carbonic anhydrase expression (Anai *et al*, 2007B). Using a similar protocol, Handrick *et al* (2009) exposed the CaP cells (LNCaP, PC-3, DU145 and DU145-Bax) to celecoxib at doses ranging from 10 μM to 75 μM for 48 hours and then irradiated the cells prior to clonogenic assay and found that the radiosensitization effect depended on the concentration of celecoxib (Handrick *et al*, 2009). Celecoxib <25 microM didn't enhance radiosensitivity in the CaP cells while celecoxib >25 microM increased radiation-induced clonogenic killing effect (Handrick *et al*, 2009). They also confirmed that clonogenic survival was less in DU145 cells transfected to overexpress Bax, but the combination effect of radiation and celecoxib was independent of Bax (Handrick *et al*, 2009). These results suggested that COX-2 expression is inversely correlated with CaP radiosensitivity. In another study, Ohneseit *et al* (2007) further confirmed that relatively low concentrations of celecoxib could not efficiently enhance radiosentsitivity of CaP cells when they treated CaP cells (PC-3, DU145, and LNCaP) and normal prostate epithelial cells (PrECs) with clinically relevant concentrations of celecoxib (5 and 10 microM) for 24 hours before irradiation (Ohneseit *et al*, 2007). The more important finding from this study is that normal PrECs were radiosensitized by celecoxib at any concentration applied (5, 10, or 25 microM celecoxib) 24 hours prior to irradiation. This study highlighted an important issue which has been ignored by most of the studies in search of effective radiosensitizers: whether the potential radiosensitizer will also increase the sensitivity of normal cells to irradiation.

Another COX-2 inhibitor (NS398) was also investigated for radiosensitization effects in CaP. Wen *et al* (2003) examined the clonogenic survival of DU145 cells treated with irradiation or NS398 combined with irradiation and found that treatment with NS398 for 48 hours before or after irradiation enhanced the clonogenic killing effect of irradiation (Wen *et al*, 2003). *In vivo* experiments also demonstrate enhanced radiosensitivity for the combination treatment, which delayed tumor growth more than any single treatment modality alone (Wen *et al*, 2003). Using western blotting, they also found that COX-2 expression was enhanced by irradiation, but this phenomenon was abolished when cells were exposed to NS398 (Wen *et al*, 2003). These results further confirmed that reduction of COX-2 expression with a COX-2 inhibitor can increase radiosensitivity in CaP cells and targeting COX-2 for radioresistance CaP cells and may have clinical significance.

In a Radiation Therapy Oncology Group (RTOG) 92-02 trial, patients enrolled were randomized into two groups to receive short-term androgen deprivation (STAD) plus radiotherapy or long-term androgen deprivation (LTAD) plus radiotherapy. Khor *et al* (2007) analyzed the data using immunohistochemical staining to assess the associations between

COX-2 expression in CaP tissues and the endpoints of this clinical trial including biochemical failure, local failure, distant metastasis, cause-specific mortality, overall mortality, and any failure. They found that the higher the expression of COX-2 in the CaP tissues, the greater the chance of failure including distant metastasis, biochemical failure or any failure (Khor *et al*, 2007). These results confirmed that COX-2 expression is associated with radiation resistance from a clinical point of view.

Combined, the above results warrant a further clinical trial to test whether COX-2 inhibition enhances the radiosensitivity of CaP, delays biochemical failure, decreases the metastatic rate and eventually improves the prognosis of the patients. One such clinical trial was begun in CaP patients who showed rising serum PSA after RP and/or radiation therapy without any radiographic evidence of metastases (Smith *et al*, 2006). Patients were assigned to celecoxib or placebo randomly. Although this trial has been aborted ahead of schedule due to concerns about the safety of celecoxib, the investigators analyzed the data of patients who had already enrolled and found that celecoxib significantly decreased mean PSA velocity compared with placebo.

4) Bcl-2 in CaP

Bcl (B-cell leukemia/lymphoma)-2 is an anti-apoptotic molecule expressed in both normal and malignant cells. It blocks apoptosis by preventing the release of pro-apoptotic factors from mitochondria and thus promotes cell survival via inhibition of the intrinsic apoptotic pathway (see Figure 2). Bcl-2 expression has been associated with worse prognostic indicators in CaP (Bubendorf *et al,* 1996).

In preclinical studies, accumulating evidence has confirmed the significance of Bcl-2 in conferring radioresistance in CaP using CaP cell lines and animal models. To elucidate the role of Bcl-2 in mediating radioresistance in CaP, Anai *et al* (2007A) exposed two CaP cell lines expressing Bcl-2 at different levels (PC-3-Bcl-2 and PC-3-Neo) to antisense Bcl-2 oligodeoxynucleotides (ODN), reverse control (CTL), or mock treatment and found that knock-down of Bcl-2 using antisense Bcl-2 ODN enhanced the radiosensitivity of both cell lines as assessed by clonogenic surviving assay (Anai *et al*, 2007A). Furthermore, they also showed that the combination of targeting Bcl-2 and irradiation inhibited the growth of CaP xenografts in nude mice accompanied by increased apoptosis, decreased angiogenesis, and decreased proliferation compared with each modality alone (Anai *et al*, 2007A). In addition to using the genomic technique to decrease the expression of Bcl-2, chemical targeting at Bcl-2 has also been investigated. (-)-Gossypol is a natural polyphenol product from cotton seed which has been identified as a potent small molecule inhibitor of both Bcl-2 and Bcl-xL. Xu L *et al* (2005) found that (-)-Gossypol enhanced radiosensitivity of CaP cells both *in vitro and in vivo*, that more apoptotic cells were induced and tumor angiogenesis was significantly inhibited in the PC-3 xenograft models treated with both modalities compared with each alone without aggravating toxicity (Xu *et al*, 2005).

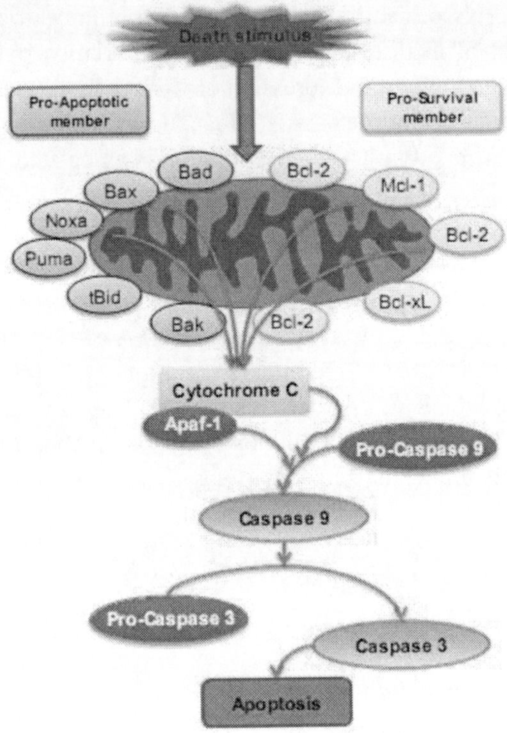

Figure 2. Intrinsic apoptotic pathway. After death stimulus, counterbalance between pro-apoptotic members including Bad, Bax, Noxa, Puma, tBid, and Bak, and pro-survival members including Bcl-2, Mcl-1, and Bcl-xL controls the release of cytochrome C from mitochondria. Once released from the mitochondria, cytochrome c binds with Apaf-1, forms apoptosome and initiates activation of the caspase cascade through caspase 9, finally inducing cell apoptosis.

In an attempt to identify the predictive value of Bcl-2 and Bax in CaP patients who underwent radiotherapy, Mackey *et al* (1998) performed a retrospective study with 41 patients who were categorized into two groups according to the clinical response to radiotherapy: radiation non-responders and radiation responders (Mackey *et al*, 1998). Immunohistochemical study of the tumor tissues from these patients showed that Bcl-2 positivity was significantly higher in CaPs of the radiation non-responders compared with the radiation responders (Mackey *et al*, 1998). They also found that a higher Bcl-2/Bax ratio was correlated with poor therapeutic responsiveness of CaP to radiotherapy, independent of age, PSA, and Gleason score (Mackey *et al*, 1998). These results suggested that the Bcl-2/Bax ratio in tumor tissue is a predictive marker for the response of CaP patients to radiotherapy. Scherr *et al* (1999) also used nadir PSA (less than 1 ng/mL) as the criterion of successful treatment to class patients into PSA nadir group or treatment failure group. The positive rate of Bcl-2 and p53 were 15.4% and 11.8% in the PSA nadir group, 84.6% and 88.2% in the treatment failure group, respectively (Scherr *et al*, 1999). They concluded that Bcl-2 and p53 expression may be helpful for predicting tumor response to definitive radiotherapy.

While Mackey's (Mackey *et al*, 1998) and Scherr's (Scherr *et al*, 1999) studies, used the clinical responses, especially serum PSA as the selection criteria for radiosensitive and radioresistant tumors,more solid evidence was reported by two other groups. Huang *et al* (1998) used immunohistochemistry to compare the expression of p53 and Bcl-2 proteins in

CaP tumor tissues from patients who failed radiotherapy to specimens from patients who had no evidence of recurrent or persistent disease at least 3 years following radiotherapy. They found that the positive rate of Bcl-2 in the treatment success group was 8% but 41% and 61% in the pre-treatment and post-treatment tissue samples of the treatment failure group, with a statistically significant difference. Thus Bcl-2 may be a useful marker to predict the outcome of CaP patients following radiotherapy (Huang *et al*, 1998). This group also found that positive rates of p53 were similar in the treatment failure group and treatment success group, and thus may not be of predictive value for the recurrence of CaP after radical radiotherapy (Huang *et al*, 1998). Rosser *et al* (2003) compared the expression of Bcl-2 in 20 recurrent CaP tissue samples (radio-recurrent group) and 20 patients' tissue samples sampled before treatment (radio-naive group) (Rosser *et al*, 2003). The median interval between the first course of full-dose EBRT and salvage surgery was 54 months (range 18-160 months) for the radio-recurrent group while the mean follow-up of the radio-naive group was 18 months (range 1-75 months) without clinical sign of recurrence (Rosser *et al*, 2003). Immunoreactivities of p53, p21, Bcl-2 and Ki-67 of these two groups were also assessed and the results showed that overexpression of Bcl-2 was detected in 55% of the tumors in the radio-recurrent group while no patient had Bcl-2 overexpression in the radio-naive group (Rosser *et al*, 2003). In contrast to the results reported by Scherr *et al* (1999), Grossfeld *et al* (1998) compared the biological phenotype of recurrent CaP after definitive radiotherapy with the pre-treatment tumor samples from the same patients and found that Bcl-2 expression rate was higher in the recurrent tumors (67% vs. 33%), but the difference didn't reach statistical significance (Grossfeld *et al*, 1998). In this study, significant differences were detected between pre-treatment tissues and recurrent tumor tissues for p53 and Ki-67 immunoreactivities (Grossfeld *et al*, 1998). The difference in results could be due to the selection criterion for patients and different antibodies and methods used for staining.

Further evidence for the importance of Bcl-2 expression in CaP radosensitivity comes from prospective clinical trials. External radiotherapy was given to 305 men with localized CaP and pretreatment tumor tissues were stained with a panel of markers from Bcl-2 family including Bcl-2, Bcl-x and Bax (Pollack *et al*, 2003). In both univariate and multivariate analysis, expression levels of Bcl-2 and Bax were confirmed as predicting factors for freedom from biochemical failure (bNED) independent of pretreatment PSA level, Gleason score and disease stage. Increased failure was found in patients with abnormally elevated Bcl-2 expression in CaP (Pollack *et al*, 2003). RTOG 86-10 (Pilepich *et al,* 2001) and RTOG 92-02 (Hanks *et al*, 2003; Horwitz *et al*, 2008) are two prominent prospective clinical trials designed to assess the role of androgen deprivation (AD) (including STAD and LTAD) combined with radiotherapy for locally advanced CaP patients. Khor *et al* (2006) assessed the association of Bcl-2 and Bax expression with CaP patient outcome in RTOG 86-10, including tumor tissues obtained from 119 patients for Bcl-2 analysis and 104 patients for Bax. They found that Bcl-2 overexpression and abnormal Bax expression existed in 26% and 47% of cases, respectively (Khor *et al,* 2006). In univariate and multivariate analyses, there was no statistically significant relationship seen between abnormal Bcl-2 or Bax expression and outcome, including local failure, distant metastasis, cause-specific mortality and overall mortality (Khor *et al*, 2006). The authors speculated that Bcl-2 and Bax would be of greater value in men with earlier-stage CaP, because patients enrolled in this trial were staged as locally-advanced. In the following study, Khor *et al* (2007) continued to examine the relationship of Bcl-2 and Bax expression with CaP patients' outcome enrolled in RTOG 92-02 including 586 high-risk CaP patients who received radical radiotherapy with either STAD or LTAD, and found that Bcl-2 was positive in 45.6% cases, and Bax expression altered in 53.9% cases (Khor *et al*, 2007). They concluded that as a single marker, Bcl-2 was not independently associated with biochemical failure, local failure, distant metastasis, cause-specific mortality or overall mortality, in agreement with the RTOG 86-10 results. In patients with negative Bcl-2/normal Bax, no statistically significant difference was noticed between STAD and LTAD groups, concerning treatment failure rates. However, less treatment failure occurred in LTAD group compared with STAD, when positive Bcl-2 and/or altered Bax were found in those patients. Thus the authors believed that LTAD may be essential for patients with abnormal expression of Bcl-2 or Bax. Vergis *et al* (2010) later reported interesting results from 201 CaP patients who were enrolled in two dose-escalation clinical trials. They found that Bcl-2 expression was predictive for 5-year freedom from biochemical failure (FFBF) independent of clinical factors and p53, MDM2 expression, both in univariate and multivariate analysis (Vergis *et al*, 2010). They also found that dose escalation from 64Gy to 74Gy improved seven-years FFBF of Bcl-2-positive patients (41% vs. 61%), but not Bcl-2-negative patients (81% vs. 87%) (Vergis *et al*, 2010). They suggested that dose escalation may be of great importance to patients with Bcl-2 expressing tumors. Regardless, Bcl-2 expression is quite probably related to poor prognosis of CaP patients treated with radiotherapy.

Thus findings from preclinical studies and clinical trials indicate that Bcl-2 plays an important role in CaP response to radiation and is a useful indicator for radiosensitivity of CaP. It is also a potential radiosensitization target, given the promising results of *in vitro* and *in vivo* results and evidence generated from several retrospective analyses of patients' cohort.

Intranuclear Factors

1. p53 in CaP

Mutations or deletion in the p53 gene located on chromosome 17p occur in approximately half of all human malignancies (Hainaut *et al*, 1998; Hollstein *et al*, 1999) and are also one of the most common genetic alterations in human primary CaP (Knillová *et al*, 2003; Quinn *et al*, 2005; Dong, 2006). p53 plays a pivotal role in multiple cellular processes such as cell cycle arrest, cell proliferation, apoptosis and the repair of DNA damage. It has been proven that p53 mutations and deletions are associated with poor prognosis and resistance to chemotherapy agents and radiotherapy in diverse tumors (Bristow *et al*, 1996; Weller, 1998; Dahm-Daphi, 2000; Bush *et al*, 2002; Bossi *et al*, 2007; Scata *et al*, 2007), due to the loss of p53-dependent apoptosis. However, whether the p53 status affects radioresistance and recurrence in CaP is still controversial.

In preclinical investigations, a study performed by Kyprianou *et al* (1998) questioned the role of p53 as an independent factor of radioresistance in a CaP cell line (Kyprianou *et al*, 1998). They transfected PC-3 cells, which are null for p53 with a plasmid encoding a mutant p53 sequence and compared the cellular response of the cells to radiation. They found no difference in apoptosis in response to irradiation between the mutant p53 transfectant and parental PC-3 cells, which suggested there was no relationship between p53 and intrinsic radiosensitivity in CaP (Kyprianou *et al*, 1998). In another study, Scott *et al* (2003) developed the PC3^{tsp53} stable transfectants by stable transfection with a human temperature-sensitive mutant p53 allele in p53-null PC-3 CaP cells and the p53 function was conditionally restored (Scott *et al*, 2003). After exposure to a single 2-Gy dose of irradiation, the maintenance of G2 arrest was significantly longer in the PC-3^{tsp53} cell line than the parental PC-3 null cell line, and clonogenic assay showed that cell survival increased slightly in the presence of functional p53 (Scott *et al*, 2003). The survival difference between PC-3^{tsp53} cells and parental PC-3 cells was more obvious when cells were exposed to three consecutive daily doses of 2Gy, which is more relevant to the clinical situation (Scott *et al*, 2003). As about two-thirds of CaP patients have wild-type p53 in their tumors, these results question whether the wild-type p53 will reduce the effectiveness of radiotherapy in CaP.

Researchers at MD Anderson Cancer Center have shown that interfering transfection of CaP with wild-type p53-cDNA affects their biological function, including resistance to ionizing irradiation (Colletier *et al*, 2000; Cowen *et al*, 2000). In this study, infection using a recombinant adenovirus-5 containing a CMV promoter and wild-type p53-cDNA (Ad5-p53) was used to facilitate p53 transgene expression in both the p53 (wild-type) LNCaP and p53 (null) PC-3 lines (Colletier *et al*, 2000). After transfection, surviving fraction after 2 Gy (SF2) was reduced more than 2.5-fold and 1.9-fold with transgene p53 expression in the LNCaP and PC-3, respectively (Colletier *et al*, 2000). SF4 was reduced over 4.5-fold and 6-fold with transgene p53 expression in the LNCaP and PC-3, respectively (Colletier *et al*, 2000). In both cell lines, combination of Ad5-p53 plus radiation (2 Gy) resulted in supra-additive apoptosis compared with each treatment alone (Colletier *et al*, 2000). Restoring the function of p53 significantly enhanced the radiosensitivity of CaP cells independent of p53 status in the parental cells. They further confirmed the *in vitro* results in PC-3 and LNCaP xenograft animal models. After treatment with radiation and intratumoral wild-type p53 injection in subcutaneous (s.c) and orthotropic tumors, the tumor growth in treated groups was slower than that in control groups (Cowen *et al*, 2000) indicating that change of p53 status can affect CaP tumor growth and increase sensitivity to radiation. Loss of endogenous p53 function is reported to decrease the cell killing effect of irradiation while inheritance of wild-type p53 increased clonogenic death significantly in CaP cells *in vitro* (Lehmann *et al*, 2007). Although several potential mechanisms may be involved in functional p53 enhancement of radiosensitivity in CaP cells, the authors concluded that increased induction of p53-dependent cellular senescence is one the main mechanisms and they suggested the p53 pathway could be used as a target for enhancing the radiosensitivity of CaP (Lehmann *et al*, 2007). In human CaP tissue studies, Stattin *et al* (1996) assessed the pre-treatment p53 status to evaluate its prognostic value in 60 CaP patients who received definitive external beam therapy, and found an inverse correlation between p53 immunoreactivity and tumor stage (Stattin *et al*, 1996). No significant difference was found in cancer-specific patient survival between the p53-positive tumors and the p53-negative tumors (109 months vs. 99 months) (Stattin *et al*, 1996). They concluded that other mechanisms may be more important in determining CaP patients' survival after radiotherapy. In another study, Huang *et al* (1998) assessed immunopositivity of p53 in CaP patients who received radiotherapy (Huang *et al*, 1998). Patients were classified into three groups: treatment success, pre-radiation failure (patients who failed after radiation and for whom the pre-radiation tumor tissue sample was available) and post-radiation failure (those for whom radiation failed and the post-radiation tumor tissue sample was available). The p53 positive rates in these groups were 75%, 67% and 58%, respectively, and without significant difference (Huang *et al*, 1998). They concluded that abnormal p53 was a less-than-useful marker to determine the radiosensitivity of CaP (Huang *et al*, 1998).

Incognito *et al* (2000) assessed p53 protein expression using immunohistochemistry and gene mutations using polymerase chain reaction (PCR)-single-strand conformation polymorphism analysis of exons 5-9 and direct DNA sequencing; and investigated associations between p53 alterations and clinico-pathological parameters, survival, and response to radiotherapy in 58 CaP patients' tissue samples (Incognito *et al*, 2000). Neither p53 overexpression nor mutation was predictive of response to radiotherapy, even though p53 protein accumulation was inversely associated with improved overall survival (Incognito *et al,* 2000). Although these results suggest that the response of CaP to radiation is independent of p53 status, more compelling data presented below illustrate that resistance to radiotherapy in human CaP may be strongly linked to the p53 protein.

Grossfeld *et al* (1998) found that p53 nuclear reactivity was significantly higher in a proportion of recurrences of CaP than in pretreatment tumors following radiation (54% vs. 8%) in primary and recurrent CaP tissues after either radiation therapy or RP (Grossfeld *et al*, 1998). Prendergast *et al* (1996) reported that in 25 stage D1 node-positive (TxN+MO) primary CaP specimens, 20% were immunoreactive for p53 and in contrast, 72% (13/18) of post-radiation locally persistent CaP specimens were immunoreactive for p53 (Prendergast *et al*, 1996). This result suggested a potential for p53 immunoreactivity to be used as a pretreatment marker that might predict local treatment failure with radiation. Relatively higher nuclear p53 accumulation rate in persistent or recurrent CaP after radiation therapy was also reported by Cheng *et al* (1999) with 91% (50/55) in CaP and 68% (19/28) in prostatic intraepithelial neoplasia (PIN) (Cheng *et al*, 1999). However, Rakozy *et al* (1999) reported a lower p53 positive rate in 33 CaP patients who failed RT, 30% (10/33) had positive p53 immunostaining and among the 10 p53 immunopositive cases, single strand conformational polymorphism (SSCP) shifts were seen in 70% (7/10) of samples with 71% (5/7) showing p53 mutations (Rakozy *et al*, 1999).

The retrospective studies described above suggest the crucial role of p53 modulating radiosensitivity in CaP. More compelling evidence comes from analysis of prospective cohorts. A subset of patients entered into the RTOG 86-10 trial who received either definitive radiation alone or definitive radiation and total androgen blockade before and during the radiation for locally advanced CaP were analyzed for the association of p53 expression and patient survival (Grignon *et al,* 1997). Abnormal nuclear expression of p53 was detected in the tumors of 18% (23/129) of these patients and was found to be related to increased incidence of distant metastases, decreased progression-free survival, and decreased overall survival, independent of the Gleason score and clinical stage (Grignon *et al*, 1997). No association was found between abnormal p53 protein expression and the time to local progression (Grignon *et al*, 1997). When patients were divided into subgroups according to assigned treatment, abnormal p53 protein expression was associated with a reduced time to development of distant metastases only in the patients receiving both radiation and hormone therapy, but not for patients treated with radiation alone (Grignon *et al,* 1997). A similar study was performed after RTOG 92-02 trial closed. Among 1514 patients who were enrolled in RTOG 92-02 trial receiving STAD with radiation or LTAD with radiation for locally advanced CaP, 777 cases had sufficient tumor tissues for p53 analysis (Che *et al*, 2007). Abnormal p53 expression was detected in 26% (168/777) of cases, which was approximate to the positive rate obtained from RTOG 86-10 (Che *et al*, 2007). Elevated p53 expression was associated with cause-specific mortality and distant metastasis (Che *et al*, 2007). Only the subgroup of patients who underwent STAD with radiation showed significant correlation between p53 status and cause-specific mortality (Che *et al*, 2007). However, after considering the prognostic value of mouse double minute 2 (MDM2) expression and Ki-67 labeling index in another study performed by Khor *et al* (2009), which also applied 478 CaP patients' data of RTOG 92-02 trial, p53 only predicted overall mortality, but lost its significance for distant metastasis and cause specific mortality by multivariate analysis (Khor *et al*, 2009). Vergis *et al* (2010) reported results that challenge the prognostic value of p53 including data from 308 patients with localized CaP that received neo-adjuvant AD and radiation in one of two dose-escalation trials. They found that expression of both Bcl-2 and p53 was significantly associated with FFBF on univariate analysis (Vergis *et al*, 2010). However, p53 was no longer statistically significant in predicting FFBF on multivariate analysis.

Studies from clinical data either support or refute a role for p53 genotype as an independent predictive factor for radiation treatment outcome in CaP treatments. Preclinical results investigating whether interfering p53 status in CaP cells would affect its radiosensitivity are controversial. Different endpoints and methodology in each study may in part account for the discordance. Nonetheless, data from RTOG 86-10 and RTOG 92-02, the prospective clinical trials with large patient' numbers, confirmed the association of p53 with patients' outcome following radiotherapy. Since p53 is categorized as a tumor suppressor gene, gene therapy to restore the normal p53 function within tumor may be a logical combination with current treatment methods to conquer radioresistance.

2. MDM2 in CaP

MDM2 is the protein product of the *mdm2* gene located at chomosome position 12q13-q14 and is an important negative regulator of p53. MDM2 represses p53 transcriptional activity by binding to and blocking the N-terminal trans-activation domain of p53, and also functions as an E3 ubiquitin ligase to facilitate nuclear export of p53 and stimulates its degradation in cytoplasm. However, when DNA damage caused by chemotherapeutic agent or irradiation, MDM2 stabilizes p53 by phosphorylating intranuclear p53 protein. Once p53 is stabilized, the transcription of MDM2 is also induced, resulting in higher MDM2 protein levels, which forms an auto-regulatory negative feedback loop (see **Figure 3**). As the most important p53 negative regulator, elevated MDM2 results in excessive inactivation of p53. MDM2 protein also affects the cell cycle, apoptosis, and tumorigenesis through interactions with other proteins, including retinoblastoma 1 (Sdek *et al*, 2004; Chang *et al*, 2007), HIF-1 α (LaRusch *et al*, 2007), and E2F1 (Ambrosini *et al*, 2007; Peirce *et al*, 2009), and affects genome stability independent of p53 (Bouska *et al*, 2009).

Zhang *et al* (2004) first reported the radiosensitization effect of antisense anti-MDM2 oligonucleotide *in vitro* and *in vivo* human cancer models by using a series of human cancer cell lines including prostate (PC-3 and LNCaP), breast (MCF-7 and MDA-MB-468), pancreas (PANC-1) and glioma (U87-MG and A172) cell lines (Zhang *et al*, 2004). In cells with at least one functional p53 allele such as LNCaP, inhibition of MDM2 with the antisense anti-MDM2 oligonucleotide lead to elevation of p53, p21 and Bax with the decrease of Bcl-2 and E2F1(Zhang *et al*, 2004). In p53 null cells such as PC-3, treatment with the antisense anti-MDM2 oligonucleotide caused elevation of Bax and p21 while E2F1 level was reduced. The ability of the antisense anti-MDM2 oligonucleotide to enhance radiosensitivity in these cell lines was proven through both the *in vitro* clonogenic assay and inhibitory effects on tumor growth in severe combined immune deficiency (SCID) or nude mice bearing xenografts, regardless the p53 status of the cell lines (Zhang *et al*, 2004). Since AD is an indispensable part of the treatment strategy for high risk CaP patients, Mu *et al* (2004) tested the combination effect of AD, radiation and antisense MDM2 (AS) in treating CaP cells *in vitro* (Mu *et al*, 2004). Only the LNCaP cell line, which has AR and functional p53 allele was used in this study. The investigators designed 18 different groups with lipofectin control, AS, antisense mismatch (ASM), AD, AD+R1881 (synthetic androgen), and radiation in all possible combinations. The results showed that AS could sensitize cells to AD, radiation, and AD+ radiation along with a reduction in MDM2 expression and an increase in p53 and p21 expression (Mu *et al*, 2004). The marked treatment effect of the triple therapy was further demonstrated by the same group in an *in vivo* orthotopic model with LNCaP cells (Stoyanova *et al*, 2007). Among different combination groups, AS-MDM2 + AD + radiation achieved the most significant inhibition of tumor growth and tumor doubling time compared with the control group, with significant down-regulation of MDM2 in the tumor tissue. These results suggest that radiation either alone or combined with AD, MDM2 is an operative target for improving the treatment results.

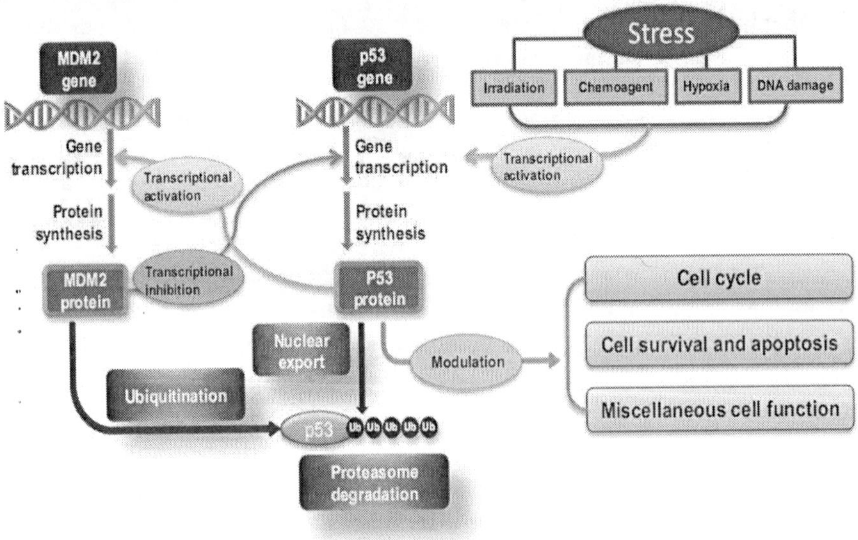

Figure 3. Negative regulation of p53 by MDM2. Under different kinds of stress, expression of p53 will be elevated following transcriptional activation. p53 protein plays important functions in cell cycle arrest, cell survival, cell apoptosis and other miscellaneous cell functions. MDM2 protein, whose transcription can be activated by p53, negatively regulates p53 expression by inhibiting p53 gene transcriptional activation and triggering ubiquitinaiton of p53 protein through recognition of the N-terminal trans-activation domain of p53 protein. The auto regulatory loop is a central mechanism for cells to maintain appropriate level of p53.

Vassiliev *et al* (2010) investigated an inhibitor of MDM2, Nutlin-3 (Nutlin), a cis-imidazoline analog, which binds MDM2 and inhibits the interaction between MDM2 and p53 leading to p53 stabilization and activation of signaling pathways involving p53. When Nutlin-3 was used alone in treating CaP cell lines (LNCaP, DU145 and PC-3), obvious inhibition of proliferation and cell cycle arrest were observed in the LNCaP cell line, which expresses wild-type p53 (Logan *et al*, 2007). Promising results have also been reported from *in vitro* studies performed on both prostate (Supiot *et al,* 2008) and lung cancer (Cao *et al*, 2006B) cell lines treated with Nutlin in combination with radiation. Supiot *et al* (2008) reported a radiosensitization effect of Nutlin-3 in three different CaP cell lines, 22RV1 (wild-type p53 (WTp53)], DU145 (mutated p53), and PC-3 (p53-null) under oxic (21% O_2), hypoxic (0.2% O_2), and anoxic (0% O_2) conditions (Supiot *et al*, 2008). As a single agent, the cytotoxicity of Nutlin-3 depended on the p53 status of the cell lines, which was the most obvious in WTp53-22RV1 cells while cytotoxicity of p53-deficient cells was minimal (Supiot *et al*, 2008). While Nutlin showed optimal activity against cancer cells that express wild-type p53, their results indicated that Nutlin can radiosensitize CaP cells independently of p53 status, although the radiosenstization effect was the most significant in WTp53-22RV1 cells among the three CaP cell lines tested (Supiot *et al*, 2008). The sensitization enhancement ratio (SER) was 1.24, 1.27 and 1.12 for 22RV1, DU145, and PC-3 under oxic condition, and 1.78, 1.31 and 1.28 under hypoxic conditions for these three cell lines, respectively (Supiot *et al*, 2008). These findings indicate that Nutlin-3 could act as a radiosensitizer via p53-independent mechanisms. It will be very interesting to investigate the combined effect of Nutlin and radiation in animal models.

MDM2 gene amplification or overexpression of MDM2 protein occur in many tumors, and correlate with poor prognosis of cancer patients (Forslund *et al*, 2008; Shinohara *et al*, 2009; Sugano *et al*, 2010). Patients enrolled in the RTOG 86-10 clinical trial were first assessed for the prognostic value of MDM2 in CaP patients receiving radiotherapy. Khor *et al* (2005) evaluated the extent and intensity of MDM2 expression in 108 patients from the cohort of the 456 CaP patients (Khor *et al*, 2005). Only the extent of MDM2 expression was marginally associated with 5-year distant metastasis rates in univariate and multivariate analysis. In a subsequent study, the same team compared the utility of immunohistochemical detection of MDM2, p53 and Ki-67 in predicting disease progression in a cohort of 478 CaP patients treated on RTOG 92-02, and found that over-expression of MDM2 was associated with increased failure rates from distant metastasis, cause-specific mortality and overall mortality, after adjusting for all markers and treatment covariates (Khor *et al*, 2009).

Apart from decreasing the cellular concentration of MDM2 with antisense oligonucleotides to block MDM2 and inhibitors to block the interaction of p53 with MDM2, other strategies which can restore the normal function of p53 are under investigation, such as inhibition of the activity of the ubiquitin ligase of MDM2 and blocking the ubiquitination of p53 by MDM2 (Lai *et al*, 2002; Yu *et al*, 2006). Some of the small molecular inhibitors have already been granted patents and are worthy of further investigation as radiosensitising agents (Weber *et al*, 2010). Targeting MDM 2 will be very promising to increase the sensitivity of radiotherapy in CaP in the future.

3. Ki-67 in CaP

Ki-67 is a protein encoded by the MKI67 gene on the long arm of human chromosome 10 (10q25) (Fonatsch *et al*, 1991). It is an important cellular marker for proliferation as it is only present during the active phases of the cell cycle (G1, S, G2, and M), but absent from resting cells (G0). Its' restricted expression in the active phases of cell cycle makes Ki-67 an enticing maker to determine the fraction of tumor tissue that is actively growing for many types of tumors. The prognostic value of Ki-67 for tumor relapse and patients' survival, including CaP patients, has been proven repeatedly by a number of studies (Scholzen *et al*, 2000; Nishimura *et al*, 2009; Broyde *et al*, 2009; Berney *et al*, 2009; Ismail *et al*, 2010; Hyun Yoon et al, 2010; Ye et al, 2010). For patients treated with radiotherapy, Ki-67 has also been confirmed as a useful marker for treatment failure (Lara *et al*, 1998; Takeuchi *et al*, 2003).

Kovarík *et al* (1996) detected kinetic alteration of Ki-67 labelling index during radiotherapy of 7 patients with different kinds of tumors (Kovarík *et al*, 1996). The change of Ki-67 was different in each patient. Some showed decrease after the first few radiation fraction followed by an increase of Ki-67 labelling index while in other patients, the Ki-67 labelling index just decreased or increased after irradiation (Kovarík *et al*, 1996). They suggested this may reflect the suppression of the original active clones and repopulation after radiation injury. Cowen *et al* (2002) performed a retrospective study to assess whether Ki-67 staining was an independent indicator of biochemical failure in CaP treated with radiotherapy and found that the dichotomized Ki-67 labelling index was an independent indicator of biochemical failure, along with pre-treatment PSA, Gleason score, and clinical stage, which meant that Ki-67 labelling index was an equally valuable prognostic factor as PSA, Gleason score, and clinical stage (Cowen *et al*, 2002).

More compelling evidence came from two studies of patients enrolled in RTOG 86-10 (Li *et al*, 2004) and RTOG 92-02 (Pollack *et al*, 2004). Of 456 patients enrolled in RTOG 86-10, CaP tissue samples were available for 108 patients of which 60 received EBRT alone and 48 patients were treated with STAD + EBRT. They found that the median Ki-67 staining index was 7.1% for the whole cohort (Pollack *et al*, 2004). Both the 3.5% and 7.1% cut-points were positively correlated with Gleason score and age by the Pearson $\chi 2$ test and with distant metastasis and disease-specific survival by univariate analysis, but not with tumor T stage and overall survival (Pollack *et al*, 2004). Multivariate analysis showed that the 3.5% cut-point for Ki-67 staining index was a relatively ideal cut-off point to determine the distant metastasis and disease-specific survival of the CaP patients while no association between Ki-67 staining index and overall survival was observed (Pollack *et al*, 2004).

Another clinical trial, RTOG 92-02, also compared the effect of STAD + radiation or LTAD + radiation in localized CaP patients (Pollack *et al*, 2004). Five-hundred and thirty-seven CaP patients in this trial had sufficient tissues for Ki-67 staining index analysis. Median Ki-67 staining index of the 537 patients was 6.5%, but they continued to use 3.5% and 7.1% as the cut-points for Ki-67 staining index as in RTOG 86-10. However, the results in this trial were inconsistent with the results of patients treated with radiation alone at M.D. Anderson Cancer Centre (Cowen *et al*, 2002) and the results from RTOG 86. When Ki-67 staining index was regarded as a continuous variable in this analysis, Ki-67 staining index was associated with local failure, biochemical failure, distant metastasis, cause-specific death, and overall death, which seems to prove the prognostic value of Ki-67 expression in CaP patients treated with radiotherapy (Pollack *et al*, 2004). When Ki-67 staining index was regarded as a categorical variable, the 7.1% Ki-67 staining index cut point was still related to biochemical failure, distant metastasis, and cause-specific death, but the 3.5% Ki-67 staining index cut point was not significant for any endpoint (Pollack *et al*, 2004). They suggested that Ki-67 staining index may be helpful for the stratification of patients in the clinic and also in future trials, but the ideal cut-point is still an issue and will not be easy to define. Despite contradictory reports on the appropriate cut-point for Ki-67 staining index, to some extent,

Ki-67 expression appears to be predictive for treatment failure of CaP patients treated with radiotherapy.

When more than one tumor marker was evaluated to predict prognosis of CaP patients, the results are more difficult to interpret. Uzoarul *et al* (1998) compared p53 and Ki-67 with age, stage, Gleason score, and ploidy for prognostic abilities in CaP patients and found that none of p53, Ki-67 and ploidy is correlated with patients' survival (Uzoarul *et al*, 1998). Pollack *et al* (2003) reported the association between expression levels of Ki-67, Bcl-2, Bax, and Bcl-x in pre-treatment tumor tissues and patients' outcome after definitive radiotherapy alone and found that, as continuous variables, Ki-67 labelling index was marginally significant for predicting biochemical failure (bNED) along with pre-treatment PSA level, Bax expression, clinical stage, and Gleason Score, but not Bcl-2 expression; as categorized variables, Ki-67 labelling index was not of predictive value (Pollack *et al*, 2003).

Khor *et al* (2009) compared the utility of expression of Ki-67, MDM2 and p53 in tumor specimens in estimating progression in patients enrolled in RTOG 92-02 and found that the overexpression of both Ki-67 and MDM2 was associated with significantly increased failure rates for all end points including overall mortality, distant metastasis and cause-specific mortality, but p53 which has been proven to be of great predictive value for CaP patients in numerous publications, was not (Khor *et al*, 2009). This may be due to the different scoring method for immunohistochemical staining in different studies. Khoo *et al* (1999) have investigated the relationship of Ki-67 labelling index to DNA-ploidy, S-phase fraction, and outcome in CaP treated with radiotherapy and found that as a continuous factor, Ki-67 labelling index was significantly associated with tumor stage, Gleason score, and pre-treatment PSA and DNA ploidy, while as a trichotomous variable (< or =1.5%, 1.5-3.5%, and >3.5%), Ki-67 labelling index correlated significantly with pre-treatment PSA, tumor stage, Gleason score and treatment failure, but not with DNA-ploidy (Khoo *et al*, 1999). Univariate analyses also proved Ki-67 labelling index as a better predictor of patient outcome than DNA-ploidy.

In addition to CaP patients undergoing definitive radiotherapy, Parker *et al* (2009) reported that Ki-67 staining level of the primary tumor tissue is also an independent biomarker for CaP patients who received salvage radiation therapy (SRT) after biochemical recurrence (Parker *et al*, 2009). Their data suggest that higher levels of Ki-67 staining are associated with increased risk of biochemical recurrence after SRT, whether adjusted for the most important three variables (pathologic tumor stage, Gleason score, and pre-SRT PSA level) or adjusted for the three features plus additional clinicopathological covariates (Parker *et al*, 2009). Thus, further study is warranted to combine Ki-67 expression level with existing predictive clinico-pathologic factors to generate more sensitive prognostic tools.

4. AR in CaP

Androgen is a vital factor in the carcinogenesis of CaP and androgen ablation is frequently used in conjunction with other treatment methods for CaP patients. CaP patients generally respond to hormone therapy at the initial treatment period, but CRPC remains a major problem in treatment failure of CaP. Hormone-resistant (HR) CaP cell lines developed by depletion of androgen from the culture medium or other methods have been utilized for exploring the difference between androgen-sensitive and androgen-refractory CaP cells with respect to ionizing radiation response. Wu *et al* (2007) established HR sub-lines-22RV1-F and 22RV1-DF from 22RV1 cells by AD for 16 weeks, and obtained HR LNCaP cell line from LNCaP with long-term bicalutamide treatment (Wu *et al*, 2007). They found faster proliferation in the HR cell lines compared with the parental cell lines, and in *in vitro* clonogenic assay and *in vivo* tumor models demonstrated comparative radiation resistance of the HR cell lines. Expression of the tumor repressor gene, p53 decreased while its negative regulator, the MDM2 oncogene, increased in the HR cells, a potential mechanism for radioresistance in the HR CaP cells (Wu *et al*, 2007). The C4-2 CaP cell line was derived from the androgen-sensitive LNCaP cell line under androgen-depleted conditions acquiring androgen-refractory characteristics as determined by clonogenic assay (Xie *et al*, 2010). Their results strongly suggested the possibility that progression to androgen-independent status may also contribute to radiation-resistant property of CaP.

While it seems the evidence is conclusive that androgen-refractory disease is more resistant to ionizing radiation, studies evaluating the therapeutic synergy between radiotherapy and androgen ablation treatment for androgen-sensitive CaP that date from the 1990s have not resolved conflicting opinions of interpretation. AD could induce increased cell quiescence, which may cause radioresistance of cancer cells, resulting in sub-additive interactions. Others also argued that supra-additive results may be generated because of the reduction of tumor burden and improved oxygenation by AD.

In one study, Pollack *et al* (1997) found that androgen ablation resulted in a maximal reduction in double thymidine analogue labeling index (10 to 1.6%) and an increase in potential doubling time (Tpot; 6-42 days), which was related to a reduction in growth fraction (65% to <10%) in a castrated male rat model (Pollack *et al*, 1997). In contrast, the length of S-phase was prolonged only from 19 hours to 23 hours and the response to androgen ablation involved little apoptosis and no necrosis (Pollack *et al*, 1997). Hence, the study suggested that the increase in Tpot was mainly caused by a shift to quiescence with minimal cell loss. With more cells at the G0 phase, which is the most resistant cell phase to radiation, the radiosensitivity will certainly be reduced. In another study, Garzotto (2000) examined the effect of AD on CaP radiosensitivity and found that androgen-sensitive CaP cells possessed increased resistance to radiation when deprived of androgenic stimuli (Garzotto, 2000). Because post-mitotic apoptosis is a dominant mechanism of radiation-induced death, the cell cycle machinery of androgen-sensitive CaP cells may be more easily halted when deprived of the androgen stimuli, giving the cells time to repair DNA before committing to mitosis and thereby avoid mitotic death. Although clinical results from both retrospective and prospective data suggest benefit from combined androgen ablation and radiotherapy in CaP, some investigators still hold the view that the benefit is not from the increased radiosensitivity of CaP cells (Hermann *et al*, 2007). However, an important caution to be kept in mind is that the cells' response to ionizing radiation will be quite different from *in vivo* models when we interpret the above study results. Zietman *et al* (1997) established an androgen dependent Shionogi CaP model in the hind limbs of NCr/Sed (nu/nu) athymic nude mice and AD was achieved by bilateral orchiectomy (Zietman *et al*, 1997). Their results indicated that orchiectomy 12 days prior to radiation (neo-adjuvant therapy) produced a significantly greater decline in the radiation dose required to control 50% of the tumors (TCD50) when compared with radiation alone or radiation combined with orchiectomy 1 day or 12 days after radiation (adjuvant therapy), with 89Gy and 42Gy in the radiation alone group and neo-adjuvant AD group, respectively (Zietman *et al*, 1997). Granfors *et al* (1997) further confirmed the above results in the Dunning R3327-PAP rat CaP model and found that castration combined with suboptimal irradiation was more efficient in delaying the re-growth of CaP tumor than each treatment modality alone (Granfors *et al*, 1997).

Hypoxia is a major problem which oncologists always confront when treating solid tumors, including CaPs (Movsas *et al*, 2001; Cvetkovic *et al*, 2001; Movsas *et al*, 2002). Androgen suppression has been shown to inhibit VEGF expression and induce tumor endothelial cell apoptosis, thereby decreasing angiogenesis in hormone-dependent CaP (Jain *et al*, 1998). Thus hormone withdrawal causes normalization of tumor vessels which may lead to tumor oxygenation and enhanced radiosensitivity. Hypoxia and radiation have been reviewed recently by Wo *et al* (2008).

Well designed prospective clinical trials have also demonstrated the benefit of neo-adjuvant hormonal deprivation therapy combined with radiation in CaP patients. Four hundred and seventy one patients categorized as bulky T2 (25 cm^2 on examination) or locally advanced T3-4 tumors with and without pelvic lymphadenopathy were enrolled in RTOG 86-10 and randomized to receive neo-adjuvant androgen deprivation 2 months prior to and during radiation, or radiation alone (Pilepich *et al*, 2001). Four hundred and fifty six patients were evaluable with 226 in the combination treatment group and 230 in radiation alone group. With a median follow-up of 6.7 years, it was reported that in patients with Gleason 2-6 tumors, the addition of AD was associated with an improvement in 8 years' local control, the incidence of distant metastases, disease free survival, biochemical disease-free survival, cause-specific survival, and overall survival (Pilepich *et al*, 2001). In patients with Gleason 7-10 tumors, no significant enhancement in either loco-regional control or survival was found with combination regimen (Pilepich *et al*, 2001). Hanks *et al* (2003) reported results from another phase III clinical trial RTOG 92-02 which tested LTAD after initial treatment with EBRT in patients with locally advanced CaP (PC; T2c-4) and with PSA level less than 150 ng/mL (Hanks *et al*, 2003). One thousand five hundred and fifty four (1,554) patients were entered into the study and randomly assigned to receive either no additional therapy (STAD-radiation therapy) or 24 months of goserelin (LTAD-radiation therapy). The LTAD-radiation therapy showed significant improvement in disease-free survival and cause-specific survival, but not in overall survival, compared with the STAD- radiation therapy arm (Hanks *et al*, 2003). However, in a subset of patients with Gleason 8-10 tumor, the LTAD-radiation therapy arm had significantly better overall survival (Hanks *et al*, 2003).

In spite of the controversies about the effect of AD on radiation response of CaP, AD has already gained momentous position in the setting of radiation when treating intermediate to high risk CaP.

Understanding Radioresistance in the Framework of Cancer Stem Cell

Definition of Cancer Stem Cells (CSCs)

CSCs are a small subset of cancer cells found within both solid tumors and hematological malignancies (Sengupta *et al*, 2010), which share signature characteristics with benign stem cells: the ability to self-renew and to differentiate. CSCs expand the CSC pool by self-renewal and also divide to generate the bulky tumors. They may also divide and differentiate into heterogeneous lineages of all nontumorigenic cancer cell types (non-CSCs) (Dick, 2008). Therefore, if CSCs survive after anti-cancer treatment, recurrence and metastasis are expected due to the ability of these cells to give rise to new tumors. If CSCs exit and are biologically different from the non-CSCs that constitute the bulky components of the tumor, this severely challenges current clinical approaches. Thus, investigation of CSCs has been a hot spot of basic cancer research and is rapidly expanding into many related aspects of cancer research, including radiosensitivity and radiosensitization.

Existence of CSCs in CaP

Although some studies suggested the cellular origins of CaP are terminally differentiated luminal cells (Nagle *et al*, 1987), evidence still supports the existence of CSCs in CaP (Gu *et al*, 2007). We have recently reviewed the literature on CSCs in CaP origin, the identification and characterization of CSCs in CaP as well as their clinical implications and therapeutic challenges (Li Y *et al*, 2010). There are also several reviews published by other authors elaborating the current status of research on CSCs in CaP, including characteristics of CSCs (Li *et al*, 2008), methodologies of assaying CSCs (Li *et al*, 2009) and the relationship of stem cells with therapy resistance (Lang *et al*, 2009). In this section, we focus on CSCs in cancer radiotherapy.

Different Response to Radiotherapy of CSCs and Non-CSCs

1. Breast Cancer

Using $CD24^{-/low}/CD44^{+}$ cancer-initiating cells isolated from MCF-7 and MDA-MB-231 breast cancer cell lines, Phillips *et al* (2006) demonstrated that surviving fraction at 2 Gy [SF (2Gy)] was elevated from 0.2 to 0.5, for monolayer cultures and mammospheres (a clump of mammary epithelial cells that form under specialized suspension culture conditions *in vitro*), that the reactive oxygen species (ROS) levels were more obvious in the monolayer cultures and that expression of the phosphorylation of H2AX, which is a standard criterion for repair of double DNA break, didn't change in the cells from mammospheres but increased in irradiated monolayer cultures (Phillips *et al*, 2006). ROS are formed during the interaction between radiation beams and intracellular water, and cause more DNA damage than direct interaction of radiation with the DNA strand. More marked ROS elevation in the monolayer cells may partially explain the relatively radioresistant response of the mammosphere cells. If CSCs are really more resistant to irradiation, sub lethal irradiation of the whole cell population will increase the number of CSCs by killing non-CSCs and leaving CSCs. In order to further confirm the relative resistance to radiation of the $CD24^{-/low}/CD44^{+}$ cancer-initiating cells, they further irradiated adherent and non-adherent cells using the clinical fractionated doses and found that irradiation of 3Gy for 5 consecutive days increased the percentage of $CD24^{-/low}/CD44^{+}$ cells in the non-adherent cell population of MCF-7 monolayer cultures, along with the induction of Jagged-1 expression and activation of Notch-1 (Phillips *et al*, 2006). These results suggest that $CD24^{-/low}/CD44^{+}$ cells are more resistant to radiation therapy. In another study, Zhang M *et al* (2008) collected tumor cells from syngeneic p53-null mouse mammary gland tumor models and identified a subpopulation of cells with $Lin^{(-)}CD29^{(H)}CD24^{(H)}$ phenotype by limiting dilution transplantation and *in vitro* mammosphere assay, which possessed tumor-initiation capacity (Zhang *et al*, 2008). After single dose irradiation from 2 Gy to 6 Gy, no significant alteration in clonogenic formation ability was observed for the cells from these mammospheres while clonogenic survival decreased significantly with the increase in radiation dose when cells were cultured on plastic in medium with serum. Gene microarray demonstrated an increased DNA damage response and expression of DNA repair genes among $Lin^{(-)}CD29^{(H)}CD24^{(H)}$ cells including Nek1, Brca1, Chek1, Hus1, Ung, Xrcc5, Sfpq, and Uhrf1, which was validated by quantitative PCR (Zhang *et al*, 2008). These results further confirmed radiation resistance exists in tumor-initiating cell-enriched mammospheres in breast cancer cells.

2. Glioma

Radiotherapy represents one of the most effective therapies for glioma (Fiveash *et al*, 2003). CD133 has been regarded as the marker for CSCs in malignant glioma in a number of studies (Beier *et al*, 2007; Günther *et al*, 2008; Liu *et al*, 2009, Annabi *et al*, 2009). Tumor cells from glioma xenografts and primary human glioblastoma samples were separated into $CD133^+$ and $CD133^-$ subgroups (Bao *et al,* 2006). *In vitro* and *in vivo* experiments demonstrated enrichment of $CD133^+$ cells after irradiation with clinically relevant doses, which represented selective survival of $CD133^+$ cells and death of $CD133^-$ populations (Bao *et al*, 2006). Clonogenic survival was assessed for $CD133^+$ and $CD133^-$ subgroups from primary culture and xenograft cells after a single dose irradiation (5 Gy) (Bao *et al*, 2006). $CD133^+$ populations displayed greater radioresistance than the corresponding $CD133^-$ populations. Irradiated $CD133^+$ cells (2 Gy) formed tumours with similar potency to untreated $CD133^+$ cells *in vivo*. By contrast, the same dose of irradiation abolished the tumorigenic capacity of $CD133^-$ cells which showed weak tumorigenicity. The relative radioresistance of $CD133^+$ cancer cells in glioma is also demonstrated in a study of clinical patients' tissue sections after high-dose irradiation (Tamura *et al*, 2010). Histological sections of 12 patients who underwent surgical removal of remnant tumors after Gamma Knife surgery (GKS) and EBRT were subjected to immunohistochemistry and data yielded from histopathological examination demonstrated marked accumulation of $CD133^+$ glioma cells, particularly in remnant tumors within the necrotic areas, while $CD133^+$ cells appeared sparse in primary sections prior to GKS and EBRT (Tamura *et al*, 2010). These results suggested that $CD133^+$ cells could survive high-dose irradiation and may account for tumor re-growth.

Most previous studies that have explored the mechanisms involved in radioresistance and searched for predictive biomarkers of radiosensitivity have used long established cell lines. Differences are expected between CSCs from patients and cell lines with regard to the response to radiation. McCord *et al* (2009) compared the survival of $CD133^+$ glioblastoma stem-like cells (TSC) with survival of three established glioma cell lines (U87, U251 and SF126) following a single dose of irradiation (up to 8 Gy) by clonogenic assay, and found that all the 6 $CD133^+$ TSCs evaluated were more sensitive to radiation than the established glioma cell lines. Neutral comet assay for detection of DNA damage, and gammaH2AX and Rad51 foci staining showed prolonged DSB repair in TSCs compared with the cell lines (McCord *et al*, 2009). These data indicated that the mechanisms through which $CD133^+$ TSCs respond to radiation are quite different from the traditional glioblastoma *in vitro* model and may also explain the reason why the previous use of radiosensitizing agents has had limited effect in improving patients' treatment response to radiotherapy.

Bao *et al* (2006) also investigated the mechanisms underlying the radioresistance of the $CD133^+$ subgroup focusing on the activation of the DNA damage checkpoint response and DNA repair capacity (Bao *et al*, 2006). Activation and phosphorylation of key mediators of cell cycle checkpoints including Rad17, Chk1 and Chk2 and DNA damage response protein ATM were more prominent in $CD133^+$ cells compared with $CD133^-$ cells after exposure to radiation, which implies effective cell cycle arrest and regulation occured in the $CD133^+$ cells ensuring efficient DNA repair before the cells divided (Bao *et al*, 2006). These results were further confirmed by the finding that the radiosensitivity enhancing effect of the Chk1 and Chk2 kinase inhibitor debromohymenialdisine is greater on the $CD133^+$ cells than on $CD133^-$ cells (Bao *et al*, 2006). Alkaline comet assay and immunofluorescent staining of γH2AX foci showed more rapid resolution of DNA damage which suggested more efficient DNA repair in the $CD133^+$ cells than $CD133^-$ cells after radiation, which may also play a critical role in the radioresistance of the CD133+ CSCs of glioblastoma. In another study, Ropolo *et al* (2009) compared the DNA repair in 5 stem glioma cell lines generated from surgery-derived tumor specimens and established the non-stem cell glioma lines (A172, D54, U87, U251 and U373) in culture. They found that the population doubling time (PDT) was significantly increased in stem cells compared with non-stem cells and that activation of the important cell cycle checkpoint kinases, Chk1 and Chk2, was also higher in untreated $CD133^+$ cells compared with $CD133^-$ cell, which was consistent with Bao's results (Bao *et al*, 2006). However, no difference in DNA damage repair was detected by single-cell gel electrophoresis and staining of γH2AX foci between $CD133^+$ and $CD133^-$ cells after 3 Gy irradiation. This was inconsistent with the increased SSB and DSB repair capacity reported by Bao *et al* (2006) in $CD133^+$ cells of primary glioma T3539 cells and D456MG xenograft cells. The authors speculated that the increased SSB and DSB repair capacity relating to radioresistance was cell line dependent instead of a common feature of the glioma CSCs, and may be attributed to prolonged cell cycle and enhanced basal activation of checkpoint proteins (Chk1 and Chk2 kinases) of glioma CSCs.

In addition to cell cycle modulation and DNA damage repair, the Notch pathway was shown to correlate with the radioresistance of glioma stem cells (Wang *et al*, 2010). Wang *et al* (2010) recently demonstrated by clonogenic survival assay that inhibition of the Notch pathway with gamma-secretase inhibitors (GSIs) renders glioma stem cells but not non-stem glioma cells more sensitive to radiation and that knockdown of Notch1 or Notch2 sensitized glioma stem cells to radiation and impaired xenograft tumor formation (Wang *et al*, 2010). Interestingly, GSI-enhanced radiation-induced cell death and impaired clonogenic survival of glioma stem cells was not accompanied by alteration of the DNA damage response, but reduced Akt activity and Mcl-1 levels. Taken together, all the data support the contribution of CSCs in glioma radioresistance, although the mechanisms through which CSCs alter radiosensitivity of glioma remain elusive.

3. Prostate Cancer

As far as we know, data related with the difference of CSC and non-CSCs in CaP haven't been published before. Both CD44 and CD133 are the most frequent CSC markers in CaP used in related research (Yang *et al*, 1999; Collins *et al*, 2005; Collins *et al*, 2006; Maitland *et al*, 2006; Patrawala *et al*, 2006; Patrawala *et al*, 2007; Wei *et al*, 2007; Tang *et al*, 2007; Hurt *et al*, 2008). In our recent study, we have used PC-3M-luc (CD44 is strongly positive) CaP cell line to explore the significance of CD44 related radiosensitivity in CaP. CD44 expression was knocked down in PC-3M-luc cell line using small hairpin RNA (shRNA) and downregulation was proven by flow cytometry, immunofluorescence staining and western blot (unpublished data). *In vitro* clone formation assay showed relative radioresistance of the $CD44^{high}$ cells compared with the $CD44^{low}$ cells (see **Figure 4**). Preliminary results suggest that more efficient DNA repair capacity in the $CD44^{high}$ cells after radiation may contribute to their survival (data not shown). Further study is warranted to explore the function of CSCs in CaP radioresistance.

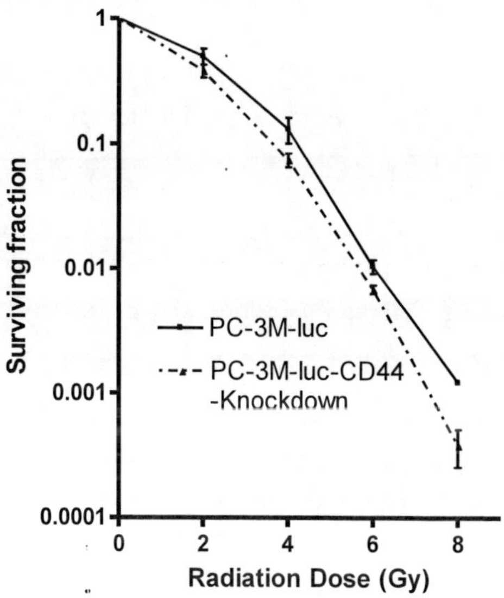

Figure 4. Surviving fraction of PC-3M-luc and a CD44-knock-down variant cell line after single dose irradiation at various doses. After a single dose of irradiation, the surviving fraction of the parental PC-3M-luc cells was significantly higher than the corresponding CD44 knock-down cells by clonogenic assay.

However, all the in vitro and in vivo experiments have tremendous limitations in evaluating the function of CSCs. The first big question to be answered is whether proposed markers such as CD133 and CD44 can be used to identify CSCs with sufficient specificity. Although the clonogenic assay has been set as the standard method to evaluate the cells' sensitivity to irradiation, Baumann et al (2009) also pointed out that this method has limitations in assessing "stemness" since it only demonstrates clonogenicity. If a proportion of early transit cells in the CSCs are greater than the non-CSC population, then the clonogenic assay will overestimate the colony forming efficiency of stem cells. By contrast, the colony forming efficiency could also be underestimated due to inappropriate culture conditions in vitro, such as the oxygenation status (Li et al, 2009; Li et al, 2010) and deficiency of microenvironment (Heddleston et al, 2009; Lin et al, 2010; Burness et al, 2010; Sottoriva et al, 2010). All the factors that may affect results on CSCs need to be taken into consideration.

Even with the state-of-the-art technologies utilized in attempting to find useful markers among genes and their expression profiles, no authoritative signature has emerged to specifically correlate with the radiation response (Begg, 2009). Although a lot of controversies still exist in the field of CSCs, future work to validate the importance of CSCs and characterize the mechanisms responsible for CSCs resistance to radiation are quite necessary and will pave the way for developing CSCs-specific radiosensitizors.

Conclusions

Radiotherapy has curative potential in treating CaP. However, tumor recurrences still frequently occur, requiring stratification of patients into different groups with distinct recurrence risk and further improvement of treatment methods to reduce the recurrence rate. If the biomarkers for predicting the treatment response of individual CaP patient and potential targets for radiosensitization are further validated, it will achieve a more favorable therapeutic ratio in the clinics.

It is increasingly clear that a dynamic and multifactorial process is involved in the response of CaP cells to radiation. All the recent studies described above suggested that abnormal expression of PI3K/Akt/PTEN, COX-2, Bcl-2, p53, MDM2, Ki-67, and AR may be related with radioresistance of CaP and targeting these molecules or their corresponding pathways by gene therapy, specific inhibitor or other methods may enhance the radiosensitivity of CaP.

The recent advances in CSCs have unlocked a new avenue for radiosensitivity research. Elucidating the role of CSCs in the cancer cells' response to radiation will enhance our understanding of CaP recurrence after radiotherapy, and may direct research towards novel and specific radiosensitiztion agents that target CSCs.

Acknowledgments

Ms WeiWei Xiao is a PhD candidate studying at the St George Clinical School, Faculty of Medicine of University of New South Wales (UNSW), Sydney, Australia and Supported by the China Scholarship Council (CSC). This study was partially funded by Cancer Care Centre Trust Fund at St George Hospital (Associate Professor Peter Graham) and National Health Medical Research Council (NHMRC) Career Development Fellowship (Dr Yong Li). We also thank Ms Jingli Hao for helping knockdown CD44 in PC-3M-luc prostate cancer cell line.

Abbreviations

AD	androgen deprivation
AdPTEN	adenoviral vector-expressed PTEN
AR	androgen receptor
Bcl-2	B-cell leukemia/lymphoma-2
C225	cetuximab

CaP	prostate cancer
COX-2	cyclooxygenase-2
CRPC	castration-resistant prostate cancer
CSCs	cancer stem cells
EBRT	external beam radiotherapy
EGFR	epidermal growth factor receptor
FFBF	freedom from biochemical failure
HR	hormone-resistant
LTAD	long-term androgen deprivation
MAPK	ras-mitogen-activated protein kinase
MDM2	mouse double minute 2
MMP-2	matrix metalloproteinase-2
MRP-1	multidrug resistance protein 1
mTOR	mammalian target of rapamycin
ODN	oligodeoxynucleotides
p-Akt	phosphorylated Akt
PCR	polymerase chain reaction
PI3K	phosphatidyl inositol 3-kinase
PIN	intraepithelial neoplasia
PrECs	prostate epithelial cells
PSA	prostate specific antigen
PTEN	phosphatase and tensin homolog
RP	prostatectomy
RTOG	Radiation Therapy Oncology Group
s.c	subcutaneous
SCID	severe combined immune deficiency
SER	sensitization enhancement ratio
shRNA	small hairpin RNA
siRNA	small interfering RNA
SRT	salvage radiation therapy
SSCP	single strand conformational polymorphism
STAD	short-term androgen deprivation
VEGF	vascular endothelial growth factor

References

Ambrosini G, Sambol EB, Carvajal D, Vassilev LT, Singer S, Schwartz GK. Mouse double minute antagonist Nutlin-3a enhances chemotherapy-induced apoptosis in cancer cells with mutant p53 by activating E2F1. *Oncogene*. 2007; 26(24):3473-3481.

Anai S, Tanaka M, Shiverick KT, Kim W, Takada S, Boehlein S, Goodison S, Mizokami A, Rosser CJ. Increased expression of cyclooxygenase-2 correlates with resistance to radiation in human prostate adenocarcinoma cells. *J Urol.* 2007A; 177(5):1913-1917.

Anai S, Goodison S, Shiverick K, Hirao Y, Brown BD, Rosser CJ. Knock-down of Bcl-2 by antisense oligodeoxynucleotides induces radiosensitization and inhibition of angiogenesis in human PC-3 prostate tumor xenografts. *Mol Cancer Ther*. 2007B; 6(1):101-111.

Anai S, Goodison S, Shiverick K, Iczkowski K, Tanaka M, Rosser CJ. Combination of PTEN gene therapy and radiation inhibits the growth of human prostate cancer xenografts. *Hum Gene Ther.* 2006; 17(10):975-984.

Annabi B, Lachambre MP, Plouffe K, Sartelet H, Béliveau R. Modulation of invasive properties of CD133+ glioblastoma stem cells: a role for MT1-MMP in bioactive lysophospholipid signaling. *Mol Carcinog*. 2009; 48(10):910-919.

Ayala G, Thompson T, Yang G, Frolov A, Li R, Scardino P, Ohori M, Wheeler T, Harper W. High levels of phosphorylated form of Akt-1 in prostate cancer and non-neoplastic prostate tissues are strong predictors of biochemical recurrence. *Clin Cancer Res*. 2004; 10(19):6572-6578.

Bao S, Wu Q, McLendon RE, Hao Y, Shi Q, Hjelmeland AB, Dewhirst MW, Bigner DD, Rich JN. Glioma stem cells promote radioresistance by preferential activation of the DNA damage response. *Nature*. 2006; 444(7120):756-760.

Baumann M, Krause M, Thames H, Trott K, Zips D. Cancer stem cells and radiotherapy. *Int J Radiat Biol*. 2009; 85(5):391-402.

Begg AC. Predicting response to radiotherapy: evolutions and revolutions. *Int J Radiat Biol*. 2009; 85(10):825-836.

Beier D, Hau P, Proescholdt M, Lohmeier A, Wischhusen J, Oefner PJ, Aigner L, Brawanski A, Bogdahn U, Beier CP. CD133(+) and CD133(-) glioblastoma-derived cancer stem cells show differential growth characteristics and molecular profiles. *Cancer Res*. 2007; 67(9):4010-4015.

Berney DM, Gopalan A, Kudahetti S, Fisher G, Ambroisine L, Foster CS, Reuter V, Eastham J, Moller H, Kattan MW, Gerald W, Cooper C, Scardino P, Cuzick J. Ki-67 and outcome in clinically localised prostate cancer: analysis of conservatively treated prostate cancer patients from the Trans-Atlantic Prostate Group study. *Br J Cancer*. 2009; 100(6):888-893.

Birck A, Ahrenkiel V, Zeuthen J, Hou-Jensen K, Guldberg P. *J Invest Dermatol. Mutation and allelic loss of the PTEN/MMAC1 gene in primary and metastatic melanoma biopsies*. 2000; 114(2):277-280.

Bossi G, Sacchi A. Restoration of wild-type p53 function in human cancer: relevance for tumor therapy. *Head Neck*. 2007; 29(3):272-284.

Bouska A, Eischen CM. Mdm2 affects genome stability independent of p53. *Cancer Res*. 2009; 69(5):1697-1701.

Breinig M, Schirmacher P, Kern MA. Cyclooxygenase-2 (COX-2)--a therapeutic target in liver cancer? *Curr Pharm Des*. 2007; 13(32):3305-3315.

Bristow RG, Benchimol S, Hill RP. The p53 gene as a modifier of intrinsic radiosensitivity: implications for radiotherapy. *Radiother Oncol*. 1996; 40(3):197-223.

Broyde A, Boycov O, Strenov Y, Okon E, Shpilberg O, Bairey O.Role and prognostic significance of the Ki-67 index in non-Hodgkin's lymphoma. *Am J Hematol*. 2009; 84(6):338-343.

Burness ML, Sipkins DA. The stem cell niche in health and malignancy. *Semin Cancer Biol*. 2010; 20(2):107-115.

Bush JA, Li G. Cancer chemoresistance: the relationship between p53 and multidrug transporters. *Int J Cancer*. 2002; 98(3):323-330.

Bussink J, Kogel AJ van der, Kaanders JH. Activation of the PI3-K/AKT pathway and implications for radioresistance mechanisms in head and neck cancer. *Lancet Oncol*. 2008; 9(3):288-296.

Byun DS, Cho K, Ryu BK, Lee MG, Park JI, Chae KS, Kim HJ, Chi SG. Frequent monoallelic deletion of PTEN and its reciprocal associatioin with PIK3CA amplification in gastric carcinoma. *Int J Cancer*. 2003; 104(3):318-327.

Cao C, Subhawong T, Albert JM, Kim KW, Geng L, Sekhar KR, Gi YJ, Lu B. Inhibition of mammalian target of rapamycin or apoptotic pathway induces autophagy and radiosensitizes PTEN null prostate cancer cells. *Cancer Res*. 2006A; 66(20):10040-10047.

Cao C, Shinohara ET, Subhawong TK, Geng L, Woon Kim K, Albert JM, Hallahan DE, Lu B. Radiosensitization of lung cancer by nutlin, an inhibitor of murine double minute 2. *Mol Cancer Ther*. 2006B; 5(2):411-417.

Chang DL, Qiu W, Ying H, Zhang Y, Chen CY, Xiao ZX. ARF promotes accumulation of retinoblastoma protein through inhibition of MDM2. *Oncogene*. 2007; 26(32):4627-4634.

Che M, DeSilvio M, Pollack A, Grignon DJ, Venkatesan VM, Hanks GE, Sandler HM; RTOG. Prognostic value of abnormal p53 expression in locally advanced prostate cancer treated with androgen deprivation and radiotherapy: a study based on RTOG 9202. *Int J Radiat Oncol Biol Phys*. 2007; 69(4):1117-1123.

Cheng L, Sebo TJ, Cheville JC, Pisansky TM, Slezak J, Bergstralh EJ, Pacelli A, Neumann RM, Zincke H, Bostwick DG. p53 protein overexpression is associated with increased cell proliferation in patients with locally recurrent prostate carcinoma after radiation therapy. *Cancer*. 1999; 85(6):1293-1299.

Colletier PJ, Ashoori F, Cowen D, Meyn RE, Tofilon P, Meistrich ME, Pollack A. Adenoviral-mediated p53 transgene expression sensitizes both wild-type and null p53 prostate cancer cells in vitro to radiation. *Int J Radiat Oncol Biol Phys*. 2000; 48(5):1507-1512.

Collins AT, Berry PA, Hyde C, Stower MJ, Maitland NJ. Prospective identification of tumorigenic prostate cancer stem cells. *Cancer Res*. 2005; 65(23):10946-10951.

Collins AT, Maitland NJ. Prostate cancer stem cells. *Eur J Cancer*. 2006; 42(9):1213-1218.

Cowen D, Salem N, Ashoori F, Meyn R, Meistrich ML, Roth JA, Pollack A. Prostate cancer radiosensitization in vivo with adenovirus-mediated p53 gene therapy. *Clin Cancer Res*. 2000; 6(11):4402-4408.

Cowen D, Troncoso P, Khoo VS, Zagars GK, von Eschenbach AC, Meistrich ML, Pollack A. Ki-67 staining is an independent correlate of biochemical failure in prostate cancer treated with radiotherapy. *Clin Cancer Res*. 2002; 8(5):1148-1154.

Cvetkovic D, Movsas B, Dicker AP, Hanlon AL, Greenberg RE, Chapman JD, Hanks GE, Tricoli JV. Increased hypoxia correlates with increased expression of the angiogenesis marker vascular endothelial growth factor in human prostate cancer. *Urology*. 2001; 57(4):821-825.

Dahm-Daphi J. p53: biology and role for cellular radiosensitivity. *Strahlenther Onkol*. 2000; 176(6):278-285.

de Muga S, Hernández S, Agell L, Salido M, Juanpere N, Lorenzo M, Lorente JA, Serrano S, Lloreta J. Molecular alterations of EGFR and PTEN in prostate cancer: association with high-grade and advanced-stage carcinomas. *Mod Pathol*. 2010; 23(5):703-712.

Diaz R, Nguewa PA, Diaz-Gonzalez JA, Hamel E, Gonzalez-Moreno O, Catena R, Serrano D, Redrado M, Sherris D, Calvo A. The novel Akt inhibitor Palomid 529 (P529) enhances the effect of radiotherapy in prostate cancer. *Br J Cancer*. 2009; 100(6):932-940.

Dick JE. Stem cell concepts renew cancer research. *Blood*. 2008; 112(13):4793-4807.

Dong JT. Prevalent mutations in prostate cancer. *J Cell Biochem*. 2006; 97(3):433-447.

Dubois A, Dorval ED, Steel L, Fiala NP, Conklin JJ. Effect of ionizing radiation on prostaglandins and gastric secretion in rhesus monkeys. *Radiat Res* 1987; 110:289-293.

Fang J, Ding M, Yang L, Liu LZ, Jiang BH. PI3K/PTEN/AKT signaling regulates prostate tumor angiogenesis.*Cell Signal*. 2007; 19(12):2487-2497.

Faratian D, Goltsov A, Lebedeva G, Sorokin A, Moodie S, Mullen P, Kay C, Um IH, Langdon S, Goryanin I, Harrison DJ. Systems biology reveals new strategies for personalizing cancer medicine and confirms the role of PTEN in resistance to trastuzumab. *Cancer Res*. 2009; 69(16):6713-6720.

Fiveash JB, Spencer SA. Role of radiation therapy and radiosurgery in glioblastoma multiforme. *Cancer J.* 2003; 9(3):222-229.

Fonatsch C, Duchrow M, Rieder H, Schlüter C, Gerdes J. Assignment of the human Ki-67 gene (MK167) to 10q25-qter. *Genomics*. 1991; 11(2):476-477.

Forslund A, Zeng Z, Qin LX, Rosenberg S, Ndubuisi M, Pincas H, Gerald W, Notterman DA, Barany F, Paty PB. MDM2 gene amplification is correlated to tumor progression but not to the presence of SNP309 or TP53 mutational status in primary colorectal cancers. *Mol Cancer Res*. 2008; 6(2):205-211.

Garzotto M. Combined androgen deprivation with radiotherapy for prostate cancer: does it make sense? *Mol Urol*. 2000; 4(3):209-213; discussion 215.

Geng L, Tan J, Himmelfarb E, Schueneman A, Niermann K, Brousal J, Fu A, Cuneo K, Kesicki EA, Treiberg J, Hayflick JS, Hallahan DE. A specific antagonist of the p110delta catalytic component of phosphatidylinositol 3'-kinase, IC486068, enhances radiation-induced tumor vascular destruction. *Cancer Res*. 2004; 64(14):4893-4899.

Gottschalk AR, Doan A, Nakamura JL, Stokoe D, Haas-Kogan DA. Inhibition of phosphatidylinositol-3-kinase causes increased sensitivity to radiation through a PKB-dependent mechanism. *Int J Radiat Oncol Biol Phys*. 2005; 63(4):1221-1227.

Gray IC, Stewart LM, Phillips SM, Hamilton JA, Gray NE, Watson GJ, Spurr NK, Snary D. Mutation and expression analysis of the putative prostate tumour-suppressor gene PTEN. *Br J Cancer*. 1998; 78(10):1296-1300.

Grignon DJ, Caplan R, Sarkar FH, Lawton CA, Hammond EH, Pilepich MV, Forman JD, Mesic J, Fu KK, Abrams RA, Pajak TF, Shipley WU, Cox JD. p53 status and prognosis of locally advanced prostatic adenocarcinoma: a study based on RTOG 8610.*J Natl Cancer Inst*. 1997; 89(2):158-165.

Grossfeld GD, Olumi AF, Connolly JA, Chew K, Gibney J, Bhargava V, Waldman FM, Carroll PR. Locally recurrent prostate tumors following either radiation therapy or radical prostatectomy have changes in Ki-67 labeling index, p53 and bcl-2 immunoreactivity. *J Urol*. 1998; 159(5):1437-1443.

Gu G, Yuan J, Wills M, Kasper S. Prostate cancer cells with stem cell characteristics reconstitute the original human tumor in vivo. *Cancer Res*. 2007; 67(10):4807-4815.

Günther HS, Schmidt NO, Phillips HS, Kemming D, Kharbanda S, Soriano R, Modrusan Z, Meissner H, Westphal M, Lamszus K. Glioblastoma-derived stem cell-enriched cultures form distinct subgroups according to molecular and phenotypic criteria. *Oncogene*. 2008; 27(20):2897-2909.

Hainaut P, Hernandez T, Robinson A, Rodriguez-Tome P, Flores T, HollsteinM, Harris CC,Montesano R. IARC database of p53 gene mutations in human tumors and cell lines:

Updated compilation, revised formats and new visualisation tools. *Nucleic Acids Res.* 1998; 26(1):205-213.

Handrick R, Ganswindt U, Faltin H, Goecke B, Daniel PT, Budach W, Belka C, Jendrossek V. Combined action of celecoxib and ionizing radiation in prostate cancer cells is independent of pro-apoptotic Bax. *Radiother Oncol.* 2009; 90(3):413-421.

Hanks GE, Pajak TF, Porter A, Grignon D, Brereton H, Venkatesan V, Horwitz EM, Lawton C, Rosenthal SA, Sandler HM, Shipley WU; Radiation Therapy Oncology Group. Phase III trial of long-term adjuvant androgen deprivation after neoadjuvant hormonal cytoreduction and radiotherapy in locally advanced carcinoma of the prostate: the Radiation Therapy Oncology Group Protocol 92-02. *J Clin Oncol.* 2003; 21(21):3972-3978.

Harima Y, Sawada S, Nagata K, Sougawa M, Ostapenko V, Ohnishi T. Mutation of the PTEN gene in advanced cervical cancer correlated with tumor progression and poor outcome after radiotherapy. *Int J Oncol.* 2001; 18(3):493-497.

Heddleston JM, Li Z, McLendon RE, Hjelmeland AB, Rich JN. The hypoxic microenvironment maintains glioblastoma stem cells and promotes reprogramming towards a cancer stem cell phenotype. *Cell Cycle*. 2009; 8(20):3274-3284.

Hermann RM, Schwarten D, Fister S, Grundker C, Rave-Frank M, Nitsche M, Hille A, Thelen P, Schmidberger H, Christiansen H. No supra-additive effects of goserelin and radiotherapy on clonogenic survival of prostate carcinoma cells in vitro. *Radiat Oncol.* 2007; 2: 31.

Hollstein M, Hergenhahn M, Yang Q, Bartsch H, Wang ZQ, Hainaut P. New approaches to understanding p53 gene tumor mutation spectra. *Mutat Res.* 1999; 431(2):199–209.

http://www.cancer.gov/cancertopics/types/prostate

http://www.prostate.org.au/articleLive/pages/Prostate-Cancer-Statistics.html

Huamani J, Willey C, Thotala D, Niermann KJ, Reyzer M, Leavitt L, Jones C, Fleishcher A, Caprioli R, Hallahan DE, Kim DW. Differential efficacy of combined therapy with radiation and AEE788 in high and low EGFR-expressing androgen-independent prostate tumor models. *Int J Radiat Oncol Biol Phys*. 2008; 71(1):237-246.

Huang A, Gandour-Edwards R, Rosenthal SA, Siders DB, Deitch AD, White RW.p53 and bcl-2 immunohistochemical alterations in prostate cancer treated with radiation therapy. *Urology*. 1998; 51(2):346-351.

Hurt EM, Kawasaki BT, Klarmann GJ, Thomas SB, Farrar WL. CD44+ CD24(-) prostate cells are early cancer progenitor/stem cells that provide a model for patients with poor prognosis. *Br J Cancer*. 2008; 98(4):756-765.

Hyun Yoon D, Ro Choi D, June Ahn H, Kim S, Ho Lee D, Kim SW, Hee Park B, Yoon SO, Huh J, Lee SW, Suh C. Ki-67 expression as a prognostic factor in diffuse large B-cell lymphoma patients treated with rituximab plus CHOP. *Eur J Haematol.* 2010; 85(2):149-157.

Incognito LS, Cazares LH, Schellhammer PF, Kuban DA, Van Dyk EO, Moriarty RP, Wright GL Jr, Somers KD. Overexpression of p53 in prostate carcinoma is associated with improved overall survival but not predictive of response to radiotherapy. *Int J Oncol.* 2000; 17(4):761-769.

Ismail FW, Shamsudin AM, Wan Z, Daud SM, Samarendra MS. Ki-67 immuno-histochemistry index in stage III giant cell tumor of the bone. *J Exp Clin Cancer Res.* 2010 doi: 10.1186/1756-9966-29-25.

Jain RK, Safabakhsh N, Sckell A, Chen Y, Jiang P, Benjamin L, Yuan F, Keshet E. *Endothelial cell death, angiogenesis, and microvascular function after castration in an androgen-dependent tumor: role of vascular endothelial growth factor*. Proc Natl Acad Sci U S A. 1998; 95(18):10820-10825.

Jani AB. Management strategies for locally advanced prostate cancer. *Drugs Aging*. 2006; 23(2):119-129.

Jemal A, Siegel R, Ward E, Hao Y, Xu J, Thun MJ. Cancer statistics, 2009. *CA Cancer J Clin*. 2009; 59(4):225-249.

Jendrossek V, Henkel M, Hennenlotter J, Vogel U, Ganswindt U, Müller I, Handrick R, Anastasiadis AG, Kuczyk M, Stenzl A, Belka C. Analysis of complex protein kinase B signalling pathways in human prostate cancer samples. *BJU Int*. 2008; 102(3):371-382.

Jiang BH, Aoki M, Zheng JZ, Li J, Vogt PK.*Myogenic signaling of phosphatidylinositol 3-kinase requires the serine-threonine kinase* Akt/protein kinase B.Proc Natl Acad Sci U S A. 1999; 96(5):2077-2081.

Joensuu G, Joensuu T, Nokisalmi P, Reddy C, Isola J, Ruutu M, Kouri M, Kupelian PA, Collan J, Pesonen S, Hemminki A. A phase I/II trial of gefitinib given concurrently with radiotherapy in patients with nonmetastatic prostate cancer. *Int J Radiat Oncol Biol Phys*. 2010;78(1):42-49.

Jones RJ. Cancer stem cells-clinical relevance. *J Mol Med*. 2009; 87(11):1105-1110.

Jung IL, Kang HJ, Kim KC, Kim IG. PTEN/pAkt/p53 signaling pathway correlates with the radioresponse of non-small cell lung cancer. *Int J Mol Med*. 2010; 25(4):517-523.

Khoo VS, Pollack A, Cowen D, Joon DL, Patel N, Terry NH, Zagars GK, von Eschenbach AC, Meistrich ML, Troncoso P. Relationship of Ki-67 labeling index to DNA-ploidy, S-phase fraction, and outcome in prostate cancer treated with radiotherapy. *Prostate*. 1999; 41(3):166-172.

Khor LY, Bae K, Paulus R, Al-Saleem T, Hammond ME, Grignon DJ, Che M, Venkatesan V, Byhardt RW, Rotman M, Hanks GE, Sandler HM, Pollack A. MDM2 and Ki-67 predict for distant metastasis and mortality in men treated with radiotherapy and androgen deprivation for prostate cancer: RTOG 92-02. *J Clin Oncol*. 2009; 27(19):3177-3384.

Khor LY, Bae K, Paulus R, Al-Saleem T, Hammond ME, Grignon DJ, Che M, Venkatesan V, Byhardt RW, Rotman M, Hanks GE, Sandler HM, Pollack A. MDM2 and Ki-67 predict for distant metastasis and mortality in men treated with radiotherapy and androgen deprivation for prostate cancer: RTOG 92-02. *J Clin Oncol*. 2009; 27(19):3177-3184.

Khor LY, Bae K, Paulus R, Al-Saleem T, Hammond ME, Grignon DJ, Che M, Venkatesan V, Byhardt RW, Rotman M, Hanks GE, Sandler HM, Pollack A. MDM2 and Ki-67 predict for distant metastasis and mortality in men treated with radiotherapy and androgen deprivation for prostate cancer: RTOG 92-02. *J Clin Oncol*. 2009; 27(19):3177-3184.

Khor LY, Bae K, Pollack A, Hammond ME, Grignon DJ, Venkatesan VM, Rosenthal SA, Ritter MA, Sandler HM, Hanks GE, Shipley WU, Dicker AP. COX-2 expression predicts prostate-cancer outcome: analysis of data from the RTOG 92-02 trial. *Lancet Oncol*. 2007; 8(10):912-920.

Khor LY, Desilvio M, Al-Saleem T, Hammond ME, Grignon DJ, Sause W, Pilepich M, Okunieff P, Sandler H, Pollack A; Radiation Therapy Oncology Group. MDM2 as a predictor of prostate carcinoma outcome: an analysis of Radiation Therapy Oncology Group Protocol 8610. *Cancer*. 2005; 104(5):962-967.

Khor LY, Moughan J, Al-Saleem T, Hammond EH, Venkatesan V, Rosenthal SA, Ritter MA, Sandler HM, Hanks GE, Shipley WU, Pollack A. Bcl-2 and Bax Expression Predict Prostate Cancer Outcome in Men Treated with Androgen Deprivation and Radiotherapy on Radiation Therapy Oncology Group Protocol 92-02. *Clin Cancer Res*. 2007; 13(12):3585-3590.

Khuri FR, Wu H, Lee JJ, Kemp BL, Lotan R, Lippman SM, et al. Cyclooxygenase-2 overexpression is a marker of poor prognosis in stage I non-small cell lung cancer. *Clin Cancer Res* 2001; 7(4):861-867.

Knillová J, Kolár Z. *The significance of key regulators of apoptosis in the development and prognosis of prostate carcinoma*. I. Proteins of the Bcl-2 family and protein p53.Biomed Pap Med Fac Univ Palacky Olomouc Czech Repub. 2003; 147(1):3-10.

Koukourakis MI, Touloupidis S. External beam radiotherapy for prostate cancer: current position and trends. *Anticancer Res*. 2006; 26(1B):485-494.

Kovarík J, Skry GD, Mikel J, Svoboda VH. Changes of Ki67 index of various tumors during radiation therapy. *Neoplasma*. 1996; 43(2):89-92.

Kwok Y, DiBiase SJ, Amin PP, Naslund M, Sklar G, Jacobs SC. Risk group stratification in patients undergoing permanent (125)I prostate brachytherapy as monotherapy. *Int J Radiat Oncol Biol Phys*. 2002; 53(3):588-594.

Lai Z, Yang T, Kim YB, Sielecki TM, Diamond MA, Strack P, Rolfe M, Caligiuri M, Benfield PA, Auger KR, Copeland RA.Differentiation of Hdm2-mediated p53 ubiquitination and Hdm2 autoubiquitination activity by small molecular weight inhibitors. *Proc Natl Acad Sci U S A*. 2002; 99(23):14734-14739.

Lang SH, Frame FM, Collins AT. Prostate cancer stem cells. *J Pathol*. 2009; 217(2):299-306.

Lara PC, Rey A, Santana C, Afonso JL, Diaz JM, González GJ, Apolinario R. The role of Ki67 proliferation assessment in predicting local control in bladder cancer patients treated by radical radiation therapy. *Radiother Oncol*. 1998; 49(2):163-167.

LaRusch GA, Jackson MW, Dunbar JD, Warren RS, Donner DB, Mayo LD. Nutlin3 blocks vascular endothelial growth factor induction by preventing the interaction between hypoxia inducible factor 1α and Hdm2. *Cancer Res*. 2007;67(2):450-454.

Lee JT Jr, Steelman LS, McCubrey JA. Phosphatidylinositol 3'-kinase activation leads to multidrug resistance protein-1 expression and chemoresistance in advanced prostate cancer cells. *Cancer Res*. 2004; 64(22):8397-8404.

Lehmann BD, McCubrey JA, Jefferson HS, Paine MS, Chappell WH, Terrian DM. A dominant role for p53-dependent cellular senescence in radiosensitization of human prostate cancer cells. *Cell Cycle*. 2007; 6(5):595-605.

Li H, Chen X, Calhoun-Davis T, Claypool K, Tang DG. PC3 human prostate carcinoma cell holoclones contain self-renewing tumor-initiating cells. *Cancer Res*. 2008; 68(6):1820-1825.

Li H, Jiang M, Honorio S, Patrawala L, Jeter CR, Calhoun-Davis T, Hayward SW, Tang DG. Methodologies in assaying prostate cancer stem cells. *Methods Mol Biol*. 2009; 568:85-138.

Li HF, Kim JS, Waldman T. Radiation-induced Akt activation modulates radioresistance in human glioblastoma cells. *Radiat Oncol*. 2009; 4:43.

Li R, Dai H, Wheeler TM, Sayeeduddin M, Scardino PT, Frolov A, Ayala GE. Prognostic value of Akt-1 in human prostate cancer: a computerized quantitative assessment with quantum dot technology. *Clin Cancer Res*. 2009; 15(10):3568-3573.

Li R, Heydon K, Hammond ME, Grignon DJ, Roach M 3rd, Wolkov HB, Sandler HM, Shipley WU, Pollack A. Ki-67 staining index predicts distant metastasis and survival in locally advanced prostate cancer treated with radiotherapy: an analysis of patients in radiation therapy oncology group protocol 86-10. *Clin Cancer Res.* 2004; 10(12 Pt 1):4118-4124.

Li Y, Cozzi PJ, Russell PJ. Promising tumor-associated antigens for future prostate cancer therapy. Med Res Rev. 2010; 30(1):67-101.

Li Z, Bao S, Wu Q, Wang H, Eyler C, Sathornsumetee S, Shi Q, Cao Y, Lathia J, McLendon RE, Hjelmeland AB, Rich JN. Hypoxia-inducible factors regulate tumorigenic capacity of glioma stem cells. *Cancer Cell.* 2009; 15(6):501-513.

Lin HK, Hu YC, Yang L, Altuwaijri S, Chen YT, Kang HY, Chang C. Suppression versus induction of androgen receptor functions by the phosphatidylinositol 3-kinase/Akt pathway in prostate cancer LNCaP cells with different passage numbers. *J Biol Chem.* 2003; 278(51):50902-50907.

Lin Q, Yun Z. Impact of the hypoxic tumor microenvironment on the regulation of cancer stem cell characteristics. *Cancer Biol Ther.* 2010; 9(12): 949-956.

Liu F, Wang JJ, You ZY, Zhang YD, Zhao Y. Radiosensitivity of prostate cancer cells is enhanced by EGFR inhibitor C225. *Urol Oncol.* 2010; 28(1):59-66.

Liu Q, Nguyen DH, Dong Q, Shitaku P, Chung K, Liu OY, Tso JL, Liu JY, Konkankit V, Cloughesy TF, Mischel PS, Lane TF, Liau LM, Nelson SF, Tso CL. Molecular properties of CD133+ glioblastoma stem cells derived from treatment-refractory recurrent brain tumors. *J Neurooncol.* 2009; 94(1):1-19.

Logan IR, McNeill HV, Cook S, Lu X, Lunec J, Robson CN. Analysis of the MDM2 antagonist nutlin-3 in human prostate cancer cells. *Prostate.* 2007; 67(8):900-906.

Loupakis F, Pollina L, Stasi I, Ruzzo A, Scartozzi M, Santini D, Masi G, Graziano F, Cremolini C, Rulli E, Canestrari E, Funel N, Schiavon G, Petrini I, Magnani M, Tonini G, Campani D, Floriani I, Cascinu S, Falcone A.PTEN expression and KRAS mutations on primary tumors and metastases in the prediction of benefit from cetuximab plus irinotecan for patients with metastatic colorectal cancer. *J Clin Oncol.* 2009; 27(16):2622-2629.

Maenhaut C, Dumont JE, Roger PP, van Staveren WC. Cancer stem cells: a reality, a myth, a fuzzy concept or a misnomer? An analysis. *Carcinogenesis.* 2010; 31(2):149-158.

Maitland NJ, Bryce SD, Stower MJ, Collins AT. Prostate cancer stem cells: a target for new therapies. *Ernst Schering Found Symp Proc.* 2006; (5):155-179.

Mao C, Liao RY, Chen Q. Loss of PTEN expression predicts resistance to EGFR-targeted monoclonal antibodies in patients with metastatic colorectal cancer. *Br J Cancer.* 2010; 102(5):940.

McCord AM, Jamal M, Williams ES, Camphausen K, Tofilon PJ. CD133+ glioblastoma stem-like cells are radiosensitive with a defective DNA damage response compared with established cell lines. *Clin Cancer Res.* 2009; 15(16):5145-53.

Menczer J. Cox-2 expression in ovarian malignancies: a review of the clinical aspects. *Eur J Obstet Gynecol Reprod Biol.* 2009; 146(2):129-132.

Michalowski AS. On radiation damage to normal tissues and its treatment. II. Anti-inflammatory drugs. *Acta Oncol.* 1994; 33(2):139-157.

Movsas B, Chapman JD, Hanlon AL, Horwitz EM, Greenberg RE, Stobbe C, Hanks GE, Pollack A. Hypoxic prostate/muscle pO2 ratio predicts for biochemical failure in patients with prostate cancer: preliminary findings. *Urology*. 2002; 60(4):634-639.

Movsas B, Chapman JD, Hanlon AL, Horwitz EM, Pinover WH, Greenberg RE, Stobbe C, Hanks GE. Hypoxia in human prostate carcinoma: an Eppendorf PO2 study. *Am J Clin Oncol.* 2001; 24(5):458-461.

Mu Z, Hachem P, Agrawal S, Pollack A. Antisense MDM2 sensitizes prostate cancer cells to androgen deprivation, radiation, and the combination. *Int J Radiat Oncol Biol Phys*. 2004; 58(2):336-343.

Nagle RB, Ahmann FR, McDaniel KM, Paquin ML, Clark VA, Celniker A. Cytokeratin characterization of human prostatic carcinoma an d its derived cell lines. *Cancer Res.* 1987; 47(1):281-286.

Negri FV, Bozzetti C, Lagrasta CA, Crafa P, Bonasoni MP, Camisa R, Pedrazzi G, Ardizzoni A. PTEN status in advanced colorectal cancer treated with cetuximab. *Br J Cancer*. 2010; 102(1):162-164.

Nguyen CT, Zelefsky MJ, Kattan MW. The current state of brachytherapy nomograms for patients with clinically localized prostate cancer. *Cancer*. 2009; 115(13 Suppl):3121-3127.

Nishimura R, Osako T, Okumura Y, Hayashi M, Arima N. Clinical significance of Ki-67 in neoadjuvant chemotherapy for primary breast cancer as a predictor for chemosensitivity and for prognosis. *Breast Cancer*. 2009 doi: 10.1007/s12282-009-0161-5.

Ohneseit PA, Krebiehl G, Dittmann K, Kehlbach R, Rodemann HP. Inhibition of cyclooxygenase-2 activity by celecoxib does not lead to radiosensitization of human prostate cancer cells in vitro. *Radiother Oncol*. 2007; 82(2):229-238.

Parker AS, Heckman MG, Wu KJ, Crook JE, Hilton TW, Pisansky TM, Bernard JR, Schild SE, Khor LY, Hammond EH, Pollack A, Buskirk SJ. Evaluation of ki-67 staining levels as an independent biomarker of biochemical recurrence after salvage radiation therapy for prostate cancer. *Int J Radiat Oncol Biol Phys.* 2009; 75(5):1364-1370.

Patrawala L, Calhoun T, Schneider-Broussard R, Li H, Bhatia B, Tang S, Reilly JG, Chandra D, Zhou J, Claypool K, Coghlan L, Tang DG. Highly purified CD44+ prostate cancer cells from xenograft human tumors are enriched in tumorigenic and metastatic progenitor cells. *Oncogene*. 2006; 25(12):1696-1708.

Patrawala L, Calhoun-Davis T, Schneider-Broussard R, Tang DG. Hierarchical organization of prostate cancer cells in xenograft tumors: the CD44+alpha2beta1+ cell population is enriched in tumor-initiating cells. *Cancer Res*. 2007; 67(14):6796-6805.

Pattje WJ, Schuuring E, Mastik MF, Slagter-Menkema L, Schrijvers ML, Alessi S, van der Laan BF, Roodenburg JL, Langendijk JA, van der Wal JE. The phosphatase and tensin homologue deleted on chromosome 10 mediates radiosensitivity in head and neck cancer. *Br J Cancer*. 2010; 102(12):1778-1785.

Pedrero JM, Carracedo DG, Pinto CM, Zapatero AH, Rodrigo JP, Nieto CS, Gonzalez MV. Frequent genetic and biochemical alterations of the PI 3-K/AKT/PTEN pathway in head and neck squamous cell carcinoma. *Int J Cancer*. 2005; 114(2):242-248.

Peirce SK, Findley HW. The MDM2 antagonist nutlin-3 sensitizes p53-null neuroblastoma cells to doxorubicin via E2F1 and TAp73. *Int J Oncol*. 2009; 34(5):1395-1402.

Petersen C, Petersen S, Milas L, Lang FF, Tofilon PJ. Enhancement of intrinsic tumor cell radiosensitivity induced by a selective cyclooxygenase-2 inhibitor. *Clin Cancer Res* 2000; 6(6):2513-2520.

Phillips TM, McBride WH, Pajonk F. The response of CD24 (-/low)/CD44+ breast cancer-initiating cells to radiation. *J Natl Cancer Inst*. 2006; 98(24):1777-1785.

Pilepich MV, Winter K, John MJ, Mesic JB, Sause W, Rubin P, Lawton C, Machtay M, Grignon D. Phase III radiation therapy oncology group (RTOG) trial 86-10 of androgen deprivation adjuvant to definitive radiotherapy in locally advanced carcinoma of the prostate. *Int J Radiat Oncol Biol Phys*. 2001; 50(5):1243-1252.

Pollack A, Cowen D, Troncoso P, Zagars GK, von Eschenbach AC, Meistrich ML, McDonnell T. Molecular markers of outcome after radiotherapy in patients with prostate carcinoma: Ki-67, bcl-2, bax, and bcl-x. *Cancer*. 2003; 97(7):1630-1638.

Pollack A, DeSilvio M, Khor LY, Li R, Al-Saleem TI, Hammond ME, Venkatesan V, Lawton CA, Roach M 3rd, Shipley WU, Hanks GE, Sandler HM. Ki-67 staining is a strong predictor of distant metastasis and mortality for men with prostate cancer treated with radiotherapy plus androgen deprivation: Radiation Therapy Oncology Group Trial 92-02. *J Clin Oncol*. 2004; 22(11):2133-2140.

Pollack A, Joon DL, Wu CS, Sikes C, Hasegawa M, Terry NH, White RA, Zagars GK, Meistrich ML. Quiescence in R3327-G rat prostate tumors after androgen ablation. *Cancer Res*. 1997; 57(12):2493-2500.

Pollack A, Joon DL, Wu CS, Sikes C, Hasegawa M, Terry NH, White RA, Zagars GK, Meistrich ML. Quiescence in R3327-G rat prostate tumors after androgen ablation. *Cancer Res*. 1997; 57(12):2493-2500.

Pommery N, Hénichart JP. Involvement of PI3K/Akt pathway in prostate cancer--potential strategies for developing targeted therapies.*Mini Rev Med Chem*. 2005; 5(12):1125-1132.

Prendergast NJ, Atkins MR, Schatte EC, Paulson DF, Walther PJ. p53 immunohistochemical and genetic alterations are associated at high incidence with post-irradiated locally persistent prostate carcinoma. *J Urol*. 1996; 155(5):1685-1692.

Quinn DI, Henshall SM, Sutherland RL. Molecular markers of prostate cancer outcome. *Eur J Cancer*. 2005; 41(6):858-887.

Rajakariar R, Yaqoob MM, Gilroy DW.COX-2 in inflammation and resolution. *Mol Interv*. 2006; 6(4):199-207.

Rakozy C, Grignon DJ, Li Y, Gheiler E, Gururajanna B, Pontes JE, Sakr W, Wood DP Jr, Sarkar FH. p53 gene alterations in prostate cancer after radiation failure, and the association with clinical outcome. A molecular and immunohistochemical analysis. *Pathol Res Pract*. 1999; 195(3):129-135.

Reid AH, Attard G, Ambroisine L, Fisher G, Kovacs G, Brewer D, Clark J, Flohr P, Edwards S, Berney DM, Foster CS, Fletcher A, Gerald WL, Møller H, Reuter VE, Scardino PT, Cuzick J, de Bono JS, Cooper CS; Transatlantic Prostate Group. Molecular characterisation of ERG, ETV1 and PTEN gene loci identifies patients at low and high risk of death from prostate cancer. *Br J Cancer*. 2010; 102(4):678-864.

Richardsen E, Uglehus RD, Due J, Busch C, Busund LT. Cancer Epidemiol. COX-2 is overexpressed in primary prostate cancer with metastatic potential and may predict survival. A comparison study between COX-2, TGF-beta, IL-10 and Ki67. *Cancer Epidemiol*. 2010; 34(3):316-322.

Ropolo M, Daga A, Griffero F, Foresta M, Casartelli G, Zunino A, Poggi A, Cappelli E, Zona G, Spaziante R, Corte G, Frosina G. Comparative analysis of DNA repair in stem and nonstem glioma cell cultures. *Mol Cancer Res.* 2009; 7(3):383-392.

Rosser CJ, Tanaka M, Pisters LL, Tanaka N, Levy LB, Hoover DC, Grossman HB, McDonnell TJ, Kuban DA, Meyn RE. Adenoviral-mediated PTEN transgene expression sensitizes Bcl-2-expressing prostate cancer cells to radiation. *Cancer Gene Ther*. 2004; 11(4):273-279.

Sandler HM, Mirhadi AJ. Radical radiotherapy for prostate cancer is the 'only way to go'. Oncology (Williston Park). 2009; 23(10):840-843.

Scata KA, El-Deiry WS. p53, BRCA1 and breast Cancer chemoresistance. *Adv Exp Med Biol.* 2007; 608:70-86.

Scholzen T, Gerdes J. The Ki-67 protein: from the known and the unknown. *J Cell Physiol.* 2000; 182(3):311-322.

Scott SL, Earle JD, Gumerlock PH. Functional p53 increases prostate cancer cell survival after exposure to fractionated doses of ionizing radiation. *Cancer Res*. 2003; 63(21):7190-7196.

Sdek P, Ying H, Zheng H, Margulis A, Tang X, Tian K, Xiao ZX.The central acidic domain of MDM2 is critical in inhibition of retinoblastoma-mediated suppression of E2F and cell growth. *J Biol Chem*. 2004; 279(51):53317-53322.

Sengupta A, Cancelas JA. Cancer Stem Cells: a stride towards cancer cure? *J Cell Physiol.* 2010; 225(1):7-14.

Sheehan KM, Sheahan K, 'Donoghue DP, MacSweeney F, Conroy RM, Fitzgerald DJ, et al. The relationship between cyclooxygenase-2 expression and colorectal cancer. *JAMA* 1999; 282(13):1254-1257.

Shinohara A, Sakano S, Hinoda Y, Nishijima J, Kawai Y, Misumi T, Nagao K, Hara T, Matsuyama H. Association of TP53 and MDM2 polymorphisms with survival in bladder cancer patients treated with chemoradiotherapy. *Cancer Sci*. 2009; 100(12):2376-2382.

Shukla S, Maclennan GT, Hartman DJ, Fu P, Resnick MI, Gupta S. Activation of PI3K-Akt signaling pathway promotes prostate cancer cell invasion.*Int J Cancer*. 2007; 121(7):1424-1432.

Sircar K, Yoshimoto M, Monzon FA, Koumakpayi IH, Katz RL, Khanna A, Alvarez K, Chen G, Darnel AD, Aprikian AG, Saad F, Bismar TA, Squire JA. PTEN genomic deletion is associated with p-Akt and AR signalling in poorer outcome, hormone refractory prostate cancer. *J Pathol.* 2009; 218(4):505-513.

Skvortsova I, Skvortsov S, Stasyk T, Raju U, Popper BA, Schiestl B, von Guggenberg E, Neher A, Bonn GK, Huber LA, Lukas P.Intracellular signaling pathways regulating radioresistance of human prostate carcinoma cells. *Proteomics*. 2008; 8(21):4521-4533.

Smith MR, Manola J, Kaufman DS, Oh WK, Bubley GJ, Kantoff PW.Celecoxib versus placebo for men with prostate cancer and a rising serum prostate-specific antigen after radical prostatectomy and/or radiation therapy. *J Clin Oncol*. 2006; 24(18):2723-2728.

Soond DR, Bjørgo E, Moltu K, Dale VQ, Patton DT, Torgersen KM, Galleway F, Twomey B, Clark J, Gaston JS, Taskén K, Bunyard P, Okkenhaug K. PI3K p110delta regulates T-cell cytokine production during primary and secondary immune responses in mice and humans. *Blood*. 2010; 115(11):2203-2213.

Sos ML, Koker M, Weir BA, Heynck S, Rabinovsky R, Zander T, Seeger JM, Weiss J, Fischer F, Frommolt P, Michel K, Peifer M, Mermel C, Girard L, Peyton M, Gazdar AF,

Minna JD, Garraway LA, Kashkar H, Pao W, Meyerson M, Thomas RK. PTEN loss contributes to erlotinib resistance in EGFR-mutant lung cancer by activation of Akt and EGFR. *Cancer Res*. 2009; 69(8):3256-3261.

Sottoriva A, Sloot PM, Medema JP, Vermeulen L. Exploring cancer stem cell niche directed tumor growth. *Cell Cycle*. 2010; 9(8): 1472-1479.

Stattin P, Damber JE, Modig H, Bergh A. Pretreatment p53 immunoreactivity does not infer radioresistance in prostate cancer patients. *Int J Radiat Oncol Biol Phys*. 1996; 35(5):885-889.

Steelman LS, Bertrand FE, McCubrey JA. The complexity of PTEN: mutation, marker and potential target for therapeutic intervention. *Expert Opin Ther Targets*. 2004; 8(6):537-550.

Steinauer KK, Gibbs I, Ning S, French JN, Armstrong J, Knox SJ. Radiation induces upregulation of cyclooxygenase-2 (COX-2) protein in PC-3 cells. *Int J Radiat Oncol Biol Phys* 2000; 48:325-328.

Stephenson AJ, Slawin KM. The value of radiotherapy in treating recurrent prostate cancer after radical prostatectomy. *Nat Clin Pract Urol*. 2004; 1(2):90-96.

Stoyanova R, Hachem P, Hensley H, Khor LY, Mu Z, Hammond ME, Agrawal S, Pollack A. Antisense-MDM2 sensitizes LNCaP prostate cancer cells to androgen deprivation, radiation, and the combination in vivo. *Int J Radiat Oncol Biol Phys*. 2007; 68(4):1151-1160.

Sugano N, Suda T, Godai TI, Tsuchida K, Shiozawa M, Sekiguchi H, Yoshihara M, Matsukuma S, Sakuma Y, Tsuchiya E, Kameda Y, Akaike M, Miyagi Y. MDM2 gene amplification in colorectal cancer is associated with disease progression at the primary site, but inversely correlated with distant metastasis.*Genes Chromosomes Cancer*. 2010; 49(7):620-629.

Supiot S, Hill RP, Bristow RG. Nutlin-3 radiosensitizes hypoxic prostate cancer cells independent of p53. *Mol Cancer Ther*. 2008; 7(4):993-999.

Takeuchi H, Ozawa S, Ando N, Kitagawa Y, Ueda M, Kitajima M. Cell-cycle regulators and the Ki-67 labeling index can predict the response to chemoradiotherapy and the survival of patients with locally advanced squamous cell carcinoma of the esophagus. *Ann Surg Oncol*. 2003; 10(7):792-800.

Tamura K, Aoyagi M, Wakimoto H, Ando N, Nariai T, Yamamoto M, Ohno K. Accumulation of CD133-positive glioma cells after high-dose irradiation by Gamma Knife surgery plus external beam radiation. *J Neurosurg*. 2010; 113(2):310-318.

Tang DG, Patrawala L, Calhoun T, Bhatia B, Choy G, Schneider-Broussard R, Jeter C. Prostate cancer stem/progenitor cells: identification, characterization, and implications. *Mol Carcinog*. 2007; 46(1):1-14.

Teng DH, Hu R, Lin H, Davis T, Iliev D, Frye C, Swedlund B, Hansen KL, Vinson VL, Gumpper KL, Ellis L, El-Naggar A, Frazier M, Jasser S, Langford LA, Lee J, Mills GB, Pershouse MA, Pollack RE, Tornos C, Troncoso P, Yung WK, Fujii G, Berson A, Steck PA. MMAC1/PTEN mutations in primary tumor specimens and tumor cell lines. *Cancer Res*. 1997; 57(23):5221-5225.

Tomioka A, Tanaka M, De Velasco MA, Anai S, Takada S, Kushibiki T, Tabata Y, Rosser CJ, Uemura H, Hirao Y. Delivery of PTEN via a novel gene microcapsule sensitizes prostate cancer cells to irradiation. *Mol Cancer Ther*. 2008; 7(7):1864-1870.

Torres-Roca JF. The role of external-beam radiation therapy in the treatment of clinically localized prostate cancer. *Cancer Control.* 2006; 13(3):188-193.

Uzoaru I, Rubenstein M, Mirochnik Y, Slobodskoy L, Shaw M, Guinan P. An evaluation of the markers p53 and Ki-67 for their predictive value in prostate cancer. *J Surg Oncol.* 1998; 67(1):33-37.

Vassilev LT, Vu BT, Graves B, Carvajal D, Podlaski F, Filipovic Z, Kong N, Kammlott U, Lukacs C, Klein C, Fotouhi N, Liu EA. In vivo activation of the p53 pathway by small-molecule antagonists of MDM2. *Science* 2004; 303 (5659): 844-848.

Vergis R, Corbishley CM, Thomas K, Horwich A, Huddart R, Khoo V, Eeles R, Sydes MR, Cooper CS, Dearnaley D, Parker C. Expression of Bcl-2, p53, and MDM2 in localized prostate cancer with respect to the outcome of radical radiotherapy dose escalation. *Int J Radiat Oncol Biol Phys.* 2010; 78(1):35-41.

Visscher DW, Pankratz VS, Santisteban M, Reynolds C, Ristimäki A, Vierkant RA, Lingle WL, Frost MH, Hartmann LC. Association between cyclooxygenase-2 expression in atypical hyperplasia and risk of breast cancer. *J Natl Cancer Inst.* 2008; 100(6):421-427.

Wagener M, Zhang X, Villarreal HG, Levy L, Allen P, Shentu S, Fang B, Krishnan S, Chang JY, Cheung MR. Effect of combining anti-epidermal growth factor receptor antibody C225 and radiation on DU145 prost ate cancer. *Oncol Rep.* 2008; 19(5):1071-1077.

Wang J, Wakeman TP, Lathia JD, Hjelmeland AB, Wang XF, White RR, Rich JN, Sullenger BA. Notch promotes radioresistance of glioma stem cells. *Stem Cells.* 2010; 28(1):17-28.

Weber L. Patented inhibitors of p53-Mdm2 interaction (2006 - 2008). *Expert Opin Ther Pat.* 2010; 20(2):179-191.

Wei C, Guomin W, Yujun L, Ruizhe Q. Cancer stem-like cells in human prostate carcinoma cells DU145: the seeds of the cell line? *Cancer Biol Ther.* 2007; 6(5):763-768.

Weller M. Predicting response to cancer chemotherapy: the role of p53. *Cell Tissue Res.* 1998; 292(3):435-445.

Wen B, Deutsch E, Eschwege P, De Crevoisier R, Nasr E, Eschwege F, Bourhis J. Cyclooxygenase-2 inhibitor NS398 enhances antitumor effect of irradiation on hormone refractory human prostate carcinoma cells. *J Urol.* 2003; 170(5):2036-2039.

Wo JY, Zietman AL. Why does androgen deprivation enhance the results of radiation therapy? *Urol Oncol.* 2008; 26(5):522-529.

Wolff H, Saukkonen K, Anttila S, Karjalainen A, Vainio H, Ristimaki A. Expression of cyclooxygenase-2 in human carcinoma. *Cancer Res* 1998; 58(22):4997-5001.

Wu CT, Chen WC, Liao SK, Hsu CL, Lee KD, Chen MF. The radiation response of hormone-resistant prostate cancer induced by long-term hormone therapy. *Endocr Relat Cancer.* 2007; 14(3):633-643.

Xie BX, Zhang H, Yu L, Wang J, Pang B, Wu RQ, Qian XL, Li SH, Shi QG, Wang LL, Zhou JG. The radiation response of androgen-refractory prostate cancer cell line C4-2 derived from androgen-sensitive cell line LNCaP. *Asian J Androl.* 2010; 12(3):405-414.

Xue Q, Hopkins B, Perruzzi C, Udayakumar D, Sherris D, Benjamin LE. Palomid 529, a novel small-molecule drug, is a TORC1/TORC2 inhibitor that reduces tumor growth, tumor angiogenesis, and vascular permeability. *Cancer Res.* 2008; 68(22):9551-9957.

Yang M, Jiang P, Sun FX, Hasegawa S, Baranov E, Chishima T, Shimada H, Moossa AR, Hoffman RM. A fluorescent orthotopic bone metastasis model of human prostate cancer. *Cancer Res.* 1999; 59(4):781-786.

Yang YM, Chang JW. Current status and issues in cancer stem cell study. *Cancer Invest.* 2008; 26(7):741-755.

Ye YK, Bi XC, He HC, Han ZD, Dai QS, Liang YX, Zeng GH, Qin WJ, Chen ZN, Zhong WD. CK20 and Ki-67 as significant prognostic factors in human bladder carcinoma. *Clin Exp Med.* 2010; 10(3):153-158.

Yoshioka Y. Current status and perspectives of brachytherapy for prostate cancer. *Int J Clin Oncol.* 2009; 14(1):31-36.

Yu GW, Rudiger S, Veprintsev D, Freund S, Fernandez-Fernandez MR, Fersht AR.*The central region of HDM2 provides a second binding site for p53*.Proc Natl Acad Sci U S A. 2006; 103(5):1227-1232.

Zhang M, Behbod F, Atkinson RL, Landis MD, Kittrell F, Edwards D, Medina D, Tsimelzon A, Hilsenbeck S, Green JE, Michalowska AM, Rosen JM. Identification of tumor-initiating cells in a p53-null mouse model of breast cancer. *Cancer Res*. 2008; 68(12):4674-4682.

Zhang XH, Huang DP, Guo GL, Chen GR, Zhang HX, Wan L, Chen SY. Coexpression of VEGF-C and COX-2 and its association with lymphangiogenesis in human breast cancer. *BMC Cancer*. 2008; 8:4.

Zhang Z, Wang H, Prasad G, Li M, Yu D, Bonner JA, Agrawal S, Zhang R. Radiosensitization by antisense anti-MDM2 mixed-backbone oligonucleotide in in vitro and in vivo human cancer models. *Clin Cancer Res.* 2004; 10(4):1263-1273.

Zietman AL, Prince EA, Nakfoor BM, Park JJ. Androgen deprivation and radiation therapy: sequencing studies using the Shionogi in vivo tumor system. *Int J Radiat Oncol Biol Phys.* 1997; 38(5):1067-1070.

Zimmermann KC, Sarbia M, Weber AA, Borchard F, Gabbert HE, Schrör K. Cyclooxygenase-2 expression in human esophageal carcinoma. *Cancer Res* 1999; 59(1):198-204.

In: Tumor Suppressors
Editor: Susan D. Nguyen

ISBN: 978-1-61761-986-1

Chapter 12

Molecular Functions of the p53 Tumor Suppressor in the Apoptotic Response to DNA Damage

Kiyotsugu Yoshida[*]
Medical Research Institute, Tokyo Medical and Dental University,
Tokyo, Japan

Abstract

The tumor suppressor p53 has been implicated in many important cellular processes, including regulation of apoptotic cell death, in the cellular response to DNA damage. When cells encounter genotoxic stress, certain sensors for DNA lesions stabilize and activate p53. Eventually, p53 exerts its tumor suppressor function by transactivating numerous target genes. Active p53 is subjected to a complex and diverse array of covalent post-translational modifications, which selectively influence the expression of p53 target genes. In this context, the molecular basis for how p53 induces apoptosis has been substantially studied; however, the relative contribution of each downstream effecter is still to be explored. Moreover, little is known about precise mechanisms by which modified p53 is capable of apoptosis induction. A thorough understanding for the whole picture of p53 modification in apoptosis will be extremely valuable in the development of highly effective and specific therapies for caner patients. This review is focused on the current views regarding the regulation of cell fate by p53 in the apoptotic response to DNA damage.

* Corresponding author: Yoshida, K. (yos.mgen@mri.tmd.ac.jp).

Introduction

Genotoxic stress that damages DNA induces cell cycle arrest, activation of DNA repair, and in the event of irreparable damage, induction of apoptosis. The decision by cells either to repair DNA lesions and continue through the cell cycle or to undergo apoptosis is relevant to the incidence of mutagenesis and, subsequently, carcinogenesis [1]. In this context, incomplete repair of DNA damage prior to replication or mitosis can result in the accumulation of heritable genetic changes. Therapeutic anti-cancer treatments that use DNA-damaging agents must strike a balance between induction of repair and apoptosis in order to maximize the therapeutic effect. However, the nature of the cellular signaling response that determines cell survival or death is far from being understood. Certain insights have been derived from the findings that the tumor suppressor p53 plays a central role in response to DNA damage. The p53 gene is one of the most common sites for genetic alterations in human solid cancers since it is mutated in more than 50% cancer cases worldwide [2]. The level of p53 protein is basically undetectable in normal cells but rapidly increases in response to a variety of stress signals. The mechanism by which the p53 protein is stabilized is not completely understood, but post-translational modification plays a pivotal role [3]. The p53 pathway can be impaired by numerous oncogenic proteins [4]. Mice engineered to have the p53 gene knocked-out develop tumors at an increased rate [5]. Subsequent research on wild-type p53 clearly demonstrates that the transcription factor is a key controller in cell cycle and determines the cell fate in response to oncogenic and to other stresses to maintain genomic integrity. The p53 has thus provided the name of "guardian of the genome" [6]. In the complexity of p53 network, there are various crucial post-translational modifications that induce p53 activation as a transcription factor. In the past 10 years, understanding of the cellular mechanisms of apoptosis mediated by p53 has advanced considerably, and the primary focus of this review is to provide an overview of p53, its mode of action and its physiological role in genotoxic stress-induced apoptosis.

Functions of p53

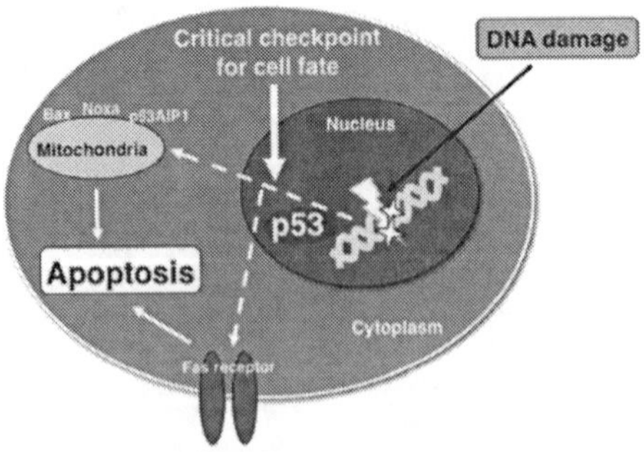

Figure 1. A hypothetical schema of a role for p53 on the critical checkpoint of cell fate in the apoptotic response to DNA damage. Following DNA damage, the cellular signaling is targeted to the nucleus, then the cell fate may be determined by p53 in the nucleus. The death signals are transmitted into the mitochondria or the receptors to induce apoptosis.

The biological role of p53 is to ensure genome integrity of cells. p53 can stimulate the repair processes and protective mechanisms, or the cessation of cell division and the induction of acquired cell death. To achieve its aims, p53 may use a wide spectrum of activities, such as its ability to function as transcription factor, by inducing or repressing different genes or as a regulatory protein, within numerous signaling pathways. The functional consequence for these different activities of p53 fits into the enforcement of genetic stability. The activity of p53 is stimulated in response to DNA damage and to various genotoxic insults that eventually compromise genome integrity [7]. Following genotoxic stress, p53 primarily determines the cell fate to induce growth arrest, DNA repair, or apoptosis. In particular, upon exposure to severe DNA damage, p53 conducts to elicit cell death by apoptosis (Fig. 1). The loss of p53 functions and the deregulated activities of p53 are involved not only in the development of malignant diseases, but also in relation to cardiovascular, neurodegenerative, infectious and metabolic diseases, as well as participate in the process of organism aging. p53 has the ability to bind specific responsive DNA elements and the specificity of the transcriptional activation depends on the ability of p53 DNA-binding domain to interact with the regulatory regions of certain genes. The transcriptional activation is determined by the N-terminus of p53, which contains several regions interacting with the transcription machinery and recruiting factors that modify local chromatin structure [8].

Stabilization of p53 in Response to DNA Damage

p53 is regulated primarily through post-translational modifications, especially phosphorylation, and the accumulation of p53 is the first step in response to cellular stress (Fig. 2) [9]. The N-terminus is heavily phosphorylated, while the C-terminus contains phosphorylated, acetylated, methylated and sumoylated residues. Post-translational modifications on the N-terminus are important for stabilizing p53 while those on the C-terminus inhibit the ability for regulation of sequence-specific DNA binding, the oligomerization state, the nuclear import/export process, and the ubiquitination [10]. The *mdm2* gene is a transcriptional target of p53, and once synthesized, the MDM2 protein can bind to p53 at the N-terminus leading to its rapid degradation through the ubiquitin-proteasome machinery [9, 11, 12]. In response to DNA damage, the ATM kinase rapidly phosphorylates p53 at Ser15. The serine/threonine kinase Chk2 acts downstream of ATM phosphorylating p53 at Ser20. These phopshorylated sites in the N-terminus of p53 are close to the Mdm2-binding region of the protein, thereby they block the interaction with Mdm2, leading to stabilization of p53, that escapes from proteasomal degradation.[10] Recent findings suggested that constitutive phosphorylation of p53 by protein kinase C (PKC) at the C-terminal domain contributes to its degradation via the ubiquitin-proteasome pathway [13].

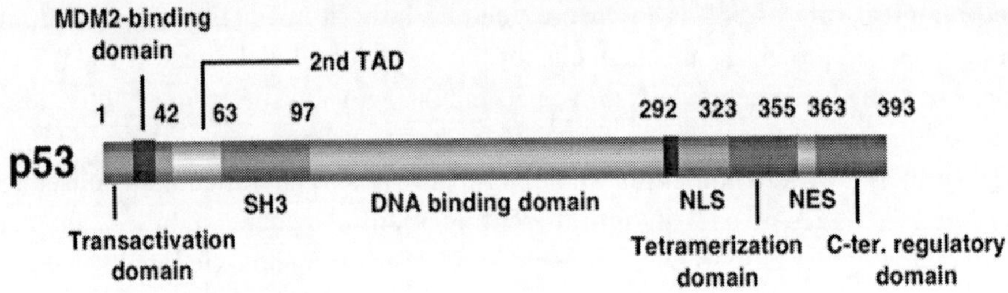

•Phosphorylation
S6, S9, S15, T18, S20, S33, S37, S46, T55, T81, S149, T150, T155, S215, S313, S314, S315, S366, S376, T377, S378, T387, S392

•Acetylation
K120, K305, K320, K370, K372, K373, K381, K382.

•Methylation
K370, K372

•Neddylation (Nedd8)
K320, K370, K372, K373

•SUMOylation
K386

•Ubiquitination
K320, K370, K372, K373, K381, K382, K386

Figure 2. Functional domain and modification residues in p53. TAD indicates transactivation domain. NLS and NES mean nuclear localization and export signals, respectively. Modifications related to apoptosis are highlighted in gray.

p53 and Apoptosis

Apoptosis is a well-studied and well-understood process that has been considered to play an important role in the tumor suppression. Apoptosis is triggered in response to a variety of signals, which can activate the extrinsic and/or intrinsic death pathways, or when cells are deprived of pro-survival signals [14]. p53 acts at multiple levels of the intrinsic and extrinsic pathways [15], via the induction of multiple apoptotic target genes, as well as via transcription-independent mechanisms [16, 17]. For example, p53 activates several important genes that are crucial for the execution of the intrinsic pathway of apoptosis including pro-apoptotic genes such as Bax, Noxa, Puma, and Apaf-1 [18-21]. When p53-dependent apoptosis is employed by cells, these cells typically undergo the intrinsic cell death pathway [16]. Further, p53 represses the apoptosis repressor with caspase recruitment domain protein, which counteracts the apoptotic functions of Puma and Bad [22]. p53 can also promote cytochrome c release by inducing the expression of the OKL38 tumor suppressor gene, which localizes to the mitochondria and augments cytochrome c release. Silencing OKL38 correlates with tumorigenesis, and its overexpression induces apoptosis in several carcinoma cell lines [23]. Among the extrinsic pathway, p53 induces the expression of the death receptor

Fas and DR5 [15]. Moreover, p53 induces the expression of the TRAIL death ligand and the Fas ligand [24, 25]. In addition to its activity as a transcriptional regulator, p53 can also induce cell death in a transcription-independent manner. It has been shown that p53 is able to physically interact with anti-apoptotic proteins including bcl-2, bcl-X_L and mcl-1 at the mitochondrial membrane [26]. When these anti-apoptotic proteins bind p53, their ability to stabilize the mitochondrial membrane is compromised resulting in permeability changes and the release of cytochrome c. Additionally, p53 can interact with bak and thus directly induce the release of cytochrome c from the intermembrane space of the mitochondrion [26]. Taken together, these studies suggest a role for mitochondrial p53 in the induction of apoptosis [27]. In addition, it should be noted that a new p53 cofactor, human cellular apoptosis susceptibility protein (hCAS/CSE1L) suppresses p53-mediated transcription by binding directly to the promoters of certain p53 target genes in a p53-independent manner [28]. The promoters bound by hCAS/CSE1L do not appear to correlate with a particular physiological outcome whereas silencing of hCAS/CSE1L inhibits ultraviolet (UV) irradiation-induced death. Finally, It was also recently shown that p53 regulates the expression of microRNAs (miRNAs), where a primary role has been attributed to the miR-34 family [29, 30]. Inactivation of miR-34 attenuates p53-mediated apoptosis in cells exposed to genotoxic stress, suggesting a role for this microRNA in regulating p53 responses.

Transcriptional Regulation of p53 in the Apoptotic Response to DNA Damage

Recent reports document that PKCδ transactivates p53 expression at the transcriptional level [1, 31, 32]. The tumor-promoting phorbol ester 12-O-tetradecanoylphorbol-13-acetate (TPA) prevents DNA damage-induced up-regulation of p53 by down-regulating PKCδ. TPA promotes tumor formation in various mice and cell culture models, and this has been correlated with the down-regulation of PKC [33]. TPA is known to activate but then down-regulate the diacylglycerol-dependent PKC isoforms [33, 34]. Previous studies demonstrated that the tumor-promoting activities of TPA are mediated at least in part by down-regulating PKCδ [35]. Moreover, transgenic mice overexpressing PKCδ in their epidermis are resistant to tumor promotion by TPA [36]. Previous studies have suggested that TPA can inhibit the DNA damage-mediated induction of p53 [37]. Moreover, other studies with protein kinase inhibitors have suggested that PKCδ regulates the p53 pathway [38]. Regulation of p53 in response to genotoxic stress commonly occurs by hampering ubiquitination and subsequent degradation of the p53 protein. By contrast, suppression of p53 expression by inhibition of PKCδ is caused by the inhibition of p53 synthesis, not increased degradation of p53 protein. Inhibiting PKCδ blocks both basal transcription of the human p53 gene and initiation of transcription from the human p53 promoter. The DNA damage-induced increase in p53 accumulation is dramatically inhibited by pretreatment of cells with the tumor promoter TPA. In addition, the PKCδ inhibitor, rottlerin, is also able to block the DNA damage-mediated induction of p53. More importantly, pretreatment of cells with TPA or with rottlerin results in the inhibition of basal p53 transcription. In this regard, accumulation of p53 can not be achieved any longer following TPA or rottlerin stimulation, because p53 transcription is blocked. It is thus conceivable that the tumor-suppressing effects of PKCδ are mediated at least in part through activating p53 transcription. Indeed, repression of the p53 promoter has been suggested as a mechanism for tumor promotion [39, 40].

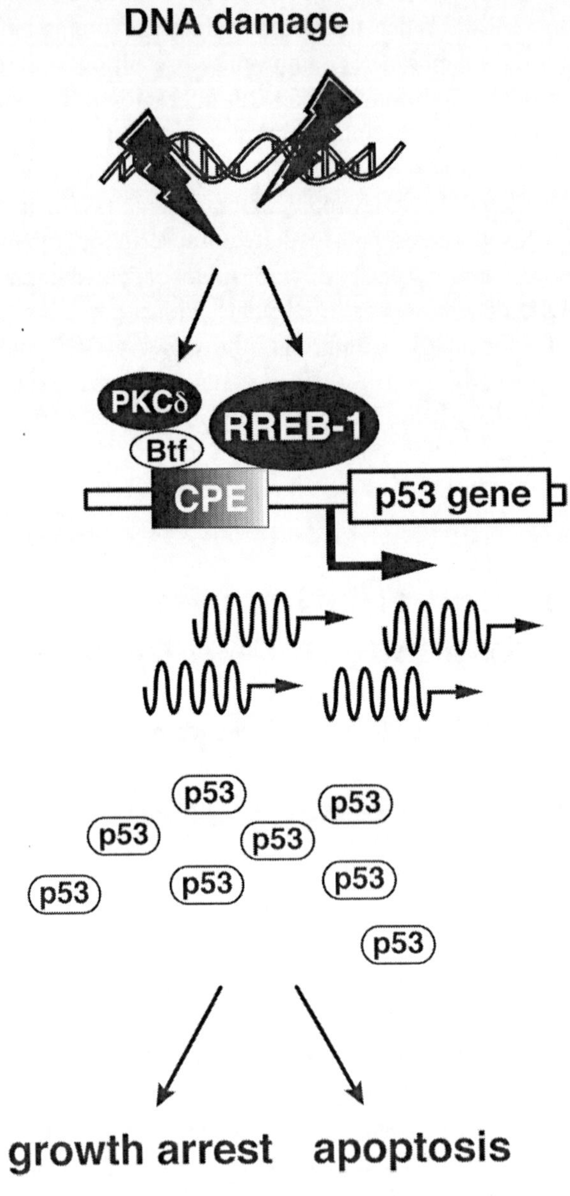

Figure 3. DNA damage-induced transcriptional regulation of p53 gene by PKCδ and Btf or RREB-1. Upon exposure to genotoxic stress, activated PKCδ induces Btf for co-occupancy to CPE-p53, thereby up-regulating the expression of p53 at mRNA levels. p53 transcription is also induced by RREB-1 via CPE-p53 in response to DNA damage.

Recent study also demonstrated that PKCδ induces the promoter activity of p53 through the p53 core promoter element (CPE-p53) and that such induction is enhanced in response to DNA damage. Upon exposure to genotoxic stress, PKCδ activates and interacts with the death-promoting transcription factor Btf (Bcl-2-associated transcription factor) to co-occupy CPE-p53. Inhibition of PKCδ activity decreases the affinity of Btf for CPE-p53, thereby reducing p53 expression at both the mRNA and protein levels. In concert with these results, disruption of Btf-mediated p53 transcription by RNA interference leads to suppression of p53-mediated apoptosis following genotoxic stress. These findings provide evidence that activation of p53 transcription by PKCδ triggers p53-dependent apoptosis in response to DNA damage (Fig. 3) [32]. Subsequently, we also found that RAS-responsive element-binding protein-1 (RREB-1) efficiently binds to the p53 promoter via CPE-p53 and transactivates p53 expression [41]. Notably, disruption of RREB-1-mediated p53 transcription suppresses the expression of the p53 target genes. We also show that, upon exposure to genotoxic stress, RREB-1 controls apoptosis in a p53-dependent manner (Fig. 3). These findings provide evidence that RREB-1 participates in modulating p53 transcription in response to DNA damage.

Post-Translational Modifications That Influence p53-Mediated Apoptosis

Accumulating studies have revealed that some of post-translational modifications are specifically linked to the apoptotic function of p53 (Fig. 2). Exploiting pathways that specifically enhance p53-mediated apoptosis have been a goal of cancer therapeutics. Some of the better-understood examples from this subset will be discussed below.

Phosphorylation of Serine at 46

Most important modification for the induction of apoptosis is the phosphorylation at serine 46 (Ser46). Enhanced apoptosis occurs as a result of this phosphorylated form of p53 selectively activating pro-apoptotic target gene transcription [42]. In response to UV irradiation, Ser46 phosphorylation is mediated by homeodomain-interacting protein kinase 2 [43, 44]. By contrast, little was known about Ser46 kinase(s) upon exposure to genotoxic stress. Recently, we found that dual-specificity tyrosine-phosphorylation-regulated kinase 2 (DYRK2) has the characteristics of an in vitro direct Ser46 kinase [45]. Moreover, our results demonstrated that DYRK2 phosphorylates p53 at Ser46 in cells exposed to genotoxic stress. Significantly, DYRK2 phosphorylation of Ser46 was associated with the induction of apoptosis following DNA damage (Fig. 4). These findings provided support a novel signaling mechanism in which phosphorylation of p53 at Ser46 by DYRK2 regulates apoptotic cell death in response to DNA damage. However, a previous study demonstrated that DYRK2 is predominantly expressed in the cytoplasm [46, 47]. We confirmed the cytoplasmic localization of DYRK2 in unstimulated cells. Furthermore, we found that DYRK2 translocates from the cytoplasm into the nucleus in response to DNA damage. The mechanism for nuclear targeting of DYRK2 is, at present, not known. Importantly, however, nuclear translocation may be required for efficient phosphorylation of p53 at Ser46 and, therefore it is conceivable that Ser46 phosphorylation occurs in relatively later periods following genotoxic stress [42, 48]. Indeed, our findings that nuclear re-distribution of

DYRK2 coincides with Ser46 phosphorylation of nuclear p53 further support the mechanism in which nuclear targeting of DYRK2 is, at least in part, required for sufficient phosphorylation of p53 at Ser46 in the nucleus [45]. Importantly, upon exposure to genotoxic stress, p53DINP1 is expressed and then recruits a kinase(s) to p53 that specifically phosphorylates Ser46 [48]. Our recent data also showed that PKCδ is, presumably indirectly, involved in phosphorylation of p53 at Ser46 [49]. PKCδ-mediated phosphorylation was required for the interaction of PKCδ with p53. The results also demonstrated that p53DINP1 associates with PKCδ upon exposure to genotoxic agents. In concert with these results, PKCδ potentiates p53-dependent apoptosis by affecting Ser46 phosphorylation in response to genotoxic stress. These findings indicate that PKCδ regulates p53 to induce apoptotic cell death in the cellular response to DNA damage [49]. Moreover, we recently found that PKCδ regulates MDM2 expression by controlling Akt-mediated phosphorylation. As a result, PKCδ could control p53 expression indirectly by modulating MDM2 function in response to DNA damage (Hew HC, et al. unpublished observation). As mentioned above, Ser46 phosphorylation occurs in the later stages of p53 activation and influences the response by specifically promoting the induction of the apoptotic gene p53AIP1 [42]. This is accompanied by downregulation of p21 expression, ultimately resulting in p53-dependent apoptosis. One possible mechanism for this enhancement is that phosphorylation of Ser46 enables prolyl isomerase Pin1-mediated conformational change and dissociation of p53 from the inhibitor of apoptosis, iASPP, thereby promoting cell death [50]. The isomerization of p53 by Pin1 facilitates the binding and acetylation of p53 by the acetyltransferase p300 [50]. However, the interaction with Pin1 is not sufficient to explain the effect of Ser46 phosphorylation on p53 function, since Pin1 loss also diminishes the ability of p53 to bind to the promoters of the non-apoptotic target genes p21 and MDM2 [51]. Further studies are definitely required toward a better understanding of how Ser46 phosphorylation confers the ability of p53 to specifically transactivate pro-apoptotic genes and to induce apoptosis. Nevertheless, a recent study demonstrated that the expression of a p53-46F mutant, in which Ser46 is replaced with phenylalanine, induces specific p53-target genes associated with apoptosis, including Noxa, p53AIP1, and p53RFP [52]. Moreover, transduction of the p53-46F enhanced apoptosis and suppressed tumor growth [52]. These findings thus provide a model in which gene-transfer of the p53-46F mutant contributes to a more effective strategy for cancer therapy. Although it is unclear whether the p53-46F is mimicked to the phosphorylation of Ser46, modification of Ser46 may be of importance for the possibility to develop a new therapeutic strategy based on the 'Super-p53' against cancer.

Modifications of Lysines at 320 and 373

Lys320 of p53 can be modified independently by both acetylation and ubiquitination to influence promoter selectivity. p53 transcriptional activity and growth arrest function is enhanced by acetylation at Lys320 by the acetyltransferase PCAF [53, 54]. On the other hand, the E3 ligase E4F1 ubiquitinates p53 at Lys320, and specifically increases the activation of cell-cycle-arrest genes, such as p21, Gadd45, and cyclin G1 while the expression of apoptotic targets remains unchanged [55]. Chromatin immunoprecipitation experiments demonstrate that Lys320-ubiquitylated p53 is bound to the p21 gene promoter, but not to that of the apoptotic target gene Noxa. Similarly, acetylation of Lys320 following drug-induced DNA-damage promotes cell survival, with Lys320-acetylated p53 binding more efficiently to the p21 promoter than does non-acetylated p53 [56]. Interestingly, for the Lys320 equivalent in mice, Lys317, mutation to an arginine leads to p53-mediated transcription of pro-apoptotic target genes, such as Puma, and Noxa [57].

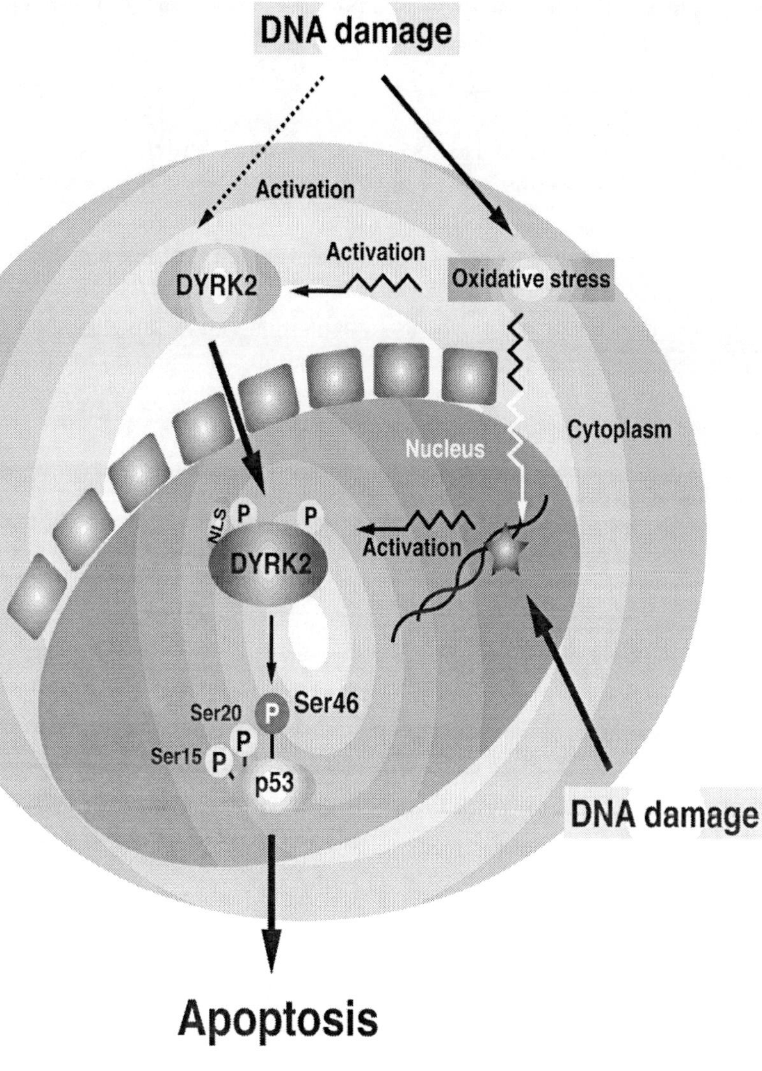

Figure 4. A proposed model for DYRK2-mediated apoptosis in the cellular response to DNA damage. Upon exposure to genotoxic stress, p53 is stabilized and activated by phosphorylation at Ser15 and Ser20. Cytoplasmic DYRK2 is activated and targeted to the nucleus, and then phosphorylates p53 at Ser46. Ser46 phosphorylation of p53 triggers induction of apoptosis by up-regulation of apoptosis-related gene expression, such as p53AIP1.

These observations are consistent with a loss of E4F1-dependent ubiquitination of Lys320, which facilitates growth arrest [55]. Furthermore, FBXO11-mediated neddylation of human p53 at Lys320 represses p53 activity and therefore the observations made in p53K317R mice are also representative of a loss of neddylation [58]. Thus, the increased apoptotic activity of mouse p53K317R may be explained by impaired acetylation, neddylation, or ubiquitination at this residue. In contrast, acetylation of Lys373, catalyzed by p300 and/or CBP, contributes to increased phosphorylation of N-terminal residues of p53, and increased ability to transactivate lower affinity binding sites including the pro-apoptotic target genes, such as PIG3, Bax, and p53AIP1 [56]. These results are consistent with a model whereby acetylation at Lys320 and Lys373 exerts as a sensor system that enables p53 to determine between growth arrest and cell death, and to coordinate gene expression patterns appropriately following DNA damage.

Acetylation of Lysine at 120

p53-dependent apoptosis is also specifically enhanced after DNA damage via acetylation at Lys120 by the MYST family acetyltransferases MOF and TIP60. Lys120 lies in the DNA-binding domain of p53, and its acetylation leads to increased recruitment of p53 specifically to pro-apoptotic target genes, such as Puma and Bax, suggesting that this modification alone can influence how p53 responds to the DNA-damaging signals. This modification seems to be required for p53-dependent apoptosis, as mutants that can no longer be modified in this way exhibit impaired apoptotic activity while maintaining the proper regulation of Mdm2 and growth-arrest genes [59, 60]. Collectively, these data indicate that a defined p53 modification can be linked to a specific cellular outcome.

Concluding Remarks

The molecular basis for how p53 induces apoptosis has been extensively studied; however, the relative contribution of each downstream effecter is still to be explored. In this regard, recent studies have shed some light on post-translational modifications and factors that can influence apoptosis whereas the answers to many questions still need to be completed. Moreover, through in vivo experimental approach, we need to verify the biological significance of each modification site both in p53 wild-type and mutant. If we could understand the whole picture of p53 modification in apoptosis, it would be then possible to develop highly effective and specific strategies for the cancer treatment.

References

[1] Yoshida, K. (2008) Nuclear trafficking of pro-apoptotic kinases in response to DNA damage. *Trends Mol Med* 14, 305-313.

[2] Hollstein, M., Sidransky, D., Vogelstein, B., & Harris, C. C. (1991) p53 mutations in human cancers. *Science* 253, 49-53.

[3] Shieh, S. Y., Ikeda, M., Taya, Y., & Prives, C. (1997) DNA damage-induced phosphorylation of p53 alleviates inhibition by MDM2. *Cell* 91, 325-334.

[4] Oren, M., Damalas, A., Gottlieb, T., Michael, D., Taplick, J., Leal, J. F., Maya, R., Moas, M., Seger, R., Taya, Y., & Ben-Ze'ev, A. (2002) Regulation of p53: intricate loops and delicate balances. *Biochem Pharmacol* 64, 865-871.

[5] Donehower, L. A., Harvey, M., Slagle, B. L., McArthur, M. J., Montgomery, C. A., Jr., Butel, J. S., & Bradley, A. (1992) Mice deficient for p53 are developmentally normal but susceptible to spontaneous tumours. *Nature* 356, 215-221.

[6] Lane, D. P. (1992) Cancer. p53, guardian of the genome. *Nature* 358, 15-16.

[7] Horn, H. F., & Vousden, K. H. (2007) Coping with stress: multiple ways to activate p53. *Oncogene* 26, 1306-1316.

[8] Harris, S. L., & Levine, A. J. (2005) The p53 pathway: positive and negative feedback loops. *Oncogene* 24, 2899-2908.

[9] Oren, M. (1999) Regulation of the p53 tumor suppressor protein. *J Biol Chem* 274, 36031-36034.

[10] Appella, E., & Anderson, C. W. (2001) Post-translational modifications and activation of p53 by genotoxic stresses. *Eur J Biochem* 268, 2764-2772.

[11] Ryan, K. M., Phillips, A. C., & Vousden, K. H. (2001) Regulation and function of the p53 tumor suppressor protein. *Curr Opin Cell Biol* 13, 332-337.

[12] Kubbutat, M. H., & Vousden, K. H. (1998) Keeping an old friend under control: regulation of p53 stability. *Mol Med Today* 4, 250-256.

[13] Chernov, M. V., Bean, L. J., Lerner, N., & Stark, G. R. (2001) Regulation of ubiquitination and degradation of p53 in unstressed cells through C-terminal phosphorylation. *J Biol Chem* 276, 31819-31824.

[14] Lowe, S. W., Cepero, E., & Evan, G. (2004) Intrinsic tumour suppression. *Nature* 432, 307-315.

[15] Haupt, S., Berger, M., Goldberg, Z., & Haupt, Y. (2003) Apoptosis - the p53 network. *J Cell Sci* 116, 4077-4085.

[16] Chipuk, J. E., & Green, D. R. (2006) Dissecting p53-dependent apoptosis. *Cell Death Differ* 13, 994-1002.

[17] Meulmeester, E., & Jochemsen, A. G. (2008) p53: a guide to apoptosis. *Curr Cancer Drug Targets* 8, 87-97.

[18] Miyashita, T., & Reed, J. C. (1995) Tumor suppressor p53 is a direct transcriptional activator of the human bax gene. *Cell* 80, 293-299.

[19] Oda, E., Ohki, R., Murasawa, H., Nemoto, J., Shibue, T., Yamashita, T., Tokino, T., Taniguchi, T., & Tanaka, N. (2000) Noxa, a BH3-only member of the Bcl-2 family and candidate mediator of p53-induced apoptosis. *Science* 288, 1053-1058.

[20] Nakano, K., & Vousden, K. H. (2001) PUMA, a novel proapoptotic gene, is induced by p53. *Mol Cell* 7, 683-694.

[21] Robles, A. I., Bemmels, N. A., Foraker, A. B., & Harris, C. C. (2001) APAF-1 is a transcriptional target of p53 in DNA damage-induced apoptosis. *Cancer Res* 61, 6660-6664.

[22] Li, Y. Z., Lu, D. Y., Tan, W. Q., Wang, J. X., & Li, P. F. (2008) p53 initiates apoptosis by transcriptionally targeting the antiapoptotic protein ARC. *Mol Cell Biol* 28, 564-574.

[23] Yao, H., Li, P., Venters, B. J., Zheng, S., Thompson, P. R., Pugh, B. F., & Wang, Y. (2008) Histone Arg modifications and p53 regulate the expression of OKL38, a mediator of apoptosis. *J Biol Chem* 283, 20060-20068.

[24] Kuribayashi, K., Krigsfeld, G., Wang, W., Xu, J., Mayes, P. A., Dicker, D. T., Wu, G. S., & El-Deiry, W. S. (2008) TNFSF10 (TRAIL), a p53 target gene that mediates p53-dependent cell death. *Cancer Biol Ther* 7, 2034-2038.

[25] Maecker, H. L., Koumenis, C., & Giaccia, A. J. (2000) p53 promotes selection for Fas-mediated apoptotic resistance. *Cancer Res* 60, 4638-4644.

[26] Wolff, S., Erster, S., Palacios, G., & Moll, U. M. (2008) p53's mitochondrial translocation and MOMP action is independent of Puma and Bax and severely disrupts mitochondrial membrane integrity. *Cell Res* 18, 733-744.

[27] Vaseva, A. V., & Moll, U. M. (2009) The mitochondrial p53 pathway. *Biochim Biophys Acta* 1787, 414-420.

[28] [28] Tanaka, T., Ohkubo, S., Tatsuno, I., & Prives, C. (2007) hCAS/CSE1L associates with chromatin and regulates expression of select p53 target genes. *Cell* 130, 638-650.

[29] Hermeking, H. (2007) p53 enters the microRNA world. *Cancer Cell* 12, 414-418.

[30] He, L., He, X., Lowe, S. W., & Hannon, G. J. (2007) microRNAs join the p53 network--another piece in the tumour-suppression puzzle. *Nat Rev Cancer* 7, 819-822.

[31] Abbas, T., White, D., Hui, L., Yoshida, K., Foster, D. A., & Bargonetti, J. (2004) Inhibition of human p53 basal transcription by down-regulation of protein kinase Cdelta. *J Biol Chem* 279, 9970-9977.

[32] Liu, H., Lu, Z. G., Miki, Y., & Yoshida, K. (2007) Protein kinase C δ induces transcription of the TP53 tumor suppressor gene by controlling death-promoting factor Btf in the apoptotic response to DNA damage. *Mol Cell Biol* 27, 8480-8491.

[33] Hansen, L. A., Monteiro-Riviere, N. A., & Smart, R. C. (1990) Differential down-regulation of epidermal protein kinase C by 12-O-tetradecanoylphorbol-13-acetate and diacylglycerol: association with epidermal hyperplasia and tumor promotion. *Cancer Res* 50, 5740-5745.

[34] Fournier, A., & Murray, A. W. (1987) Application of phorbol ester to mouse skin causes a rapid and sustained loss of protein kinase C. *Nature* 330, 767-769.

[35] Lu, Z., Hornia, A., Jiang, Y. W., Zang, Q., Ohno, S., & Foster, D. A. (1997) Tumor promotion by depleting cells of protein kinase C δ. *Mol Cell Biol* 17, 3418-3428.

[36] Reddig, P. J., Dreckschmidt, N. E., Ahrens, H., Simsiman, R., Tseng, C. P., Zou, J., Oberley, T. D., & Verma, A. K. (1999) Transgenic mice overexpressing protein kinase Cδ in the epidermis are resistant to skin tumor promotion by 12-O-tetradecanoylphorbol-13-acetate. *Cancer Res* 59, 5710-5718.

[37] Magnelli, L., Cinelli, M., & Chiarugi, V. (1995) Phorbol esters attenuate the expression of p53 in cells treated with doxorubicin and protect TS-P53/K562 from apoptosis. *Biochem Biophys Res Commun* 215, 641-645.

[38] Ghosh, J. C., Suzuki, K., Kodama, S., & Watanabe, M. (1999) Effects of protein kinase inhibitors on the accumulation kinetics of p53 protein in normal human embryo cells following X-irradiation. *J Radiat Res (Tokyo)* 40, 23-37.

[39] Raman, V., Martensen, S. A., Reisman, D., Evron, E., Odenwald, W. F., Jaffee, E., Marks, J., & Sukumar, S. (2000) Compromised HOXA5 function can limit p53 expression in human breast tumours. *Nature* 405, 974-978.

[40] Stuart, E. T., Haffner, R., Oren, M., & Gruss, P. (1995) Loss of p53 function through PAX-mediated transcriptional repression. *EMBO J* 14, 5638-5645.

[41] Liu, H., Hew, H. C., Lu, Z. G., Yamaguchi, T., Miki, Y., & Yoshida, K. (2009) DNA damage signalling recruits RREB-1 to the p53 tumour suppressor promoter. *Biochem J* 422, 543-551.

[42] Oda, K., Arakawa, H., Tanaka, T., Matsuda, K., Tanikawa, C., Mori, T., Nishimori, H., Tamai, K., Tokino, T., Nakamura, Y., & Taya, Y. (2000) p53AIP1, a potential mediator of p53-dependent apoptosis, and its regulation by Ser-46-phosphorylated p53. *Cell* 102, 849-862.

[43] Hofmann, T. G., Moller, A., Sirma, H., Zentgraf, H., Taya, Y., Droge, W., Will, H., & Schmitz, M. L. (2002) Regulation of p53 activity by its interaction with homeodomain-interacting protein kinase-2. *Nat Cell Biol* 4, 1-10.

[44] D'Orazi, G., Cecchinelli, B., Bruno, T., Manni, I., Higashimoto, Y., Saito, S., Gostissa, M., Coen, S., Marchetti, A., Del Sal, G., Piaggio, G., Fanciulli, M., Appella, E., & Soddu, S. (2002) Homeodomain-interacting protein kinase-2 phosphorylates p53 at Ser 46 and mediates apoptosis. *Nat Cell Biol* 4, 11-19.

[45] Taira, N., Nihira, K., Yamaguchi, T., Miki, Y., & Yoshida, K. (2007) DYRK2 is targeted to the nucleus and controls p53 via Ser46 phosphorylation in the apoptotic response to DNA damage. *Mol Cell* 25, 725-738.

[46] Becker, W., Weber, Y., Wetzel, K., Eirmbter, K., Tejedor, F. J., & Joost, H. G. (1998) Sequence characteristics, subcellular localization, and substrate specificity of DYRK-related kinases, a novel family of dual specificity protein kinases. *J Biol Chem* 273, 25893-25902.

[47] Yoshida, K. (2008) Role for DYRK family kinases on regulation of apoptosis. *Biochem Pharmacol* 76, 1389-1394.

[48] Okamura, S., Arakawa, H., Tanaka, T., Nakanishi, H., Ng, C. C., Taya, Y., Monden, M., & Nakamura, Y. (2001) p53DINP1, a p53-inducible gene, regulates p53-dependent apoptosis. *Mol Cell* 8, 85-94.

[49] Yoshida, K., Liu, H., & Miki, Y. (2006) Protein Kinase C δ regulates Ser46 phosphorylation of p53 tumor suppressor in the apoptotic response to DNA damage. *J Biol Chem* 281, 5734-5740.

[50] Mantovani, F., Tocco, F., Girardini, J., Smith, P., Gasco, M., Lu, X., Crook, T., & Del Sal, G. (2007) The prolyl isomerase Pin1 orchestrates p53 acetylation and dissociation from the apoptosis inhibitor iASPP. *Nat Struct Mol Biol* 14, 912-920.

[51] Zheng, H., You, H., Zhou, X. Z., Murray, S. A., Uchida, T., Wulf, G., Gu, L., Tang, X., Lu, K. P., & Xiao, Z. X. (2002) The prolyl isomerase Pin1 is a regulator of p53 in genotoxic response. *Nature* 419, 849-853.

[52] Nakamura, Y., Futamura, M., Kamino, H., Yoshida, K., Nakamura, Y., & Arakawa, H. (2006) Identification of p53-46F as a super p53 with an enhanced ability to induce p53-dependent apoptosis. *Cancer Sci* 97, 633-641.

[53] Liu, L., Scolnick, D. M., Trievel, R. C., Zhang, H. B., Marmorstein, R., Halazonetis, T. D., & Berger, S. L. (1999) p53 sites acetylated in vitro by PCAF and p300 are acetylated in vivo in response to DNA damage. *Mol Cell Biol* 19, 1202-1209.

[54] Barlev, N. A., Liu, L., Chehab, N. H., Mansfield, K., Harris, K. G., Halazonetis, T. D., & Berger, S. L. (2001) Acetylation of p53 activates transcription through recruitment of coactivators/histone acetyltransferases. *Mol Cell* 8, 1243-1254.

[55] Le Cam, L., Linares, L. K., Paul, C., Julien, E., Lacroix, M., Hatchi, E., Triboulet, R., Bossis, G., Shmueli, A., Rodriguez, M. S., Coux, O., & Sardet, C. (2006) E4F1 is an atypical ubiquitin ligase that modulates p53 effector functions independently of degradation. *Cell* 127, 775-788.

[56] Knights, C. D., Catania, J., Di Giovanni, S., Muratoglu, S., Perez, R., Swartzbeck, A., Quong, A. A., Zhang, X., Beerman, T., Pestell, R. G., & Avantaggiati, M. L. (2006) Distinct p53 acetylation cassettes differentially influence gene-expression patterns and cell fate. *J Cell Biol* 173, 533-544.
[57] Chao, C., Wu, Z., Mazur, S. J., Borges, H., Rossi, M., Lin, T., Wang, J. Y., Anderson, C. W., Appella, E., & Xu, Y. (2006) Acetylation of mouse p53 at lysine 317 negatively regulates p53 apoptotic activities after DNA damage. *Mol Cell Biol* 26, 6859-6869.
[58] Abida, W. M., Nikolaev, A., Zhao, W., Zhang, W., & Gu, W. (2007) FBXO11 promotes the Neddylation of p53 and inhibits its transcriptional activity. *J Biol Chem* 282, 1797-1804.
[59] Sykes, S. M., Mellert, H. S., Holbert, M. A., Li, K., Marmorstein, R., Lane, W. S., & McMahon, S. B. (2006) Acetylation of the p53 DNA-binding domain regulates apoptosis induction. *Mol Cell* 24, 841-851.
[60] Tang, Y., Luo, J., Zhang, W., & Gu, W. (2006) Tip60-dependent acetylation of p53 modulates the decision between cell-cycle arrest and apoptosis. *Mol Cell* 24, 827-839.

In: Tumor Suppressors
Editor: Susan D. Nguyen
ISBN: 978-1-61761-986-1

Chapter 13

How does Tumor Suppressor FHIT Modulate Oxidative Stress and DNA Damage Checkpoints in Early Cancer?*

Hideshi Ishii[1,2] and Toshiyuki Saito[2]
[1]Center for Molecular Medicine, Jichi Medical University, Tochigi, Japan
[2]National Institute of Radiological Science, Chiba, Japan

Abstract

Oxidative stress, a biochemical condition that is characterized by an imbalance between the presence of relatively high levels of toxic reactive species and antioxidative defense mechanisms, has been linked to various cellular philology and disorders characterized by cell death, such as stem cells of neural and hematopoietic systems. Recent studies indicate that common chromosome fragile sites, non-random targets of double stranded breaks under replication perturbation that are characteristic of tumors, paradoxically encode the tumor suppressor FHIT gene, which modulates response to oxidative stress and DNA damage. Since it is inactivated in precancer or early stages of carcinogenesis, we propose that the FHIT gene plays a role in the creation of cancer initiating cells. Mechanistic roles of FHIT in modulating oxidative stress and DNA damage checkpoints of cancer initiating cells are also discussed.

Key words: tumor suppressor, ROS, DNA damage, oxidative stress, genotoxin.

1. Oxidative Stress in Cancer

During natural aging, adult stem cells are known to have a reduced restorative capacity and are more vulnerable to oxidative stress resulting from exogenous and endogenous insults

* Author Correspondence: Center for Molecular Medicine, Jichi Medical University, Yakushiji 3311-1, Tochigi, Japan (hishii@ms.jichi.ac.jp)

[1]. Oxidative stress has been linked to several disorders characterized by cell death, such as stem cells of neural and hematopoietic systems. Apoptosis and necrosis are the two major forms of cell death that have been described in tumors, and stimuli inducing oxidative stress can cause both types of death, depending on the intensity and the duration of the insult. Oxidative stress is a biochemical condition that is characterized by an imbalance between the presence of relatively high levels of toxic reactive species, principally consisting of reactive oxygen species (ROS), reactive nitrogen species (RNS), and antioxidative defense mechanisms [2]. ROS and RNS are organic or inorganic molecules that have an odd number of electrons, which can be formed through oxidation-reduction reactions and are highly reactive. ROS, including free radicals, such as hydroxyl and superoxide radicals, and nonradicals, such as hydrogen peroxide and singlet oxygen, are essential for life because of their role in many vital processes such as signal transduction [2, 3]. Reactive species can interact with cellular macromolecules, including lipids, proteins, and DNA to promote irreversible oxidative damage and interfere with vital cellular functions. ROS and RNS can attack DNA directly and form mutagenic lesions [2, 4, 5]. ROS are a significant source of DNA damage under physiological conditions and play important roles in aging and diseases, including cancer.

It is reported that cancer cells themselves induce oxidative stress [2]. Actually ROS levels have been found to be significantly higher, and glutathione peroxidase (GPX) and superoxidase dismutase (SOD) activities, which are anti-oxidant enzyme systems, significantly lower in cancer patients [2]. Metabolically active cancer cells require a high level of ATP supply to maintain uncontrolled cell growth and proliferation [2]. The high-energy demand in the mitochondrial respiration chain contributes to ROS generation [2]. It was shown that excess concentrations of oxidant not only could depress proliferation, but also may increase apoptosis [2].

On the other hand, a small fraction of tumors, cancer initiating cells which are in dormancy at G0 or slow cycling, or resister side population in flow-cytometry, was documented to have self-renewal and tumorigenicity, characterization of cancer stem cells of the gastro-intestinal system [6] and were protected from ROS-induced damages [7]. Although further investigation will be necessary for ROS in cancer initiating cells, the low level of ROS in dormancy mimics somatic stem or precursor cells, such as hematopoietic organs [7]. The low ROS will be beneficial for the survival of cancer cells against various stresses such as chemotherapy and radiation therapy, and such dormant stem-like cells presumably are early deviations or at least indistinguishable from cancer initiating cells. Actually, many anticancer drugs work by affecting DNA synthesis and they do not kill resting cells in dormancy unless those cells divide soon after exposure to the drugs [2, 8]. The efficacy of anticancer drugs used in chemotherapy is limited by the fraction of actively dividing cells [2, 8].

2. Genetic Alterations

A double stranded break, which can be induced by various genotoxic insults, such as stalling replication forks by replication inhibition and oxidative stress/ROS, induces a break in a chromosome causing translocations, inversions, insertions, breaks, and deletions, all of which are common characteristics of tumors. Genetic as well as epigenetic alterations are fundamental hallmarks of cancer. Genomic alterations at critical loci that inactivate tumor suppressors and activate proto-oncogenes are accumulated in cancerous cells; classical tumor suppressor genes such as retinoblastoma 1 and TP53, and oncogenes such as RAS and MYC, have been extensively studied [9, 10]. The accumulations occur in a stepwise manner in the course of carcinogenesis, which progresses from early stages with a few or several alterations to advanced stages with numerous alterations, leading to aggressive, biological behaviors. The mechanism of multi-step carcinogenesis of the colon has been shown involving the Apc gene and is considered to be a model for human familial adenomatous polyposis [11]. Also, stepwise development of chromosome aberrations was reported in the pathogenesis of therapy-related myelodysplasia (t-MDS) and acute myeloid leukemia (t-AML) based on cytogenetic characteristics [12]. Alternative genetic pathways include the recurrent balanced translocations or inversions, which directly result in chimeric rearrangement of genes for hematopoietic transcription factors (class II mutations) that disturb cellular differentiation; and activating point mutations or internal tandem duplications of genes involved in signal transduction as tyrosine kinase receptors or genes more downstream in the RAS-BRAF pathway (class I mutations). Therapy-related and de novo myelodysplasia and acute myeloid leukemia seem to share genetic pathways.

Previous studies suggest that genomic alterations, which non-randomly occur at early stages, might play a role in progression of multi-step carcinogenesis [11, 12]. Previous studies indicated that alterations of common chromosome fragile sites at specific loci, such as most active fragile FRA3B/FHIT and FRA16D/WWOX, are induced; those alterations are observed frequently in cancer and detectable from precancer or very early to advanced stages of cancer [13]. The fragile FHIT gene is among the first targets of induced DNA damage in precancer and significant fractions of solid tumors and hematopoietic malignancies. Moreover, recent studies have shown that Fhit is involved in cellular response after genotoxin exposure, and resultant surveillance of genome integrity.

3. Tumor Suppressor FHIT

Common chromosome fragile sites are large regions that preferentially exhibit gaps or breaks, visible in metaphase chromosomes, when cells are exposed to replicative stress conditions by carcinogens and DNA synthesis is partially perturbed [13-17]. Fragile site instability in cultured cells is well documented and includes occurrence of gaps and breaks on metaphase chromosomes, translocation and deletions breakpoints, and sister chromosome exchanges [17]. FRA3B and FRA16D, at chromosome regions 3p14.2 and 16q23.3, are the two most active or most fragile of the common human fragile sites, and are frequently deleted or altered in environmental carcinogen-associated cancers and also in hematopoietic disorders [13-17]. Genomic sequences at fragile sites [18, 19] and protein signal pathways that monitor their stability, including Atr [20], Brca1 [21], Smc1 [22], Fanconi anemia pathway proteins [23], Chk1 [24], Hus1 [25] and Rad51 [26] have been characterized [17]. Both homologous or homology-dependent recombination and non-homologous end-joining repair pathways regulate the stability of FRA3B and FRA16D fragile sites, indicating that double-strand breaks are formed at common fragile sites as a result of replication perturbation [26]. It is proposed that the fragile sites are so called replication difficult zones susceptible to delay of

DNA replication, which would be monitored by cellular responses, such as DNA damage checkpoints [16].

The FHIT gene is inactivated or altered in a large fraction of tumors by homo- or hemizygous deletions [13, 27], by translocations [13], and/or by the involvement of methylation of 5' CpG islands [28-32]. Those genomic deletions and possibly methylation are involved in FHIT inactivation by environmental carcinogens. Loss of Fhit expression in lung cancer is related to smoking even in early stages of cancer [33-38] and a possible correlation between loss of Fhit expression in epithelial cells and smoking was also shown in early stages of esophageal cancer [39]. Similar to gastrointestinal organs and lungs, the urinary bladder is an organ which can be exposed to environmental carcinogens and their metabolites. Fhit expression was altered in 61% [40] and > 50% [41] of bladder cancer. FHIT allelic losses were shown in 22% [42] and > 50% [43] of bladder cancer.

4. Inadequate DNA Damage Response in Fhit Deficiency

Recent studies have indicated that Fhit has a role in the elimination of cells with alterations in checkpoint response, ie, a role in surveillance of genome integrity [44-47], suggesting that the DNA-damage susceptible FRA3B/FHIT common chromosome fragile region, paradoxically, encodes a protein that is necessary for protecting cells from accumulation of this type of damage through its role in the modulation of DNA damage response proteins; and that inactivation of Fhit contributes to accumulation of abnormal checkpoint phenotypes in cancer development. It was reported that Fhit is involved in the maintenance of genome integrity at the mid-S checkpoint, through the Atr/Chk1 pathway, and that Fhit deficiency altered the response to DNA damaging genotoxins [44-46]. The introduction of exogenous Fhit into cells in vitro led to the modulation of expression of checkpoint proteins Hus1 and Chk1 at the mid-S checkpoint, modulation that led to induction of apoptosis in esophageal cancer cells, but not in non-cancerous primary cells [47]. Mutation of the conserved Fhit tyrosine 114 within the sequence DSIY114EEL, which can be phosphorylated by Src tyrosine kinase family members [48], resulted in failure of this function, suggesting the importance of this residue. Sequence analysis of reporter vectors harboring the p16INK4A genomic region indicated that short homology dependent repairs resulted in mis-repairs with internal deletions in not a few cases of Fhit deficient cells (submitted), indicating that loss of Fhit elicits inadequate repairs of DNA damages.

5. Impaired ROS Reaction in Fhit Deficiency

Animal experiments show that exposure to benzene is characterized by multi-site carcinogenicity, ie, development of tumors in various glandular tissues and organs, including hematopoietic cells, Zymbal gland, Harderian gland, preputial gland, mammary gland, ovary and lung [49, 50]. The role of benzene toxicity in carcinogenicity is shown by the previous investigations. The well-established course of chronic benzene toxicity resulting from excessive workplace exposure includes decreases in circulating erythrocytes, leukocytes and platelets and, if exposure continues, to pancytopenia, which may accompany bone marrow aplasia and myelodysplastic syndrome (MDS); an alternative result is the development of acute myelogenous leukemia [51].

Benzene and its major metabolites are not mutagenic in the Ames Salmonella test [52], but they induce chromosomal aberration in vitro and in vivo [52-54]. The metabolism of benzene to reactive metabolites such as benzene oxide by hepatic enzymes, mainly cytochrome P450-2E1 (CYP2E1), is a prerequisite for the cyto- and genotoxicities after benzene exposure [51]. It is likely that hydroquinone and catechol, two major down-stream metabolites of benzene, can be metabolically activated to reactive species, semiquinones or quinones, which rapidly bind proteins or nucleotides as a result of the peroxidiatic action of bone marrow myeloperoxidase, or prostaglandin H synthase of bone marrow macrophages [51]. The metabolic actions are considered relevant to the hematological toxicity of benzene, suggesting that benzene metabolites direct benzene-induced disorders.

Recently it was observed that absence of Fhit expression in hematopoietic cells exposed to hydroquinone, a metabolite of benzene, leads to resistance to induction of cell death, assessed by in vitro and in vivo transplantation of hydroquinone-exposed Fhit-deficient bone marrow stem cells [55]. Transplantation of hydroquinone-exposed Fhit-deficient bone marrow stem cells resulted in inhibition of the bone marrow suppression exhibited by wild type transplanted bone marrow [55]. Immunohistochemical analyses of bone marrow transplants showed insensitivity to apoptosis in Fhit-deficient bone marrow; assessment of DNA damage showed that occurrence of the oxidized base was reduced in Fhit-deficient bone marrow. Treatment with antioxidant N-acetyl-l-cysteine indicated that that the decreased oxidative damage to Fhit-deficient (relative to wild type) hematopoietic cells accounts for the survival advantage of Fhit-deficient bone marrow. Homology-dependent recombination repair predominated in Fhit-deficient cells, though not error-free repair. It is proposed that reduced oxidative stress, coupled with efficient but error-prone DNA damage repair, allows unscheduled, long-term survival of genotoxin-exposed Fhit-deficient hematopoietic stem cells carrying deleterious mutations.

It is hypothesized that Fhit deficiency resulted in reduced ROS production in hematopoietic cells and consequent reduced apoptosis, as observed in epithelial cancer-derived cells lacking Fhit and thus lacking the Fhit-Fdxr complex involved in ROS production during oxidative stress [55, 56]. The survival advantage of Fhit-deficient cells during post-hydroquinone hemopoiesis is offset by the efficient, but imperfect repair of DNA damage caused by severe oxidative stress, leading inevitably to further accumulation of genomic damage [55]. The increased expression of a marker of DNA double-strand breaks in spleens of hydroquinone-treated Fhit-deficient cell transplanted mice suggests accumulation of DNA damage that could lead to genomic instability.

References

[1] Matheu, A., Maraver, A., Klatt, P., Flores, I., Garcia-Cao, I., Borras, C., Flores, J.M., Vina, J., Blasco, M.A., & Serrano, M. (2007). *Delayed ageing through damage protection by the Arf/p53 pathway. Nature*, 448;375-379.

[2] Ozben, T. (2007) *Oxidative stress and apoptosis: Impact on cancer therapy. J. Pharma. Sci.*, 96, in press.

[3] Conklin, K.A. (2004). *Chemotherapy-associated oxidative stress: Impact on chemotherapeutic effectiveness. Integr. Cancer Ther.* 3;294-300.

[4] Aydin, A., Arsova-Sarafinovska, Z., Sayal, A., Eken, A., Erdem, O., Erten, K., Ozgok, Y., & Dimovski, A. (2006). *Oxidative stress and antioxidant status in non-metastatic prostate cancer and benign prostatic hyperplasia. Clin. Biochem.* 39;176-179.

[5] Dotan, Y., Lichtenberg, D., & Pinchuk, I. (2004). *Lipid peroxidation cannot be used as a universal criterion of oxidative stress. Prog. Lipid Res.*, 43;200-227.

[6] Haraguchi, N., Utsunomiya, T., Inoue, H., Tanaka, F., Mimori, K., Barnard, G.F., & Mori, M. (2006). *Characterization of a side population of cancer cells from human gastrointestinal system. Stem Cell.*, 24;506-13.

[7] Jang, Y.Y., & Sharkis, S.J. (2007). *A low level of reactive oxygen species selects for primitive hematopoietic stem cells that may reside in the low-oxygenic niche. Blood*, in press.

[8] Borek, C. (2004). *Dietary antioxidants and human cancer. Integr. Cancer Ther.*, 3;333-341.

[9] Hickman, E.S., Moroni, M.C., & Helin, K. (2002). *The role of p53 and pRB in apoptosis and cancer. Curr. Opin. Genet. Dev.*, 12;60–66.

[10] Malumbres, M., & Barbacid, M. (2003). *RAS oncogenes: the first 30 years. Nat. Rev. Cancer,* 3;459–465.

[11] Yamada, Y., & Mori, H. (2007). *Multistep carcinogenesis of the colon in Apc(Min/+) mouse. Cancer Sci.,* 98;6-10.

[12] Pedersen-Bjergaard, J., Christiansen, D.H., Desta, F., & Andersen, M.K. (2006). *Alternative genetic pathways and cooperating genetic abnormalities in the pathogenesis of therapy-related myelodysplasia and acute myeloid leukemia. Leukemia*, 20;1943-1949.

[13] Huebner, K., & Croce, C.M. (2001). *FRA3B and other common fragile sites: the weakest link. Nat. Rev. Cancer*, 1;214-221.

[14] Glover, T.W., Berger, C., Coyle, J., & Echo, B. (1984). *DNA polymerase alpha inhibition by aphidicolin induces gaps and breaks at common fragile sites in human chromosomes. Hum. Genet.,* 67;136-142.

[15] Glover, T.W., & Stein, C.K. (1988). *Chromosome breakage and recombination at fragile sites. Am. J. Hum. Genet.,* 43;265-73.

[16] Zlotorynski, E., Rahat, A., Skaug, J., Ben-Porat, N., Ozeri, E., Hershberg, R., Levi, A., Scherer, S.W., Margalit, H., & Kerem, B. (2003). *Molecular basis for expression of common and rare fragile sites. Mol Cell Biol.,* 23;7143-7151.

[17] Arlt, M.F., Durkin, S.G., Ragland, R.L., & Glover, T.W. (2006). *Common fragile sites as targets for chromosome rearrangements. DNA Repair (Amst),* 5(9-10);1126-1135.

[18] Inoue, H., Ishii, H., Alder, H., Snyder, E., Druck, T., Huebner, K., & Croce, C.M. (1997). *Sequence of the FRA3B common fragile region: implications for the mechanism of FHIT deletion. Proc. Natl. Acad. Sci. USA*, 94;14584-14589.

[19] Mimori, K., Druck, T., Inoue, H., Alder, H., Berk, L., Mori, M., Huebner, K., & Croce, C.M. (1999). *Cancer-specific chromosome alterations in the constitutive fragile region FRA3B. Proc. Natl. Acad. Sci. USA,* 96:7456-7461.

[20] Casper, A.M., Nghiem, P., Arlt, M.F., & Glover, T.W. (2002). *ATR regulates fragile site stability. Cell,* 111;779-789.

[21] Arlt, M.F., Xu, B., Durkin, S.G., Casper, A.M., Kastan, M.B., & Glover. T.W. (2004). *BRCA1 is required for common-fragile-site stability via its G2/M checkpoint function. Mol Cell Biol.,* 24;6701-6709.

[22] Musio, A., Montagna, C., Mariani, T., Tilenni, M., Focarelli, M.L., Brait, L., Indino, E., Benedetti, P.A., Chessa, L., Albertini, A., Ried, T., & Vezzoni, P. (2005). *SMC1 involvement in fragile site expression. Hum. Mol. Genet.,* 14;525-533.

[23] Howlett, N.G., Taniguchi, T., Durkin, S.G., & D'Andrea, A.D., Glover, T.W. (2005). *The Fanconi anemia pathway is required for the DNA replication stress response and for the regulation of common fragile site stability. Hum. Mol. Genet.,* 14;693-701.

[24] Durkin, S.G., Arlt, M.F., Howlett, N.G., & Glover, T.W. (2006). *Depletion of CHK1, but not CHK2, induces chromosomal instability and breaks at common fragile sites. Oncogene,* 25;4381-4388.

[25] Zhu, M., & Weiss, R.S. (2007). *Increased common fragile site expression, cell proliferation defects, and apoptosis following conditional inactivation of mouse Hus1 in primary cultured cells. Mol. Biol. Cell.,*18;1044-1055.

[26] Schwartz, M., Zlotorynski, E., Goldberg, M., Ozeri, E., Rahat, A., le Sage, C., Chen, B.P., Chen, D.J., Agami, R., & Kerem, B. (2005). *Homologous recombination and nonhomologous end-joining repair pathways regulate fragile site stability. Gene. Dev.,* 19:2715-2726.

[27] Sozzi, G., Huebner, K., & Croce, C.M. (1998). *FHIT in human cancer. Adv. Cancer Res*., 74;141-166.

[28] Chang, K.W., Kao, S.Y., Tzeng, R.J., Liu, C.J., Cheng, A.J., Yang, S.C., Wong, Y.K., & Lin, S.C. (2002). *Multiple molecular alterations of FHIT in betel-associated oral carcinoma. J. Pathol.,* 196;300-306.

[29] Maruyama, R., Toyooka, S., Toyooka, K.O., Virmani, A.K., Zochbauer-Muller, S., Farinas, A.J., Minna, J.D., McConnell, J., Frenkel, E.P., & Gazdar, A.F. (2002). *Aberrant promoter methylation profile of prostate cancers and its relationship to clinicopathological features. Clin. Cancer Res.,* 8;514-519.

[30] Maruyama, R., Toyooka, S., Toyooka, K.O., Harada, K., Virmani, A.K., Zochbauer-Muller, S., Farinas, A.J., Vakar-Lopez, F., Minna, J.D., Sagalowsky, A., Czerniak, B., & Gazdar, A.F. (2001). *Aberrant promoter methylation profile of bladder cancer and its relationship to clinicopathological features. Cancer Res.,* 61;8659-8663.

[31] Zochbauer-Muller, S., Fong, K.M., Maitra, A., Lam, S., Geradts, J., Ashfaq, R., Virmani, A.K., Milchgrub, S., Gazdar, A.F., & Minna, J.D. (2001). *5′ CpG island methylation of the FHIT gene is correlated with loss of gene expression in lung and breast cancer. Cancer Res.,* 61;3581-3585.

[32] Tanaka, H., Shimada, Y., Harada, H., Shinoda, M., Hatooka, S., Imamura, M., & Ishizaki, K. (1998). *Methylation of the 5′ CpG island of the FHIT gene is closely associated with transcriptional inactivation in esophageal squamous cell carcinomas. Cancer Res.,* 58;3429-3434.

[33] Sozzi, G., Pastorino, U., Moiraghi, L., Tagliabue, E., Pezzella, F., Ghirelli, C., Tornielli, S., Sard, L., Huebner, K., Pierotti, M.A., Croce, C.M., & Pilotti, S. (1998). *Loss of FHIT function in lung cancer and preinvasive bronchial lesions. Cancer Res.,* 58;5032-5037.

[34] Tseng, J.E., Kemp, B.L., Khuri, F.R., Kurie, J.M., Lee, J.S., Zhou, X., Liu, D., Hong, W.K., & Mao, L. (1999). *Loss of Fhit is frequent in stage I non-small cell lung cancer and in the lungs of chronic smokers. Cancer Res.*, 59;4798-4803.

[35] Tomizawa, Y., Nakajima, T., Kohno, T., Saito, R., Yamaguchi, N., & Yokota, J. (1998). *Clinicopathological significance of Fhit protein expression in stage I non-small cell lung carcinoma. Cancer Res.*, 58;5478-5483.

[36] Sozzi, G., Sard, L., De Gregorio, L., Marchetti, A., Musso, K., Buttitta, F., Tornielli, S., Pellegrini, S., Veronese, M.L., Manenti, G., Incarbone, M., Chella, A., Angeletti, C.A., Pastorino, U., Huebner, K., Bevilaqua, G., Pilotti, S., Croce, C.M., & Pierotti, M.A. (1997). *Association between cigarette smoking and FHIT gene alterations in lung cancer. Cancer Res.*, 57;2121-2123.

[37] Nelson, H.H., Wiencke, J.K., Gunn, L., Wain, J.C., Christiani, D.C., & Kelsey, K.T. (1998). *Chromosome 3p14 alterations in lung cancer: evidence that FHIT exon deletion is a target of tobacco carcinogens and asbestos. Cancer Res.*, 58;1804-1807.

[38] Stein, C.K., Glover, T.W., Palmer, J.L., & Glisson, B.S. (2002). *Direct correlation between FRA3B expression and cigarette smoking. Gene., Chrom. Cancer,* 34;333-340.

[39] Mori, M., Mimori, K., Shiraishi, T., Alder, H., Inoue, H., Tanaka, Y., Sugimachi, K., Huebner, K., & Croce, C.M. (2000). *Altered expression of Fhit in carcinoma and precarcinomatous lesions of the esophagus. Cancer Res.*, 60;1177-1182.

[40] Baffa, R., Gomella, L.G., Vecchione, A., Bassi, P., Mimori, K., Sedor, J., Calviello, C.M., Gardiman, M., Minimo, C., Strup, S.E., McCue, P.A., Kovatich, A.J., Pagano, F., Huebner, K., & Croce, C.M. (2000). *Loss of FHIT expression in trasitional cell carcinoma of the urinary bladder. Am. J. Pathol.*, 156;419-424.

[41] Skopelitou, A.S., Gloustianou, G., Bai, M., & Huebner, K. (2001). *FHIT gene expression in human urinary bladder transitional cell carcinomas. In Vivo*, 15;169-173.

[42] Wada, T., Louhelainen, J., Hemminki, K., Adolfsson, J., Wijkstrom, H., Norming, U., Borgstrom, E., Hansson, J., & Steineck, G. (2001). *The prevalence of loss of heterozygosity in chromosome 3, including FHIT, in bladder cancer, using the fluorescent multiplex polymerase chain reaction. BJU Intern.*, 87;876-881.

[43] Louhelainen, J., Wijkstrom, H., & Hemminki, K. (2001). *Multiple regions with allelic loss at chromosome 3 in superficial multifocal bladder tumors. International J. Oncol.*, 18;203-210.

[44] Ottey, M., Han, S.Y., Druck, T., Barnoski, B.L., McCorkell, K.A., Croce, C.M., Raventos-Suarez, C., Fairchild, C.R., Wang, Y., & Huebner, K. (2004). *Fhit-deficient normal and cancer cells are mitomycin C and UVC resistant. Br. J. Cancer,* 91;1669-1677.

[45] Hu, B., Han, S.Y., Wang, X., Ottey, M., Potoczek, M.B., Dicker, A., Huebner, K., & Wang, Y. (2005). *Involvement of the Fhit gene in the ionizing radiation-activated ATR/CHK1 pathway. J. Cell Physiol.*, 202.518-523.

[46] Hu, B., Wang, H., Wang, X., Lu, H.R., Huang, C., Powell, S.N., Huebner, K., & Wang, Y. (2005). *Fhit and CHK1 have opposing effects on homologous recombination repair. Cancer Res.*, 65;8613-8616.

[47] Ishii, H., Mimori, K., Inoue, H., Inageta, T., Ishikawa, K., Semba, S., Druck, T., Trapasso, F., Tani, K., Vecchione, A., Croce, C.M., Mori, M., & Huebner, K. (2006). *Fhit modulates the DNA damage checkpoint response. Cancer Res.*, 66;11287-11292.

[48] Pekarsky, Y., Garrison, P.N., Palamarchuk, A., Zanesi, N., Aqeilan, R.I., Huebner, K., Barnes, L.D., & Croce, C.M. (2004). *Fhit is a physiological target of the protein kinase Src. Proc Natl Acad Sci U S A.,* 101;3775-3779.

[49] Huff, J.E., Haseman, J.K., DeMarini, D.M., Eustis, S., Maronpot, R.R., Peters, A.C., Persing, R.L., Chrisp, C.E., & Jacobs, A.C. (1989). *Multiple-site carcinogenicity of benzene in Fischer 344 rats and B6C3F1 mice. Environ Health Perspect.,* 82;125-163.

[50] Maltoni, C., Ciliberti, A., Cotti, G., Conti, B., & Belpoggi, F. (1989). *Benzene, an experimental multipotential carcinogen: results of the long-term bioassays performed at the Bologna Institute of Oncology. Environ Health Perspect.,* 82;109-124.

[51] Snyder, R. (2002). *Benzene and leukemia. Crit. Rev. Toxicol.,* 32;155-210.

[52] Dean, B.J. (1985). *Recent findings on the genetic toxicology of benzene, toluene, xylenes and phenols. Mutat. Res.,* 154;153-181.

[53] Yager, J.W., Eastmond, D.A., Robertson, M.L., Paradisin, W.M., Smith, M.T. (1990). *Characterization of micronuclei induced in human lymphocytes by benzene metabolites. Cancer Res.,* 50;393-399.

[54] Wolman, S.R. (1977). *Cytologic and cytogenetic effects of benzene. J. Toxicol. Environ. Health. Suppl.,* 2;63-68.

[55] Ishii, H., Mimori, K., Ishikawa, K., Okumura, H., Pichiorri, F., Druck, T., Inoue, H., Vecchione, A., Croce, C.M., Saito, T., Mori, M., & Huebner, K. (2008), *Fhit-deficient hematopoietic stem cells survive hydroquinone treatment long-term, carrying precancerous alterations.* in press.

[56] Trapasso, F., Pichiorri, F., Gasparo, M., Palumbo, T., Raso, C., Aqeilan, R.I., Gaudio, E., Iuliano, R., Okumura, H., Di Leva, G., Fabbri, M., Birk, D.E., Green-Church, K., Spagnoli, L.G., Venuta, S., Huebner, K., & Croce, C.M. (2008). *Fhit interaction with ferredoxin reductase triggers generation of reactive oxygen species and apoptosis.* in press.

In: Tumor Suppressors
Editor: Susan D. Nguyen
ISBN: 978-1-61761-986-1

Chapter 14

Role of the Tumor Suppressor PDCD4 in the Differentiation of the Skin

***Sachiko Matsuhashi*[1], *Takeshi Okawa*[2] *and Yutaka Narisawa*[2]**
[1]Department of Internal Medicine and
[2]Department of Dermatology, Saga Medical School, Saga University,
Saga 849-8501, Japan.

Abstract

First isolated as an antigen gene involved in the cell cycle, the human programmed cell death 4 (PDCD4) gene mapped at 10q24. Mouse Pdcd4 was shown to suppress the transformation of JB6 mouse epidermal cells exposed to promoters such as TPA, inhibiting AP-1 transactivation. PDCD4 expression was down-regulated in many tumor tissues. PDCD4/Pdcd4 was classified as a protein synthesis regulator, because the protein associates with eIF4A, a component of the initiation complex of protein synthesis, thereby inhibiting cap-dependent translations. When cells are stimulated by mitogens, the PDCD4-protein is phosphorylated by S6K activated through Akt-mTOR signal transduction pathway and degraded in an ubiquitin-proteasome system, stimulating protein synthesis and carcinogenesis. Besides the regulation of translation, PDCD4/Pdcd4 also regulates transcriptions and induces apoptosis as it is over-expressed in tumor cells by plasmid transfection.

In the normal skin, PDCD4 expression was localized in differentiating cell layers of epidermis but was absent or less extent in PCNA-positive cell layers such as basal cell layers of epidermis or bulbar area of hair follicles. Apoptotic casepase systems were shown to be activated on the cornification of epidermis and on the induction of apoptosis by UVB irradiation which induced PDCD4 expression in HaCaT cells. These results indicates that PDCD4 may contribute for the differentiation of epidermal cells and hair follicles. In the transgenic mice specifically expressing Pdcd4 in epidermal cell lineages, the epidermis was resistant to carcinogenesis and the hair follicles underwent earlier catagen to show a shorter hair phenotype than the normal skin. This results support the idea that PDCD4 may contribute to the differentiation on the hair follicles. However, Pdcd4 nock-down mice showed normal development although the animals were more sensitive to carcinogenesis than normal siblings. PDCD4 might partly contribute to the differentiation of the skin.

Introduction

The human programmed cell death 4 (PDCD4) gene (H731) was first isolated as an antigen gene involved in the cell cycle [Matsuhashi et al. 1997, Yoshinaga et al. 1999] and mapped at 10q24 [Soejima et al. 1999]. Expression of the human gene (197/15a) was modulated by interleukins: up-regulated by IL12 and down-regulated by IL2 and IL15 in NK and T cells [Azzoni et al. 1998]. The mouse homolog (Pdcd4) was isolated as a gene (MA-3) that was up-regulated in association with apoptosis [Shibahara et al. 1995] and the same gene (TIS) was down-regulated by a treatment of cells with topoisomerase inhibitors [Onishi et al. 1998]. The chicken homolog was also isolated and shown to be regulated by the transcription factor myb [Schlichter et al. 2001a,b]. The isolation of rat homolog (DUG) also has been reported [Goke et al. 2002]. The amino acid sequence of the gene was well conserved between animal species (>90%). Since the mouse Pdcd4 was shown to suppress the neoplastic transformation of JB6 mouse epidermal cells exposed to the tumor promoter 12-O-tetradecanoylphorbol 13 acetate (TPA) [Cmarik et al. 1999], the functions of PDCD4/Pdcd4 to suppress neoplastic transformation and carcinogenesis have been investigated by many scientists and well established both in vitro and in vivo. PDCD4 expression has been shown to be suppressed in many tumor tissues such as lung cancers [Chen et al. 2003], pancreatic cancers [Ma et al. 2005], hepatocellular carcinomas [Zhang et al 2006], colon cancers [Lee et al. 2006], skin carcinomas [Matsuhashi et al. 2007], breast cancers [Wen et al. 2007] and glioma tissues [Gao et al. 2007]. PDCD4 expression was suppressed at mRNA levels in some tumor tissues while the protein levels were down-regulated without changing the mRNA levels in other cases, indicating that PDCD4 expression is controlled at both levels of transcription and translation. Recently, it has been reported that microRNA-21 targets PDCD4/Pdcd4 mRNA regulating PDCD4 expression [Asangani et al. 2008, Frankel et al. 2008, Zhu et al. 2008, Lu et al. 2008, Chen et al. 2008, Talotta et al. 2009]. We discuss, in this report, the molecular mechanisms and functions of PDCD4/Pdcd4 and propose a possibility that PDCD4 may function in the differentiation of the skin.

Molecular Mechanisms and Functions of PDCD4

PDCD4/Pdcd4-protein possesses two MA-3 domains homologous to the M1 domain of eukaryotic translation initiation factor 4G (eIF4G), a component of the translation initiation complex eIF4F [Aravind and Koonin, 2000] and potential nuclear localization signals as shown in Figure 1. The mouse Pdcd4-protein associates with eIF4A which binds to eIF4G in the initiation complex eIF4F and inhibits the RNA helicase activity of eIF4A, thereby inhibiting cap-dependent translation (Figure 2) [Yang et al. 2003a, 2004] including insulin-like-growth factor II, transforming growth factor-β, androgen receptor, CDK4, cyclin D1, p53 and ornithine decarboxylase (ODC) [reviewed in Clemens and Bommer 1999]. The binding function of the MA-3 domains with eIF4A has been well investigated [Zakowicz et al. 2005, LaRonde-LeBlanc et al. 2007, Waters et al.2007, Suzuki et al. 2008, Loh et al. 2009, Chang et al. 2009]. In response to growth factors, in cells, PDCD4-protein was rapidly phosphorylated on S^{67}, by the protein kinase S6K1 which is activated through the mitogen-activated Akt-mammalian target of rapamycin (mTOR) signaling pathway (Figure 2). The phosphorylation of S^{67} promotes the phosphorylation of S^{71} and S^{76} in the canonical $SCF^{\beta TRCP}$ ubiquitin ligase binding motif $D^{70}SGRGDS^{76}$ of PDCD4, resulting in the degradation of PDCD4 in the ubiquitin-proteasome system [Dorrello et al. 2006, Sonenberg and Pause 2006, Frescas and Pagano 2008]. Loss of PDCD4 stimulated protein synthesis, subsequently cell growth and proliferation led to carcinogenesis of cells (Figure 2).

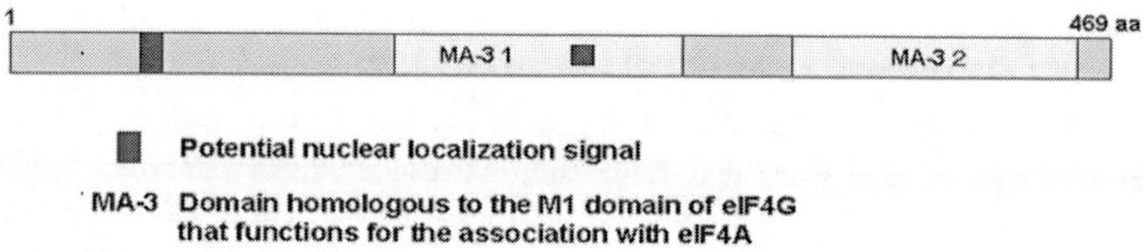

Figure 1. Schematic sequence of PDCD4.

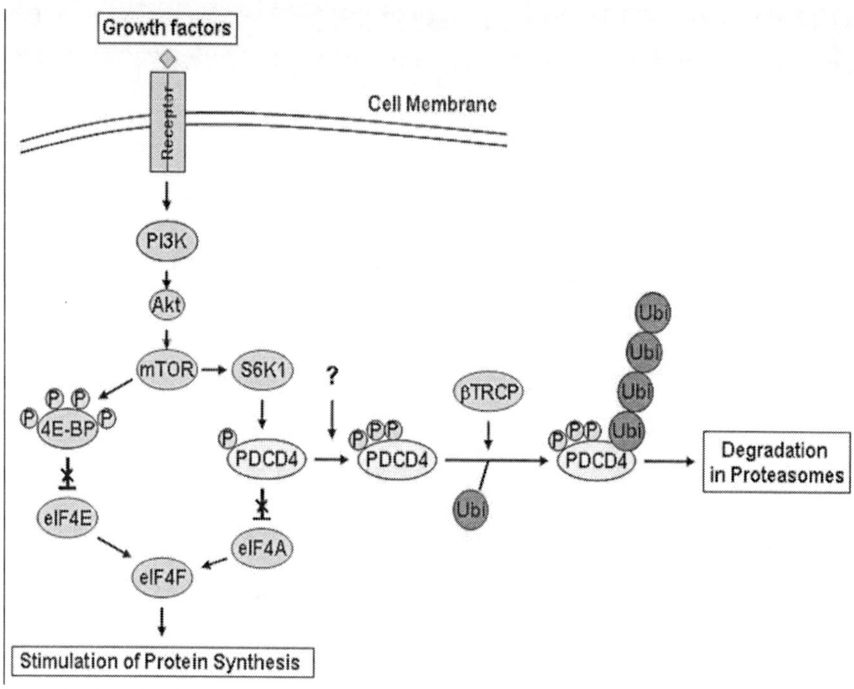

PDCD4 and 4E-BP inhibit cap-dependent protein syntheeis by binding to eIF4A and eIF4E, components of the translation initiation complex eIF4F, respectively. On the induction of cells by mitogens, both inhibitors, PDCD4 and 4E-BP were phosphorylated through the activated PI3K-Akt-mTOR signaling pathway. Consequently, PDCD4 is degraded in the ubiquitin-proteasome system, and the phosphorylated 4E-BP dissociates from eIF4E and the free eIF4E binds with the cap-structure of mRNA, stimulating cap-dependent protein synthesis in both ways.

Figure 2. Schematic pathway of PDCD4 degradation and targeting protein synthesis.

It was demonstrated that Pdcd4 inhibits activator protein 1 (AP-1) transactivation but not nuclear factor-kB (NF-kB) or ODC transactivation in the mouse epidermal JB6 cells [Yang et al 2001, 2003b] and that Pdcd4 interferes with the phosphorylation of c-Jun by Jun N-terminal kinase (JNK) [Bitomsky et al. 2004]. Ectopic expression of Pdcd4 in metastatic colon carcinoma cells suppressed invasion and inhibited the transcription of mitogen-activated protein kinase kinase kinase kinase 1 (MAP4K1)/hematopoietic progenitor kinase 1 which is a upstream kinase of JNK activation [Yang et al. 2006] and is involved in the transforming growth facter-β (TGF-β)-induced JNK signaling pathway (Figure 3) [Zhou et al. 1999]. Consequently, suppression of MAP4K1 inhibits c-Jun phosphorylation and consequent AP-1 transactivities led to cell proliferation and invasion (Figure 3). The regulation of AP-1 activities by Pdcd4 in vivo was shown by generating transgenic mice that over-express Pdcd4 in the epidermis [Jansen et al. 2005]. As an another regulation of transcription by Pdcd4, it was reported that Pdcd4 nock-down by short hairpin RNA (shRNA) stimulated invasion of colon tumor HT29 cells and inhibited cadherin expression resulting in the accumulation of active β-catenin in nuclei and stimulation of β-catenin/T cell factor (Tcf)-dependent transcription as well as AP-1 dependent transcription [Wang et al. 2008].

We have shown that PDCD4 is involved in the signaling pathway of TGF-β1-induced apoptosis in the hepatoma cell line Huh7 [Zhang et al. 2006]. Activated-TGF-β1 receptors up-regulated PDCD4 mRNA levels through the activation of Smad system (Figure 3) and activated caspases 8, 9 and 3 led to apoptosis. On PDCD4 overexpression in tumor cells by the transfection of plasmid, PDCD4-protein is accumulated in the nuclei and induces apoptosis of the cells [Afonia et al. 2004, Zhang et al. 2006]. The mechanisms by which PDCD4/Pdcd4 regulates transcriptions or induces apoptosis are not yet clear and must be elucidated in the future.

Role of PDCD4 in the Differentiation of the Skin

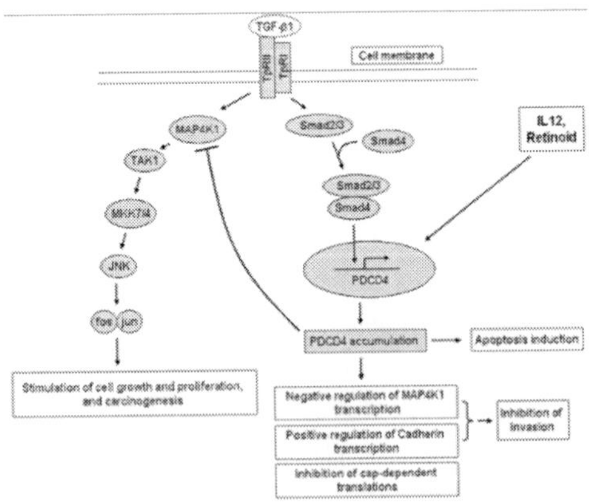

TGF-β1-activated Smad-signaling system stimulates PDCD4 expression and apoptosis of Huh7 hepatoma cells. TGF-β1 also activates TAK1-JNK signaling pathway. PDCD4 inhibits the transcription of MAP4K1 that is the upstream kinase of TAK1 resulting in the inhibition of AP-1 (Jun-Fos) activity. The MAP4K1-TAK1-JNK signaling pathway may be not activated in the Huh7 because MAP4K1 and TAK1 are little expressed in the cells.

Figure 3. Schematic signaling pathways of PDCD4 functions.

Histochemical analyses of the human skin (Figure 4) [Matsuhashi et al. 2007] demonstrated that PDCD4-positive cells were localized in the differentiating keratinocyte cell layers in the epidermis. PDCD4-protein was detected particularly in the suprabasal cell layers and mostly localized in the nuclei (Figure 4a). The basal cell layer including PCNA-positive cells was negatively or less stained and the cornified layer was not (Figure 4a,b). In the hair follicles, the outer root sheath (ORS) was entirely stained with weakly or negatively stained cell layers in the inner portion, while the PCNA positive basal cell layer was almost PDCD4-negative (Figure 4e,f). The cells of the inner root sheath (IRS) surrounding the hair shaft also was PDCD4-positive although the fused IRS was not stained. In the hair bulb, the dermal papilla and the PCNA-positive basal cells surrounding the dermal papilla were not stained while suprabasal cells including proliferating and undifferentiated cells were weakly or moderately stained (Figure 4c,d). The cells before cornification in the hair shaft were PDCD4-positive. The mature cells of the sebaceous gland containing lipid droplets were weakly or negatively stained while the peripherally located immature cells without lipid droplets were strongly stained. The sweat gland was also PDCD4-positive. These staining patterns of the skin indicated that the PDCD4 might function for the differentiation of epidermis and hair follicle. PDCD4 may contribute to the differentiation of the skin by inhibiting AP-1 activity that otherwise would induce cells to proliferate as mentioned before. The regression of the hair follicle during catagen requires apoptosis [Muller-Rover et al. 2001]. The apoptotic caspases were activated on cornification in human epidermal equivalents [Chaturvedi et al. 2006] and on the induction of apoptosis by PDCD4 overexpression in the human hepatoma Huh7 cells [Zhang et al. 2006]. Therefore, PDCD4 also may contribute to the cornification of the epidermis or to the catagen of the hair follicle by activating the caspase cascade. The activation of a apoptotic caspase cascade also was reported in the ultraviolet B (UVB)-induced apoptosis of HPV-immortalized human keratinocytes in death receptor-independent manner [Daher et al. 2006]. We have observed UVB-irradiation stimulated PDCD4 expression in the human keratinocyte HaCaT cells (Figure 5). Overexpression of PDCD4 does not always induce apoptosis; it depends on cell-types, physiology and what induces PDCD4-expression. For example, we and others [Shibahara et al. 1995, Yang et al. 2006] observed that PDCD4/Pdcd4-overexpression by the transfection of plasmid can not induce apoptosis of NIH3T3 cells but do that of the mouse transformed fibroblast cell line L cells.

Jansen et al [2005] have generated transgenic mice over-expressing Pdcd4 in the epidermis (K14-Pdcd4). K14-regulated Pdcd4 expression not only suppressed the carcinogenesis of epidermis induced by 7,12-dimethylbenz(a)authracene (DMBA)/TPA, but also caused a neonatal short-hair phenotype due to early catagen entry compared with matched wild siblings, indicating that Pdcd4 overexpression stimulates the differentiation of the hair follicles [Jansen et al. 2005]. This results support the idea that PDCD4 may function for the differentiation of the skin. However, Pdcd4 nock-out mice apparently exhibit no abnormality in the skin although they developed spontaneous lymphomas, mostly B lymphoma origin tumors with a reduced life span [Hilliard et al. 2006]. Altogether, these results indicate that different signaling systems contribute to the differentiation of the skin, for

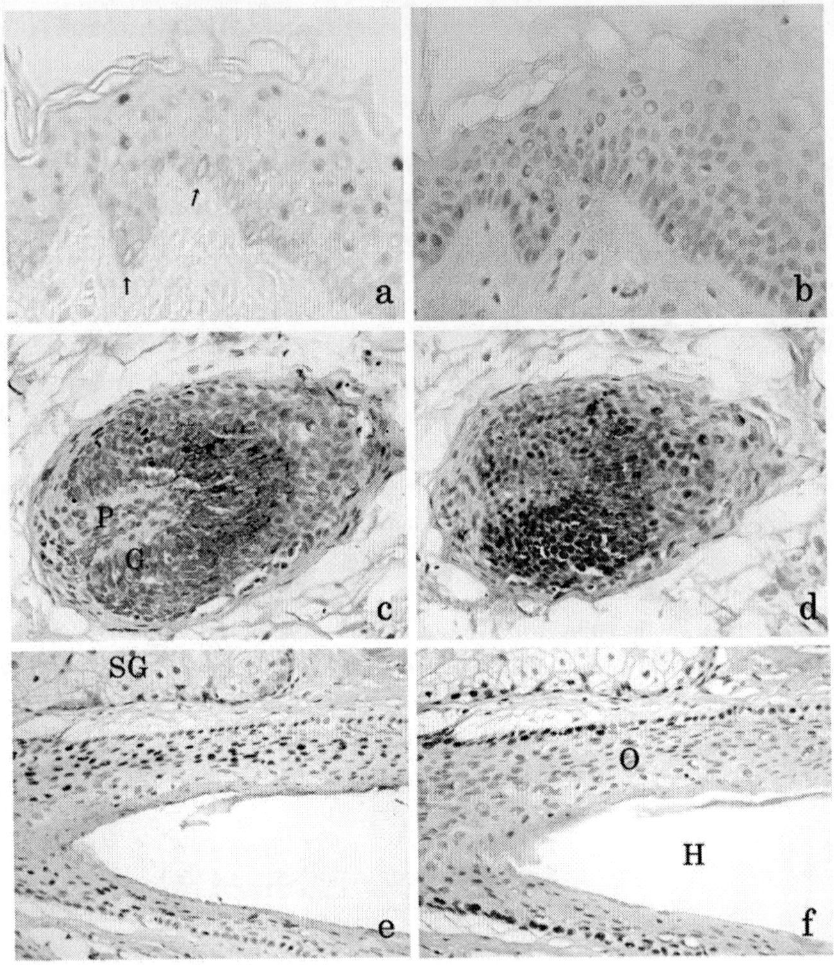

a and b, Scalp skin; PDCD4-positive cells (a) are localized in the suprabasal layers while PCNA-positive cells (b) are localized in the basal and lower suprabasal layers of epidermis. Arrows show melanocytes. c and d, Hair follicle of scalp skin; Matrix cells are strongly stained with anti-PCNA antibody (d) but rarely stained with anti-PDCD4 antibody (c). e and f, Hair follicle of Scalp skin; PCNA-positive cells (f) are localized in the outside basal layers and PDCD4-positive cells (e) in the inside layers of the outer root sheath (ORS). P, dermal papilla, G, germinal cells, SG, sebaceous gland, O, ORS, H, hair.

Figure 4. Staining patterns of serial sections obtained by simultaneous staining with either anti-PDCD4 antibody (a, c and e) or anti-PCNA antibody (b, d and f) in skin.

example, such as co-operation of TGF-β and Wnt signaling pathways [Edlund et al. 2005], while TGF–β1 did not stimulate PDCD4 expression of the human keratinocyte HaCaT cells. PDCD4 may at least partly contribute to the differentiation of the skin. As a PDCD4 function in differentiation, involvement in granulocytic differentiation of promyelocyte leukemia cells, has been reported [Ozpolat et al. 2007]. The function of PDCD4 in differentiation is a next coming interesting problem in the future.

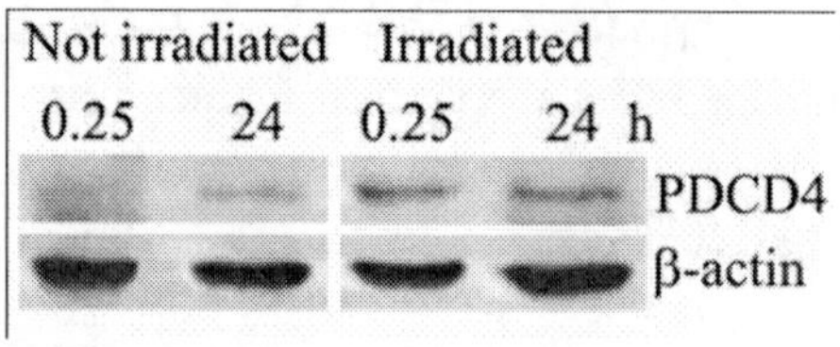

HaCaT cell cultures were irradiated with 48J UVB and analyzed by Western blotting after culturing for indicated times in the figure.

Figure 5. UVB irradiation stimulates PDCD4 expression.

Conclusion

The anti-neoplastic activity of PDCD4/Pdcd4 was well established in vitro and in vivo: PDCD4/Pdcd4 1) inhibits cap-dependent translation resulting in the inhibition of protein syntheses which stimulate cell growth and proliferation, 2) inhibits AP-1 transactivations by a mechanism that PDCD4 inhibits the transcription of MAP4K1, an upstream kinase of c-jun activation and 3) positively regulates cadherin expression of which loss stimulates invasion. Overexpression of PDCD4 induces the apoptosis of tumor cells. We have proposed evidences that the tumor suppressor PDCD4 may at least partly function in the differentiation of keratinocytes and hair follicles inhibiting AP-1 activity and/or inducing apoptosis.

References

Afonia, O., Juste, D., Das, S., Matsuhashi, S. & Samuels, H. H. (2004). Induction of PDCD4 tumor suppressor gene expression by RAR agonists, antiestrogen and HER-2/neu antagonist in breast cancer cells. Evidence for a role in apoptosis. *Oncogene*, *23*, 8135-8145.

Aravind, L. & Koonin, E. V. (2000). Eukaryote-specific domains in translation initiation factors: Implications for translation regulation and evolution of the translation system. *Genome Res*, *10*, 1172-1184.

Asangani, I. A., Rasheed, S. A., Nikolova, D. A., Leupold, J. H., Colburn, N. H., Post, S. & Allgayer, H. (2008). MicroRNA-21 (miR-21) post-trancriptionally downregulates tumor suppressor Pdcd4 and stimulates invasion, intravasation and metastasis in colorectal cancer. *Oncogene*, *27*, 2128-2136.

Azzoni, L., Zatsepina, O., Abebe, B., Bennett, I. M., Kanakaraj, P. & Perussia, B. (1998). Differential transcriptional regulation of CD161 and a novel gene, 197/15a, by IL-2, IL-15, and IL-12 in NK and T cells. *J Immunol*, *161*, 3493-3500.

Bitomsky, N., Bohm, M. & Klempnauer K. H. (2004). Transformation suppressor protein Pdcd4 interferes with JNK-mediated phosphorylation of c-Jun and recruitment of the coactivator p300 by c-Jun. *Oncogene*, *23*, 7484-7493.

Chang, J. H., Cho, Y. H., Sohn, S. Y., Choi, J. M., Kim, A., Kim, Y. C., Jang, S. K. & Cho, Y. (2009). Crystal structure of the eIF4A-PDCD4 complex. *Proc Natl Acad Sci U S A*, *106*, 3148-3153.

Chaturvedi, V., Sitailo, L. A., Bodner, B., Denning, M. F. & Nickoloff, B. J. (2006). Defining the caspase-containing apoptotic machinery contributing to cornification in human epidermal equivalents. *Exp Dermatol*, *15*, 14-22.

Chen, Y., Knosel, T., Kristiansen, G., Pietas, A., Garber, M. E., Matsuhashi, S., Ozaki, I. & Petersen, I. (2003). Loss of PDCD4 expression in human lung cancer correlates with tumour progression and prognosis. *J Pathol*, *200,* 640-646.

Chen, Y., Liu, W., Chao, T., Zhang, Y., Yan, X., Gong, Y., Qiang, B., Yuan, J., Sun, M. & Peng, X. (2008). MicroRNA-21 down-regulates the expression of tumor suppressor PDCD4 in human glioblastoma cell T98G. *Cancer Lett*, *272*, 197-205.

Clemens, M. J. & Bommer, U. A. (1999). Translational control: the cancer connection. *Int J Biochem Cell Biol*, *31*, 1-23.

Cmarik, J. L., Min, H., Hegamyer, G., Zhan, S., Kulesz-Martin, M., Yoshinaga, H., Matsuhashi, S. & Colburn, N. H. (1999). Differentially expressed protein Pdcd4 inhibits tumor pormoter-induced neoplastic transformation. *Proc Natl Acad Sci U S A*, *96*, 14037-14042.

Daher, A., Simbulan-Rosenthal, C. M. & Rosenthal, D. S. (2006). Apoptosis induced by ultraviolet B in HPV-immortalized human keratinocytes requires caspase-9 and is death receptor independent. *Exp Dermatol*, *15*, 23-34.

Dorrello, N. V., Peschiaroli, A., Guardavaccaro, D., Colburn, N. H., Sherman, N. E. & Pagano, M. (2006). S6K1- and betaTRCP-mediated degradation of PDCD4 promotes protein translation and cell growth. *Science*, 314, 467-471.

Edlund, S., Lee, S. Y., Grimsby, S., Zhang, S., Aspenstrom, P., Heldin, C. H. & Landstrom, M. (2005). Interaction between Smad7 and β-catenin: Importance for transforming growth factor β-induced apoptosis. *Mol Cell Biol*, *25*, 1475-1488.

Frankel, L. B., Christoffersen, N. R., Jacobsen, A., Lindow, M., Krogh, A. & Lund, A. H. (2008). Programmed cell death 4 (PDCD4) is an important functional target of the microRNA miR-21 in breast cancer cells. *J Biol Chem*, *283*, 1026-1033.

Frescas, D. & Pagano, M. (2008). Deregulated proteolysis by the F-box proteins SKP2 and beta-TrCP: tipping the scales of cancer. *Nat Rev Cancer*, *8*, 438-449.

Gao, F., Zhang, P., Zhou, C., Li, J., Wang, Q., Zhu, F., Ma, C., Sun, W. & Zhang, L. (2007). Frequent loss of PDCD4 expression in human glioma: Possible role in the tumorigenesis of glioma. *Oncol Rep*, *17*, 123-128.

Goke, A., Goke, R., Knolle A., Trusheim, H., Schmidt, H., Wilmen, A., Carmody, R., Goke, B. & Chen, Y. H. (2002). DUG is a novel homologue of translation initiation factor 4G that binds eIF4A. *Biochem Biophys Res Commun*, *297*, 78-82.

Hilliard, A., Hilliard, B., Zheng, S. T., Sun, H., Miwa, T., Song, W., Goke, R. & Chen, Y. H. (2006). Translational regulation of autoimmune inflammation and lymphoma genesis by programmed cell death 4. *J Immunol*, *177*, 8095-8102.

Jansen, A. P., Corinne, E., Camalier, C. E. & Colburn, N. H. (2005). Epidermal expression of the translation inhibitor programmed cell death 4 suppresses tumorigenesis. *Cancer Res*, *65*, 6034-6041.

LaRonde-LeBlanc, N., Santhanam, A. N., Baker, A. R., Wlodawer, A. & Colburn, N. H. (2007). Structural basis for inhibition of translation by the tumor suppressor Pdcd4. *Mol Cell Biol*, *27*, 147-156.

Lee, S., Bang, S., Song, K. & Lee, I. (2006). Differential expression in normal-adenoma-carcinoma sequence suggests complex molecular carcinogenesis in colon. *Oncol Rep*, *16*, 747-754.

Loh, P. G., Yang, H. S., Walsh, M. A., Wang, Q., Wang, X., Cheng, Z., Liu, D. & Song, H. (2009). Structural basis for translational inhibition by the tumour suppressor Pdcd4. *EMBO J*, *28*, 274-285.

Lu, Z., Liu, M., Stribinskis, V., Kinge, C. M., Ramos K. S., Colburn N. H. & Li, Y. (2008). MicroRNA-21 promotes cell transformation by targeting the programmed cell death 4 gene. *Oncogene*, *27*, 4373-4379.

Ma, G., Guo, K. J., Zhang, H., Ozaki, I., Matsuhashi, S., Zheng, X. Y. & Dong, M. (2005). Expression of programmed cell death 4 and its clinicopathological significance in human pancreatic cancer. *Zhongguo Yi Xue Ke Xue Yuan Xue Bao*, *27*, 597-600.

Matsuhashi, S., Narisawa, Y., Ozaki, I. & Mizuta, T. (2007). Expression patterns of programmed cell death 4 protein in normal skin and some representative skin lesions. *Exp Dermatol*, *16*, 179-184.

Matsuhashi, S., Yoshinaga, H., Yatsuki, H., Tsugita, A. & Hori, K. (1997). Isolation of a novel gene from a human cell line with Pr-28 MAb which recognizes a nuclear antigen involved in the cell cycle. *Res Commun Biochem Cell Mol Biol.*, *1*, 109-120.

Muller-Rover, S., Handjiski, B., van der Veen, C., Eichmuller, S., Foitzik, K., Mckay, I. A., Stenn, K. S. & Paus, R. (2001). A comprehensive guide for the accurate classification of murine hair follicles in distinct hair cycle stages. *J Invest Dermatol*, *117*, 3-15.

Onishi, Y., Hashimoto, S. & Kizaki, H. (1998). Cloning of the TIS gene suppressed by topoisomerase inhibitors. *Gene*, *215*, 453-459

Ozpolat, B., Akar, U., Steiner, M., Zorrilla-Calancha, I., Tirado-Gomez, M., Colburn, N. H., Danilenko, M., Kornblau, S. & Berestein, G. L. (2007). Programmed cell death-4 tumor suppressor protein contributes to retinoic acid-induced terminal granulocytic differentiation of human myeloid leukemia cells. *Mol Cancer Res*, *5*, 95-108.

Schlichter, U., Burk, O., Worpenberg, S. & Klempnauer, K. H. (2001a). The chicken Pdcd4 gene is regulated by v-Myb. *Oncogene*, *20*, 231-239.

Schlichter, U., Kattmann, D., Appl, H., Miethe, J., Brehmer-Fastnacht, A. & Klempnauer, K. H. (2001b). Identification of the myb-inducible promoter of the chicken Pdcd4 gene. *Biochem Biophys Acta*, *1520*, 99-104.

Shibahara, K., Asano, M., Ishida, Y., Aoki, T., Koike, T. & Honjo, T. (1995). Isolation of novel mouse gene MA-3 that is induced upon programmed cell death. *Gene*, *166*, 297-301.

Soejima, H., Miyoshi, O., Yoshinaga, H., Masaki, Z., Ozaki, I., Kajiwara, S., Niikawa, N., Matsuhashi, S. & Mukai, T. (1999). Assignment of the programmed cell death 4 gene (PDCD4) to human chromosome band 10q24 by in situ hybridization. *Cytogenet Cell Genet*, *87,* 113-114.

Sonenberg, N. and Pause, A. (2006). Signal transduction, Protein synthesis and oncogenesis meet again. *Science, 314,* 428-429.

Suzuki, C., Garces, R. G., Edmonds, K. A., Hiller, S., Hyberts, S. G., Marintchev, A. & Wagner, G. (2008). PDCD4 inhibits translation initiation by binding to eIF4A using both its MA3 domains. *Proc Natl Acad Sci U S A*, *105*, 3274-3279.

Talotta, F., Cimmino, A., Matarazzo, M. R., Casalino, L., De Vita, G., D'Esposito, M., Di Lauro, R. & Verde, P. (2009). An autoregulatory loop mediated by miR-21 and PDCD4 controls the AP-1 activity in RAS transformation. *Oncogene*, *28*, 73-84.

Wang, Q., Sun, Z. & Yang, H. S. (2008). Downregulation of tumor suppressor Pdcd4 promotes invasion and activates both beta-catenin/Tcf and AP-1-dependent transcription in colon carcinoma cells. *Oncogene*, *27*, 1527-1535.

Waters, L. C., Veverka, V., Bohm, M, Schmedt, T., Choong, P. T., Muskett, F. W., Klempnauer, K. H. & Carr, M. D. (2007). Structure of the C-terminal MA-3 domain of the tumour suppressor protein Pdcd4 and characterization of its interaction with eIF4A. *Oncogene*, *26*, 4941-4950.

Wen, Y. H., Shi, X., Chiriboga, L., Matsuhashi, S., Yee, H. & Afonia, O. (2007). Alterations in the expression of PDCD4 in ductal carcinoma of the breast. *Oncol Rep*, *18*, 1387-1393.

Yang, H. S., Cho, M. H., Zakowicz, H., Hegamyer, G., Sonenberg, N. & Colburn, N. H. (2004). A novel function of the MA-3 domains in transformation and translation suppressor Pdcd4 is essential for its binding to eukaryotic translation initiation factor 4A. *Mol Cell Biol*, *24*, 3894-3906.

Yang, H. S., Jansen, A. P., Nair, R., Shibahara, K., Verma, A. K., Cmarik, J. L. & Colburn,N. H. (2001). A novel transformation suppressor, Pdcd4, inhibits AP-1 transactivation but not NF-kappaB or ODC transactivation. *Oncogene*, *20*, 669-676.

Yang, H. S., Jansen, A. P., Komar, A. A., Zheng, X., Merrick, W. C., Costes, S., Lockett, S. J., Sonenberg, N. & Colburn, N. H. (2003a). The transformation suppressor Pdcd4 is a novel eukaryotic translation Initiation factor 4A binding protein that inhibits translation. *Mol Cell Biol*, *23,* 26-37.

Yang, H. S., Knies, J. L., Stark, C. & Colburn, N. H. (2003b). Pdcd4 suppresses tumor phenotype in JB6 cells by inhibiting AP-1 transactivation. *Oncogene*, *22*, 3712-3720.

Yang, H. S., Matthews, C. P., Clair, T., Wang, Q., Baker, A. R., Li, C. C. H., Tan, T. H. & Colburn, N. H. (2006). Tumorigenesis suppressor Pdcd4 down-regulates mitogen-activated protein kinase kinase kinase kinase 1 expression to suppress colon carcinoma cell invasion. *Mol Cell Biol*, *26*, 1297-1306.

Yoshinaga, H., Matsuhashi, S., Fujiyama, C. & Masaki, Z. (1999). Novel human PDCD4 (H731) gene expressed in proliferative cells is expressed in the samll duct epithelial cells of the breast as revealed by an anti-H731 antibody. *Pathol Int*, *49*, 1067-1077.

Zakowicz, H., Yang, H. S., Stark, C., Wlodawer, A., Laronde-Leblanc, N. & Colburn, N. H. (2005). Mutational analysis of the DEAD-box RNA helicase eIF4AII characterizes its interaction with transformation suppressor Pdcd4 and eIF4GI. *RNA*, *11*, 261-274.

Zhang, H., Ozaki, I., Mizuta, T., Hamajima, H., Yasutake, T., Eguchi, Y., Ideguchi, H., Yamamoto, K. & Matsuhashi, S. (2006). Involvement of programmed cell death 4 in transforming growth factor β1-induced apoptosis in human hepatocellular carcinoma. *Oncogene*, *25*, 6101-6112.

Zhou, G., Lee, S. C., Yao, Z. & Tan, T. H. (1999). Hematopoietic progenitor kinase 1 is a component of transforming growth factor β-induced c-Jun N-terminal kinase signaling cascade. *J Biol Chem*, *274*, 13133-13138.

Zhu, S., Wu, H., Wu, F., Nie, D., Sheng, S. & Mo, Y. Y. (2008). MicroRNA-21 targets tumor suppressor genes in invasion and metastasis. *Cell Res*, *18*, 350-359.

Chapter Sources

The following chapters have been previously published:

Chapter 13 – A version of this chapter was also published in *Progress in DNA Damage Research*, edited by Souta Miura and Shouta Nakano, published by Nova Science Publishers, Inc. It was submitted for appropriate modifications in an effort to encourage wider dissemination of research.

Chapter 14 – A version of this chapter was also published in *Dermatology Research Focus on Acne, Melanoma and Psoriasis,* edited by David E. Roth, published by Nova Science Publishers, Inc. It was submitted for appropriate modifications in an effort to encourage wider dissemination of research.

Index

1

10q23, ix, 89
10q24, xii, 253, 254, 261

9

9p24, x, 161, 162, 169

A

A>G mutations, vii, 2
accessibility, 143, 151
acetaldehyde, vii, 1, 2, 3, 4, 6, 7, 8, 12, 13, 16, 17, 18, 19, 20, 21, 22, 23
acetate, 254
acetylated levels, x, 150, 156
acetylation, x, 47, 97, 144, 149, 150, 151, 152, 153, 157, 236, 238, 241, 242
acid, vii, ix, 9, 10, 12, 14, 22, 25, 26, 27, 28, 29, 30, 31, 32, 33, 38, 40, 49, 106, 117, 133, 153, 157, 254, 261
acidity, 39
activation, 256, 257, 259
active site, x, 90, 149, 154, 156
acute lymphoblastic leukemia, 35, 37
acute myelogenous leukemia, 247
acute myeloid leukemia, 245, 248
acute promyelocytic leukemia, 158
adenine, 5
adenocarcinoma, 39, 74, 87, 182, 215, 218
adenoma, 23, 40, 74, 75, 125, 261
adenomatous polyposis coli, ix, 105, 106, 120, 121, 122, 123, 124, 125, 126, 127, 128, 129, 130, 131
adenovirus, 193, 201, 217
ADH, 3, 53, 54
adhesion, ix, 48, 71, 76, 79, 82, 90, 92, 93, 95, 102, 103, 109, 115, 122, 123, 124, 127, 128, 163, 165, 168, 172, 191, 192
adhesion properties, 93
adhesions, 103, 170
adult stem cells, 41, 243
aerodigestive tract, 22
AFB1, vii, 1, 2, 3, 4, 6, 7, 8, 9, 11, 12, 15, 16, 18
aflatoxin, vii, 1, 2, 19, 20, 21, 22, 23, 24
Africa, 19
aggressiveness, viii, 71, 75, 78, 83
aging process, 34, 35
airway hyperresponsiveness, 100
Akt-mTOR signal transduction, xii, 253
alcohol abuse, 22
alcohol consumption, 3
alcoholism, 22
alkaloids, 116
alkylation, 15, 118
allele, 92, 106, 124, 193, 201, 203
allelic loss, x, 161, 216, 246, 250
alopecia, 27, 28
alpha, 248
alternative, 247
alters, 38, 91, 186
amino, 254
amino acid, vii, ix, 25, 26, 27, 28, 29, 30, 33, 40, 106, 114, 117, 133, 254
amino acids, 26, 28, 29, 30, 33, 114
AML, 245
amoeboid, 93
ANC, 203
anchoring, 115, 128
androgen, 79, 179, 190, 196, 199, 202, 204, 207, 208, 209, 214, 215, 217, 218, 219, 220, 222, 223, 224, 226, 227, 254
anemia, 26, 27, 30, 245, 249
aneuploidy, 116, 119, 141

angiogenesis, 79, 176, 191, 197, 209, 215, 217, 218, 220, 227
anhydrase, 196
animals, xii, 254
anorexia, 33
antagonism, 81
antagonist, 259
antibody, 137, 168, 195, 227, 258, 262
anticancer, 244
anti-cancer, xi, 159, 189, 210, 230
anticancer drug, 159, 183, 244
antigen, xii, 73, 117, 195, 215, 225, 253, 254, 261
antioxidant, 247, 248
anti-oxidant, 244
antioxidants, 248
antioxidative, xii, 243, 244
antisense, 197, 203, 205, 215, 228
antisense oligonucleotides, 205
antitumor, 156, 227
anxiety, 25, 34
AP, xii, 253, 256, 257, 259, 262
APC, v, viii, ix, 41, 44, 48, 50, 51, 53, 54, 56, 57, 64, 105, 106, 107, 108, 109, 110, 111, 112, 113, 114, 115, 116, 117, 118, 119, 121, 122, 123, 124, 125, 126, 127, 128, 129, 130, 131, 132
APC-deficient cancers, ix, 105, 119, 120
aplasia, 247
apoptosis pathways, xi, 142, 189
apoptotic, 257, 260
Apoptotic, xii, 253
apoptotic pathways, x, 149, 153
Arabidopsis thaliana, 179
ARC, 7, 13, 239
architecture, 86, 124, 125
arginine, 2, 12, 237
arrest, x, 12, 49, 94, 95, 100, 109, 110, 116, 117, 130, 137, 141, 149, 153, 156, 183, 195, 200, 201, 204, 205, 212, 230, 231, 236, 237, 238, 242
arthritis, 98
asbestos, 250
ascorbic acid, vii, 25, 27, 29, 30
Asia, 40
aspartate, 94
aspirate, 56
aspiration, viii, 43, 45, 52, 53, 54, 55
assessment, viii, 43, 57, 221, 247
asthma, 100
astrocytes, 110, 114
ataxia, 135
atherosclerosis, 33, 40
atherosclerotic plaque, 33, 40
ATP, 47, 138, 139, 146, 244
attachment, 72, 115
autoimmune, 260
autoimmunity, 91, 98, 187
autosomal dominant, 91, 106
autosomal recessive, x, 80, 133
axons, 114, 167

B

B1 (AFB1), vii, 1, 2
bacteria, 39, 95, 96
basal layer, 258
basal metabolic rate, 33
base pair, 15, 16, 151
basement membrane, 93
Bcl-2 proteins, 198
beneficial effect, xi, 47, 190
benign, 28, 33, 34, 55, 56, 57, 75, 106, 134, 192, 194, 209, 248
benign prostatic hyperplasia, 248
benzene, 246, 247, 251
benzo(a)pyrene, 2
beriberi, 26, 30
beverages, 31
bias, vii, 2, 16, 18
binding, 255, 261, 262
bioassays, 251
biochemical, xii, 243, 244
biochemistry, 26
bioinformatics, 180, 186
biological, 245
biological behavior, 245
biological processes, 15, 106
biomarkers, xi, 181, 186, 189, 190, 191, 211, 214
biomass, 26, 27
biopsy, 54, 56
biotin, 27, 29
bladder, 246, 249, 250
bladder cancer, 152, 162, 169, 221, 225, 246, 249, 250
bone, 26, 51, 219, 227, 247
bone marrow, 26, 247
bone marrow transplant, 247
brachytherapy, 190, 221, 223, 228
brain, ix, x, 51, 80, 81, 84, 89, 100, 133, 137, 144, 222
brain cancer, ix, 81, 89
brain size, x, 133
brain tumor, 222
BRCA1, 249
BRCT-Repeat Inhibitor, ix, 133
breast cancer, viii, 28, 35, 38, 39, 44, 45, 48, 49, 50, 51, 52, 54, 55, 56, 57, 58, 74, 75, 78, 79, 83, 85, 87, 90, 93, 103, 124, 134, 136, 154, 160, 176,

177, 178, 184, 185, 210, 223, 224, 227, 228, 249, 254, 259, 260
breast carcinoma, 50, 124, 176
BRIT1, v, ix, 133, 134, 135, 136, 137, 138, 139, 140, 141, 142, 143, 144, 145, 146
bronchial asthma, 100
budding, 82
bulbar, xii, 253
Butcher, 98

C

Ca^{2+}, 102
cachexia, 33
cadherin, 256, 259
caloric restriction, 33, 41
cancer death, viii, xi, 43, 44, 189
cancer progression, 93, 111, 118
cancer screening, viii, 44
cancerous cells, viii, 43, 245
cancers, 245
candidates, 4, 183
CaP, xi, 189, 190, 191, 192, 193, 194, 195, 196, 197, 198, 199, 200, 201, 202, 203, 204, 205, 206, 207, 208, 209, 210, 212, 214, 215
capacity, 243
cap-dependent translations, xii, 253
capillary, 52, 53
carbon, 46, 151
carcinogen, vii, 1, 2, 12, 18, 23, 34, 245, 251
carcinogenesis, vii, xi, xii, 2, 3, 4, 12, 16, 18, 19, 21, 22, 23, 35, 40, 41, 45, 47, 50, 52, 56, 125, 151, 152, 154, 161, 162, 175, 183, 207, 230, 243, 245, 248, 253, 254, 255, 257, 261
carcinogenicity, 246, 251
carcinogens, 245, 246, 250
, carcinoma, vii, x, 1, 2, 3, 15, 17, 19, 20, 21, 23, 54, 55, 56, 74, 75, 78, 81, 82, 83, 84, 85, 121, 124, 125, 150, 154, 155, 156, 158, 159, 161, 162, 169, 176, 177, 181, 184, 185, 195, 217, 219, 220, 221, 223, 224, 225226, 227, 228, 232, 249, 250, 256, 261, 262
carcinomas, 254
casein, 107, 109, 117, 130
caspase, 257, 260
caspases, 94, 101, 102, 131, 256, 257
castration, 191, 209, 215, 220
catechol, 247
catheter, 52
CCND2, viii, 44, 48, 50, 51, 53, 54, 55, 56, 57
CDK inhibitor, x, 149, 153
CDK4, 254
cDNA, 5, 193, 201
CEC, 82
cell, xii, 243, 244, 247, 249, 250, 253, 254, 255, 256, 257, 259, 260, 261, 262
cell body, 164
cell culture, 4, 225, 233, 259
cell cycle, xii, 4, 94, 100, 101, 103, 109, 110, 113, 115, 116, 117, 119, 123, 126, 128, 129, 130, 135, 137, 138, 139, 141, 143, 152, 156, 162, 163, 167, 168, 171, 173, 177, 183, 200, 203, 204, 205, 208, 212, 230, 253, 254, 261
cell death, x, xi, xii, 39, 94, 95, 98, 99, 119, 149, 152, 153, 195, 212, 220, 229, 231, 232, 235, 238, 239, 243, 244, 247, 253, 254, 260, 261, 262
cell differentiation, 110, 154
cell fate, xi, 153, 154, 159, 229, 230, 231, 242
cell growth, 244, 255, 259, 260
cell invasion, 78, 80, 93, 99, 225, 262
cell killing, 195, 201
cell lines, ix, 2, 16, 20, 21, 23, 74, 75, 78, 79, 81, 89, 90, 93, 101, 116, 130, 134, 135, 137, 157, 158, 162, 169, 177, 178, 179, 180, 183, 190, 193, 194, 195, 197, 201, 203, 204, 207, 210, 211, 212, 218, 222, 223, 226, 232
cell metabolism, 39
cell signaling, xi, 189
cell surface, 76
cellular maintenance, viii, 43
cellular philology, xii, 243
central nervous system, 106, 111, 114
centromere, 116
centrosome, 108, 114, 115, 117, 124, 138, 145, 171, 172
cerebral cortex, 114, 127
cervical cancer, 153, 219
CGC, 9, 10, 14
chemokine receptor, 95
chemokines, 96
chemoprevention, 57
chemopreventive agents, 183
chemotaxis, 91, 92, 98, 99, 100
chemotherapeutic agent, 39, 116, 203
chemotherapy, viii, 25, 26, 32, 33, 34, 39, 40, 41, 52, 101, 190, 200, 215, 223, 227, 244
Chemotherapy, 248
chicken, 137, 138, 254, 261
childhood, 34, 35
China, 22, 189, 214
cholangiocarcinoma, 101
choline, vii, 25, 27, 28, 29, 30, 33, 38
chromatin modifiers, x, 47, 149, 158
chromosomal instability, 52, 116, 128, 249
chromosome, ix, x, xii, 47, 77, 89, 101, 102, 103, 106, 115, 120, 128, 129, 134, 137, 140, 141, 145,

146, 161, 193, 200, 205, 223, 243, 244, 245, 246, 248, 250, 261
chromosome 10, ix, 89, 101, 103, 205, 223
chromosomes, 245, 248
cigarette smoking, 250
circulation, 39, 95
class, 94, 152, 153, 154, 159, 163, 198, 245
classification, 261
cleavage, 94, 108, 118, 131, 167, 172
clinical syndrome, 136
clinical trials, 34, 41, 153, 156, 159, 193, 199, 200, 203, 209
clone, 213
cloning, 106, 168
clusters, 47, 109, 113
coding, x, 106, 119, 134, 149, 150, 156, 176, 179, 180, 183, 184
codon, vii, 1, 2, 11, 12, 15, 16, 18, 19, 134
codon 245, vii, 2
codon 249, vii, 1, 2, 11, 12, 15, 16, 18, 19
collagen, 93
colon, 35, 41, 49, 90, 106, 109, 120, 121, 122, 125, 130, 131, 152, 154, 158, 178, 184, 245, 248, 254, 256, 261, 262
colon cancer, 41, 49, 90, 109, 120, 121, 122, 130, 131, 152, 178, 184, 254
color, iv
colorectal cancer, ix, 35, 105, 106, 109, 111, 113, 117, 118, 120, 130, 132, 159, 218, 222, 223, 225, 226, 259
combination therapy, 193
combined effect, 144, 205
common findings, 154
compensation, 140
competition, 80
compilation, 219
complexity, 39, 119, 226, 230
compliance, 30, 31, 186
components, 255
composition, 3
compounds, 4, 6, 96
condensation, 16, 94, 137, 140, 145, 146
conflict, 19, 82
conflict of interest, 19, 82
consciousness, 34
consensus, 90, 117
consumption, 3, 20, 21, 23, 29, 31, 32
control group, 44, 201, 204
controversies, vii, 1, 4, 209, 214
corepressor, 111
correlation, 48, 50, 51, 54, 58, 79, 90, 176, 201, 203, 246, 250
correlation analysis, 54
correlation coefficient, 50
correlations, 31
cortex, 114, 115, 127
counterbalance, 198
CpG islands, 246
CpG sites, vii, 2, 7, 15, 16, 151
criticism, 36
cross links, 16
CSCs, xi, 189, 190, 209, 210, 211, 212, 213, 214, 215
CSF, 129
CTA, 10
C-terminal, 262
cues, 114
culture, 4, 5, 6, 23, 29, 114, 207, 210, 211, 212, 213, 233
culture conditions, 210, 213
cycles, 4, 5, 138
cyclin D1, 254
cycling, 164, 167, 244
cyclooxygenase, 215, 223, 224, 225, 226, 227
cysteine, vii, 25, 29, 32, 247
cytochrome, 20, 21, 94, 198, 232, 247
cytogenetic, 245, 251
cytogenetics, 169
cytokines, 91, 94, 96, 176
cytokinesis, xi, 115, 127, 161, 162, 163, 167, 168, 171, 172
cytologic examination, 57
cytology, 52, 56, 57
cytomegalovirus, 193
cytometry, 213, 244
cytoplasm, 94, 96, 167, 203, 235
cytosine, viii, 15, 43, 46, 47, 48, 151
cytoskeleton, ix, 71, 92, 105, 108, 109, 110, 111, 112, 114, 119, 122, 126, 163, 164
cytotoxicity, 4, 6, 23, 39, 205

D

database, vii, 1, 4, 6, 7, 11, 13, 16, 17, 20, 22, 218
de novo, 245
deacetylation, x, 149, 150, 152, 155, 158
death, xii, 244, 253, 254, 257, 260, 261, 262
deaths, 195
defects, 80, 84, 91, 92, 115, 119, 122, 128, 129, 140, 249
defense, xii, 243, 244
defense mechanisms, xii, 243, 244
deficiencies, 29, 30, 40
deficiency, vii, ix, x, 25, 27, 28, 29, 32, 37, 38, 73, 86, 105, 121, 122, 133, 134, 136, 204, 213, 215, 246, 247

degradation, ix, 76, 82, 105, 107, 109, 111, 117, 124, 129, 136, 156, 203, 231, 233, 239, 241, 255, 260
dendrites, 114, 164
deoxyribonucleic acid, 22
deoxyribose, 26, 27
depolymerization, 113
depression, 25, 33, 34
deprivation, 26, 32, 33, 94, 196, 199, 209, 214, 215, 217, 218, 219, 220, 223, 224, 226, 227, 228
deregulation, ix, 71, 77, 78, 79, 150, 153, 192
destruction, viii, ix, 25, 29, 32, 105, 107, 109, 119, 123, 218
detachment, 163
detection, 20, 23, 45, 48, 50, 52, 56, 57, 58, 139, 205, 211
detoxification, 3
developmental disorder, 91
diacylglycerol, 233, 240
diagnosis, 39, 44, 51, 161, 184, 191
diapedesis, 95
dicentric chromosome, 134
diet, 27, 28, 29, 30, 37, 40
differentiation, xii, 245, 253, 254, 257, 259, 261
digestion, 48
diploid, 4
directionality, 100
discordance, 203
discs, 110, 123, 125
disease gene, x, 133, 146
disease progression, 150, 205, 226
disorder, x, 80, 133, 163
displacement, 72, 130
dissociation, 72, 86, 236, 241
DNA damage, x, xi, xii, 12, 20, 22, 35, 38, 118, 133, 134, 135, 136, 137, 139, 140, 141, 142, 143, 144, 145, 146, 147, 160, 200, 203, 210, 211, 212, 216, 222, 229, 230, 231, 233, 234, 235, 237, 238, 239, 240, 241, 242, 243, 244, 245, 246, 247, 250
DNA lesions, xi, 135, 137, 139, 143, 229, 230
DNA ligase, 139
DNA ploidy, 207
DNA polymerase, 5, 24, 117, 130, 248
DNA repair, ix, x, 12, 48, 49, 105, 117, 130, 133, 135, 136, 138, 139, 140, 141, 143, 144, 145, 146, 147, 211, 212, 213, 225, 230, 231
DNA sequencing, 5, 19, 202
donors, 29, 33
dosage, 135, 182
down-regulation, x, 95, 124, 150, 195, 196, 204, 233, 240
Drosophila, 49, 80, 111, 122, 123, 124, 125, 132, 138, 145, 146, 186
drugs, 26, 27, 32, 94, 119, 135, 140, 162, 167, 182, 183, 222, 244

E

E.coli, 96
East Asia, 40
E-cadherin, x, 48, 109, 110, 122, 125, 149, 150, 155, 156, 160
ectoderm, 153
eczema, 27, 28, 30
edema, 96, 226
EGF, 76, 82, 164
egg, 27
Egypt, 12
eIF4A, xii, 253, 254, 255, 259, 260, 261, 262
electrons, 244
electrophoresis, 23, 212
embryogenesis, 167
emotion, 34
encoding, 73, 86, 114, 162, 176, 177, 181, 200
endogenous, 243
endometrial carcinoma, 90, 159
endonuclease, 117
endoscopy, 54
endothelial cells, 102
endothelium, 95
enlargement, 91
environmental, 245, 246
environmental factors, 182
environmental stimuli, 139
enzymatic activity, 153
enzyme, 244
enzymes, 46, 47, 48, 111, 150, 152, 154, 156, 247
epidemiology, 21
epidermal cells, xii, 253, 254
epidermis, xii, 122, 233, 240, 253, 256, 257, 258
epigenetic, 244
epigenetic alterations, 162, 244
epigenetic modification, x, 150, 157, 161
epigenetic silencing, x, 149, 150, 152, 154, 156
epigenetics, 157, 158, 160
epithelia, 109, 110
epithelial cell, 262
epithelial cells, viii, 19, 43, 45, 74, 75, 78, 79, 109, 110, 111, 112, 114, 119, 123, 124, 130, 131, 134, 154, 160, 196, 210, 215, 246, 262
epithelial ovarian cancer, 77, 87, 134
epithelium, 26, 106, 111, 115, 119, 122, 124
erythrocytes, 247
esophageal, 246, 249
esophageal cancer, 3, 22, 246
esophageal squamous cell carcinoma, 249
esophagus, 2, 3, 17, 182, 185, 226, 250

essential fatty acids, vii, 25, 28, 30
ester, 233, 240
estrogen, 49
ethanol, vii, 2, 3, 12, 20, 21, 22
ethanol metabolism, 22
euchromatin, 117, 139, 184
eukaryotic cell, viii, 71
excision, 108, 117, 130
execution, 232
exercise, viii, 25, 39
exocytosis, 73, 74
exogenous, 243, 246
exons, 6, 7, 8, 9, 106, 202
exploration, 28
exposure, vii, 1, 2, 3, 4, 6, 7, 12, 15, 16, 17, 18, 35, 94, 135, 137, 191, 201, 212, 225, 231, 234, 235, 237, 244, 245, 246, 247
extracellular matrix, 93, 103, 163
extraction, 5
extraocular muscles, 163, 169, 170, 171
extravasation, 38
eye movement, 163
EZH2, v, x, 149, 150, 152, 153, 154, 155, 156, 157, 159, 160

F

failure, 246
faith, 34
false positive, 48
familial, 245
family, 246
family history, 44
family members, viii, 42, 71, 72, 73, 78, 125, 162, 246
FASAY, vii, 1, 2, 4, 6, 11, 12, 16, 17, 18, 19, 22
fasting, 32
fat, 28
fatty acids, vii, 25, 27, 28, 30, 31, 32
F-box, 260
feedback, 98, 165, 203, 239
FHIT gene, xii, 243, 245, 246, 249, 250
fibers, 162, 163, 164, 165, 169, 170, 171
fibroblast, 257
fibroblast growth factor, 76, 87
fibroblasts, vii, 1, 4, 6, 7, 9, 13, 15, 18, 77, 94, 110, 115, 117
fibrosis, 163, 169, 170, 171
fidelity, 143
field defect, viii, 43
fluid, viii, 43, 44, 45, 50, 52, 53, 54, 55, 56, 57, 58
folate, 27, 37, 40
folic acid, vii, 25, 26, 27, 29, 30, 33, 40
follicle, 257, 258
follicles, xii, 253, 257, 259, 261
formaldehyde, 48
fragile site, xii, 243, 245, 248, 249
fragments, 94, 113, 179
frameshift mutation, 7
France, 1, 4, 5, 19
free radical, 244
free radicals, 244
freedom, 199, 215
frequencies, 51, 57, 106
functional analysis, 19, 22
Functional Analysis of Separated Alleles in Yeast, vii, 1, 4, 22
fungi, 2, 95
fusion, 72, 73, 74, 82, 158

G

G>A transitions, vii, 2, 7, 12, 15, 17, 18
G>T mutations, 17
G>T transversion, vii, 1, 2, 7, 12, 15, 16, 17, 18
gallbladder, 154, 159
gastritis, 75, 81, 85
gastrointestinal, 246, 248
gastrulation, 124, 170
GC/CG sequence, vii, 2, 15
gel, 5, 23, 50, 212
gene, xii, 243, 245, 246, 249, 250, 253, 254, 259, 261, 262
gene amplification, 205, 218, 226
gene expression, x, 47, 75, 81, 84, 85, 130, 144, 149, 150, 152, 154, 155, 176, 237, 238, 249, 250, 259
gene promoter, 150, 236
gene silencing, 152, 154, 157, 158
gene therapy, 193, 203, 214, 215, 217
gene transfer, 98, 193
generation, 244, 251
genetic, 245, 248, 251
genetic abnormalities, 248
genetic alteration, 2, 3, 16, 106, 120, 134, 150, 154, 200, 224, 230
genetic disease, x, 133, 136
genetic disorders, 73
genetic information, 135, 143
genetic programs, 176
genome, ix, 46, 47, 51, 73, 106, 133, 134, 135, 136, 138, 139, 141, 144, 146, 147, 150, 157, 183, 184, 203, 216, 230, 231, 239, 245, 246
genomic, 245, 246, 247
genomic instability, x, 133, 134, 135, 137, 152, 247
genomic regions, 186
genomic stability, x, 133, 135, 141, 145, 146
genomics, 81, 84, 184
genotoxic, 244

genotoxic stresses, x, 133, 239
genotoxin, vii, 1, 2, 4, 18, 243, 245, 247
genotoxins, 246
genotype, 203
germ line, 44
germline mutations, 91
GG sequence, 15
gland, 109, 122, 123, 170, 211, 246, 257, 258
glial cells, 110
glioblastoma, ix, 89, 98, 100, 211, 212, 216, 218, 219, 221, 222, 260
glioblastoma multiforme, 218
glioma, 203, 211, 212, 222, 225, 226, 227, 254, 260
glucose, vii, 25, 32, 39
glucose tolerance, 32
glucose tolerance test, 32
glutamic acid, 157
glutathione, 29, 32, 244
glutathione peroxidase, 244
glycogen, 127
growth, 254, 256, 259, 260, 262
growth arrest, x, 130, 149, 153, 231, 236, 237
growth factor, ix, 71, 75, 76, 77, 78, 79, 80, 81, 82, 84, 85, 86, 87, 94, 99, 100, 164, 165, 170, 171, 176, 190, 193, 215, 217, 220, 221, 227, 254, 260, 262
growth factors, 255
GTPases, v, viii, 71, 72, 82, 83, 85, 86, 92, 100, 112, 164, 170, 171
Guangdong, 189
Guangzhou, 189
guanine, 2, 12, 15, 16, 21, 49, 72, 112, 125
guardian, 135, 230, 239

H

HaCaT cells, xii, 253, 257, 258
hair, xii, 253, 257, 258, 259, 261
hair follicle, xii, 253, 257, 259, 261
half-life, 97
HBV, 2, 16
HCC, vii, 1, 2, 7, 11, 12, 15, 16, 18, 75
HDAC, v, x, 46, 149, 150, 151, 152, 153, 154, 155, 156, 157, 159
HE, 65, 228
head and neck cancer, 24, 41, 216, 223
heat treatment, 94
hematological, 247
hematopoietic, xii, 243, 244, 245, 246, 247, 248, 251, 256
hematopoietic cells, 246, 247
hematopoietic stem cells, 247, 248, 251
hematopoietic system, xii, 243, 244
hepatitis, 2, 22, 23
hepatocarcinogen, 3, 12
hepatocarcinogenesis, 22, 23
hepatocellular, 254, 262
hepatocellular carcinoma, vii, 1, 19, 21, 23, 74, 75, 81, 84, 85, 184, 254, 262
hepatocytes, 2, 19
hepatoma, 256, 257
herbal teas, viii, 25, 32
heterochromatin, 139, 143, 152
high-risk women, viii, 44, 52, 56, 57, 58
histidine, 49
histochemistry, 219
histology, 56
histone, x, 47, 117, 118, 129, 131, 135, 137, 147, 149, 150, 151, 152, 153, 154, 155, 156, 157, 158, 159, 160, 181, 241
histone deacetylase, x, 47, 118, 129, 131, 149, 151, 152, 157, 158, 159
histones, x, 47, 147, 149, 151, 152, 153, 155
homeostasis, ix, 29, 105, 106, 119
homocysteine, 38
homolog, 254
honesty, 26
Hong Kong, 175
host, 26, 38, 91, 96, 100, 182, 186
hTERT, ix, 133
hub, 141, 147
human, xii, 245, 248, 249, 250, 251, 253, 254, 257, 258, 260, 261, 262
human brain, 100, 144
human genome, 47, 106, 151, 157, 183, 184
human papilloma virus, 111
human tumours, vii, 1, 4, 7, 17, 18
Hunter, 76, 82, 171
hybrid, 110, 113, 163
hybridization, 73, 261
hydrogels, 193
hydrogen, 244
hydrogen peroxide, 244
hydroquinone, 247, 251
hydroxyl, 244
hygiene, 3
hyperglycemia, 31, 32, 33, 39
hypermethylation, viii, x, 40, 43, 45, 46, 47, 48, 49, 50, 51, 52, 53, 55, 56, 57, 149, 150, 151, 152, 159
hyperplasia, 54, 227, 240, 248
hypersensitivity, 130, 140
hyperthermia, 36, 39
hypertrophy, 106, 134
hypoglycemia, 32, 33
hypothesis, 3, 12, 106, 111, 118, 154, 192
hypoxia, 31, 37, 192, 217, 221
hypoxic cells, 33

I

IARC database, vii, 1, 4, 6, 7, 11, 13, 16, 17, 218
ideal, 34, 91, 206
IL-1, 259
IL-15, 259
IL-2, 259
imbalances, 169
immature cell, 257
immune regulation, 91
immune response, 225
immune system, 96
immunity, 91, 99
immunoglobulins, 91
immunohistochemistry, 198, 202, 211
immunoprecipitation, 236
immunoreactivity, 201, 202, 218, 226
impacts, 108
imprinting, 47
in situ, 261
in situ hybridization, 261
in vitro, 246, 247, 254, 259
in vitro exposure, vii, 1, 4
in vitro pattern, vii, 2, 4
in vivo, xi, 15, 21, 23, 29, 78, 90, 95, 100, 102, 107, 109, 114, 115, 116, 117, 121, 126, 129, 134, 135, 154, 156, 159, 172, 190, 193, 195, 197, 200, 203, 208, 211, 213, 217, 218, 226, 228, 238, 241, 247, 254, 256, 259
incidence, 3, 34, 38, 44, 102, 136, 202, 209, 224, 230
incubation time, 4
independence, 176
India, 65
induction, xi, xii, 91, 119, 171, 179, 183, 186, 195, 201, 210, 221, 222, 229, 230, 231, 232, 233, 234, 235, 237, 242, 246, 247, 253, 255, 257
infants, 20, 22
inflammation, 91, 94, 95, 96, 98, 99, 100, 102, 195, 224, 260
inhibition, xi, 6, 20, 26, 38, 39, 49, 94, 95, 97, 102, 114, 155, 160, 161, 163, 164, 165, 166, 168, 176, 177, 183, 192, 195, 197, 203, 204, 205, 212, 215, 217, 225, 233, 238, 244, 247, 248, 256, 259, 260, 261
inhibitor, ix, x, 40, 48, 49, 86, 94, 107, 118, 131, 133, 149, 150, 153, 154, 155, 156, 157, 159, 167, 172, 173, 192, 193, 194, 195, 196, 197, 204, 212, 214, 217, 222, 224, 227, 233, 236, 241, 260
inhibitors, 254, 255, 261
initiation, viii, xii, 43, 45, 47, 78, 94, 111, 120, 125, 134, 143, 144, 164, 165, 211, 233, 253, 254, 255, 259, 260, 261, 262
innate immunity, 91, 99
inoculation, 193
inositol, 27, 28, 30, 38, 90, 92, 99, 102, 190, 215
insertion, 6, 7, 8, 9, 14, 90
instability, 245
insulin, 32, 33, 74, 85, 102, 163, 164, 254
insulin dependent diabetes, 33
insulin signaling, 102
insulinoma, 74
insults, 243, 244
integrin, 76, 78, 81, 82, 95, 99, 164, 165
integrins, ix, 71, 171
integrity, 245, 246
intensity, 244
interaction, 251, 262
interference, 115, 235
interleukins, 254
internalization, 84, 87
internists, 37
intervention, 31, 33, 40, 191, 226
intestinal flora, 27
intestinal villi, 109
intestine, 109, 119, 121, 131
invasive lesions, 50
inversions, 244
invertebrates, 170
ionizing radiation, 27, 135, 145, 192, 208, 218, 219, 225, 250
irradiation, xii, 2, 135, 137, 190, 192, 193, 195, 196, 197, 200, 201, 203, 206, 209, 210, 211, 212, 213, 226, 227, 233, 235, 240, 253, 257, 259
IRS, 163, 257
isolation, 110, 254
isoleucine, 28
isomerization, 236

J

Japan, 84, 149, 161, 169, 229, 243, 253
JNK, 256, 259
Jordan, 21, 39
Jun, 256, 259, 262

K

Kank1 gene, x, 161, 162, 165, 168
Kank1 protein, xi, 161, 163
keratinocyte, 257, 258
keratinocytes, 257, 259, 260
kidney, 33, 78, 84, 87, 90
kidney stones, 33
kinase, 245, 246, 251, 255, 256, 259, 262
kinase activity, 95, 121
kinetics, 240
kinetochore, 115, 116

Korea, 40

L

labeling, 203, 208, 218, 220, 226
lactic acid, 31, 33
lesions, xi, 22, 28, 50, 56, 57, 73, 83, 134, 135, 137, 139, 143, 150, 229, 230, 244, 249, 250, 261
leucine, 5, 28
leukemia, 26, 27, 28, 29, 31, 35, 37, 136, 153, 156, 158, 177, 178, 197, 214, 245, 247, 248, 251, 258, 261
leukemia cells, 258, 261
ligand, 76, 84, 94, 107, 233
lipid, 257
Lipid, 248
lipids, 27, 28, 244
lithium, 5
liver, 2, 3, 4, 12, 16, 21, 23, 27, 30, 40, 41, 106, 195, 216
liver cancer, 21, 216
localization, 74, 85, 92, 109, 110, 111, 112, 113, 114, 115, 116, 123, 124, 129, 145, 157, 172, 232, 235, 241, 254
locus, 50, 80, 100, 106, 120, 154, 159, 160, 162, 165
LOH analysis, ix, 89
loneliness, 34
long-term, 247, 251
loss of heterozygosity, 250
lung, 246, 249, 250, 254, 260
lung cancer, vii, 1, 3, 17, 20, 34, 90, 162, 169, 176, 177, 182, 185, 187, 195, 205, 217, 220, 221, 226, 246, 249, 250, 254, 260
Luo, v, 89, 95, 99, 100, 102, 103, 158, 167, 171, 242
lymph, 51, 91, 209
lymph node, 51, 91
lymphadenopathy, 209
lymphangiogenesis, 228
lymphocytes, 22, 23, 73, 74, 91, 187, 251
lymphoid, 107
lymphoma, 37, 134, 144, 179, 181, 185, 197, 214, 216, 219, 257, 260
lymphomas, 257
lysine, 28, 47, 151, 152, 153, 154, 157, 158, 242
lysis, 29, 33, 38
lysosome, 74

M

M1, 254
machinery, ix, x, 98, 105, 141, 150, 151, 154, 208, 231, 260
macromolecules, 244
macrophages, 92, 102, 247
maintenance, 246
majority, 15, 16, 33, 48
malignancy, 56, 74, 216
malignant cells, x, 150, 154, 197
malignant tissues, x, 57, 149
malignant tumors, 150
malnutrition, 28, 30
mammography, 44, 57
mammoplasty, 51
manipulation, viii, 25, 26, 30, 31, 33, 34, 183
mantle, 134, 144
MAP kinases, 170
MAPK/ERK, xi, 189
mapping, 20
markers, xi, 38, 57, 80, 185, 190, 191, 194, 199, 205, 212, 213, 214, 224, 227
marrow, 26, 247
mast cells, 102
mastectomy, 44, 54, 56
matrix, 78, 93, 96, 103, 110, 115, 163, 193, 215
matrix metalloproteinase, 93, 96, 193, 215
MBP, 46
MCPH1, v, x, 133, 144, 145, 146
median, 54, 55, 193, 195, 199, 206, 209
medical care, 37
melanoma, 74, 75, 87, 90, 216
membranes, 27, 28, 72, 73
mental health, 37
mental retardation, 73, 83
mesothelioma, 184
metabolism, 12, 20, 22, 26, 31, 38, 39, 40, 49, 90, 117, 176, 247
metabolite, 247
metabolites, 32, 246, 247, 251
metabolizing, 90
metalloproteinase, 40, 49, 93, 99, 121, 193, 215
metaphase, 128, 245
metastasis, ix, xi, 29, 39, 51, 71, 75, 76, 79, 87, 93, 120, 134, 161, 165, 168, 170, 176, 185, 190, 197, 199, 203, 205, 206, 207, 210, 220, 222, 224, 226, 227, 259, 262
metastatic, 248, 256
methodology, 203
methyl group, viii, 43, 47, 151
methylation, viii, x, 15, 33, 40, 43, 44, 45, 46, 47, 48, 49, 50, 51, 52, 53, 54, 55, 56, 57, 58, 106, 129, 149, 150, 151, 152, 153, 154, 155, 156, 157, 158, 159, 160, 181, 246, 249
Methylation, 249
mice, vii, ix, xii, 2, 3, 7, 15, 18, 20, 38, 77, 78, 89, 91, 92, 94, 95, 96, 97, 98, 101, 102, 111, 115, 119, 121, 123, 128, 129, 135, 140, 145, 162, 170,

177, 178, 182, 187, 193, 197, 204, 208, 225, 233, 237, 240, 247, 251, 254, 256, 257
microcephalin, x, 133, 144, 145
microcephaly, x, 133, 137, 138, 144, 146
microenvironments, 82
micronucleus, 22
microRNA, xi, 99, 175, 176, 177, 178, 179, 180, 181, 182, 183, 184, 185, 186, 187, 233, 240, 254, 260
migration, ix, xi, 48, 71, 78, 79, 81, 82, 90, 92, 93, 95, 102, 103, 105, 106, 108, 109, 110, 112, 114, 115, 119, 121, 122, 123, 124, 126, 127, 161, 162, 163, 164, 165, 166, 168, 169, 170, 172, 191, 192
MIP, 95
mitochondria, 40, 197, 198, 230, 232
mitochondrial, 244
mitogen, 99, 190, 215, 255, 256, 262
mitogen-activated protein kinase, 256, 262
mitogens, xii, 253, 255
mitosis, ix, 105, 108, 109, 115, 116, 117, 128, 137, 138, 145, 167, 208, 230
mitotic cell death, x, 149, 153
MMP, 93, 96, 107, 193, 215, 216
MMP-2, 193, 215
MMP-9, 93, 96, 193
MMPs, 93
model system, 87, 109, 110, 111, 115, 138, 183
modeling, 41
modification, x, xi, 30, 47, 144, 149, 150, 151, 152, 153, 157, 161, 229, 230, 232, 235, 238
modulation, 246
modules, 134, 179
molecular mechanisms, 254
molecular weight, 221
molecules, 28, 72, 77, 79, 94, 115, 135, 162, 164, 167, 176, 183, 187, 214, 244
monitoring, 29, 194
monoclonal antibody, 168, 195
morphogenesis, 49, 109, 110, 114, 127, 163, 171
morphology, 109, 112, 113, 193
mortality rate, 96
motif, 89, 90, 97, 112, 163, 164, 165, 166, 255
mouse, xii, 253, 254, 256, 257, 261
MRI, 44, 57, 58
mRNA, 97, 131, 134, 176, 179, 234, 235, 254, 255, 256
mucin, 124
mucosa, 21, 78, 84, 125
multicellular organisms, 163
multiple factors, 78
multipotential, 251
multi-protein complexes, ix, 105
muscles, 163, 167, 169, 170, 171
mutagenesis, 23, 230
mutant, 12, 41, 77, 78, 79, 80, 84, 92, 107, 109, 115, 116, 117, 118, 119, 123, 126, 127, 129, 146, 163, 180, 181, 185, 200, 215, 226, 236, 238
mutation, vii, x, 1, 2, 4, 6, 7, 8, 9, 10, 12, 14, 15, 16, 17, 21, 22, 44, 51, 55, 57, 80, 91, 102, 106, 107, 109, 111, 113, 118, 119, 122, 129, 131, 150, 152, 161, 167, 169, 171, 181, 202, 219, 226, 237
mutations, vii, 1, 2, 3, 4, 6, 7, 8, 9, 11, 12, 13, 14, 15, 16, 17, 18, 19, 20, 21, 22, 23, 35, 36, 73, 75, 76, 78, 79, 80, 84, 87, 90, 91, 100, 101, 102, 103, 106, 118, 119, 120, 121, 128, 129, 130, 131, 136, 139, 163, 167, 170, 193, 200, 202, 218, 222, 226, 238, 245, 247
MYC, 245
myelodysplasia, 245, 248
myeloid, 245, 261
myeloperoxidase, 247
myosin, 73, 86, 167, 168, 172

N

NAD, 152
NADH, 27
natural selection, 33
nausea, 25, 34
neck cancer, 24, 41, 216, 223
necrosis, 38, 101, 208, 244
negative feedback, 203, 239
neocortex, 127
neonatal, 257
neoplastic, 254, 259, 260
neoplastic tissue, 194
nerve, 27, 167, 171
nervous system, 74, 102, 106, 111, 114
nested PCR, 55
Netherlands, 57, 58
neural development, 74
neuroblastoma, 34, 178, 179, 187, 223
neuroendocrine cells, 74, 83
neuronal apoptosis, 132
neuronal cells, 110, 114, 167
neuronal development disorder, x, 133
neurons, 115
neuropathy, 27, 73, 87
neurotransmitter, 86
neutropenia, 96, 100
neutrophils, 91, 92, 94, 95, 96, 97, 99, 103
New England, 39
New South Wales, 189, 214
NF-kB, 256
niacin, vii, 25, 27, 29, 30
niacin deficiency, 29
Nigeria, 12

nipple fluid, viii, 43, 44, 45, 50, 52, 53, 54, 55, 57, 58
nitrogen, 244
nitrosamines, 3
NK, 254, 259
nodes, 51, 91
non-cancerous cells, viii, 43
non-insulin dependent diabetes, 33
non-random, xii, 243, 245
nonsense mutation, 80, 109
non-smokers, 7, 13, 17
normal, xii, 253, 261
normal development, xii, 254
novel screening, viii, 43, 45
N-terminal, 256, 262
nuclear, 254, 256, 261
nucleation, 112
nuclei, 154, 158, 256, 257
nucleic acid, 27, 32
nucleoprotein, 141
nucleosome, 47, 151, 181
nucleotide sequence, viii, 43
nucleotides, 32, 247
nucleus, 74, 94, 96, 119, 230, 235, 237, 241
nutrient manipulation, viii, 25, 26, 29, 30, 31, 32, 33, 34
nutrients, vii, 25, 26, 29, 30, 31, 32, 33
nutrition, 30, 33, 40

O

obesity, 33, 84
objective criteria, 31
oculomotor, 167
oculomotor nerve, 167
oesophageal, vii, 2, 17, 18, 21
oligomerization, 137, 231
Oncogene, 249, 259, 261, 262
oncogenes, viii, xi, 23, 71, 73, 79, 161, 169, 175, 176, 182, 245, 248
oncogenesis, x, 75, 77, 150, 261
Oncology, 251
oncoproteins, xi, 189
oophorectomy, 44
opportunities, 32, 120
Opportunities, 45
oral cancers, 34
oral cavity, 3, 21
organ, 45, 101, 246
organic chemicals, 26
organism, 231
organizing, 115, 165, 166
ornithine, 255
ovarian cancer, viii, 71, 78, 79, 86, 87, 103, 134, 136, 178
ovary, 246
overlap, 118, 145
oxidation, 3, 32, 97, 244
oxidative, xii, 243, 244, 247, 248
oxidative damage, 244, 247
oxidative stress, xii, 243, 244, 247, 248
oxide, 247
oxygen, 3, 92, 95, 135, 210, 244, 248, 251
oxytocin nasal spray, viii, 44, 52

P

p16INK4A, x, 48, 149, 150, 155, 156, 246
p21WAF1/CIP1, x, 149, 153, 155
Pacific, 40
pain, 25, 36
palliative, 25
pancreas, 3, 41, 84, 203
pancreatic, 254, 261
pancreatic cancer, 124, 176, 186, 254, 261
parallel, 51, 111, 123, 152
parathyroid, 106
patents, 205
pathogenesis, ix, x, 21, 105, 133, 156, 158, 245, 248
pathogens, 95, 96
pathways, ix, x, xi, 3, 32, 71, 72, 73, 77, 78, 80, 92, 94, 98, 99, 117, 130, 135, 137, 139, 141, 142, 144, 147, 149, 153, 158, 159, 162, 164, 179, 183, 185, 189, 190, 191, 204, 214, 220, 225, 231, 232, 235, 245, 248, 249, 256, 258
patients, 244
PCR, viii, 5, 8, 44, 48, 50, 54, 55, 56, 60, 63, 83, 202, 211, 215
PDGF, 102
pellagra, 27, 30
peptidase, 49
peptides, 40, 90
perfusion, vii, 25, 27, 31
peripheral blood, 83
peripheral blood mononuclear cell, 83
peripheral neuropathy, 27, 73
peritoneal cavity, 95
permeability, 227, 233
permission, iv, 30, 34, 35, 46
permit, 7, 31, 33
pernicious anemia, 27, 30
peroxidation, 248
peroxide, 244
perturbation, xii, 243, 245
pH, 39
phagocytosis, 49, 91
pharynx, 3

phenotype, xii, 77, 80, 81, 111, 116, 119, 140, 186, 199, 211, 219, 253, 257, 262
phenotypes, x, 33, 78, 79, 106, 109, 119, 134, 140, 149, 153, 246
phenylalanine, 28, 29, 236
phosphoinositides, 99
phospholipids, 28
phosphorylation, 47, 78, 90, 92, 93, 94, 96, 97, 98, 107, 108, 109, 113, 114, 115, 116, 117, 118, 126, 127, 129, 137, 139, 140, 144, 163, 167, 172, 191, 210, 212, 231, 235, 237, 238, 239, 241, 255, 256, 259
physiology, 191, 257
PI3K, ix, xi, 86, 89, 91, 92, 95, 98, 99, 114, 163, 164, 165, 169, 189, 190, 191, 192, 193, 194, 195, 214, 215, 218, 224, 225, 255
PI3K/AKT, xi, 189
pilot study, 52
placebo, viii, 25, 26, 30, 31, 34, 36, 37, 41, 197, 225
plaque, 33, 40
plasma membrane, 74, 78, 79, 94, 111, 112, 114, 126
plasmid, xii, 5, 193, 200, 253, 256, 257
platelets, 247
ploidy, 207, 220
PM, 59, 61, 62, 66, 226
pneumonia, 96, 100
point mutation, 245
polarity, ix, 92, 105, 108, 109, 110, 111, 114, 115, 119, 124, 125, 127, 128, 163
polarization, 91, 106, 109, 110, 111, 112, 114, 119, 123, 124, 126, 128
polycomb repressive complex, x, 149
polymerase, 5, 24, 117, 130, 146, 202, 215, 248, 250
polymerase chain reaction, 202, 215, 250
polymerization, 92, 93, 113, 126, 164, 165, 166, 168, 171
polymorphism, 22, 202, 215
polymorphisms, 24, 225
polyploid, 167, 171
polyploidy, 128
polyps, 106, 120
polyunsaturated fat, 28
polyunsaturated fatty acids, 28
pools, 113
population, 244, 248
pRB, 248
precancer, xii, 243, 245
precursor cells, 244
prevention, iv, 38, 44, 183
primary cells, 246
primary tumor, 51, 207, 222, 226
priming, 115
probands, 44
producers, 3
production, 247
progenitor cells, ix, 71, 81, 223, 226
prognosis, 31, 38, 52, 81, 154, 159, 184, 191, 194, 195, 197, 200, 205, 207, 218, 219, 221, 223, 260
programming, 82
proliferation, x, 28, 31, 33, 37, 49, 75, 76, 77, 78, 79, 81, 86, 90, 91, 93, 106, 110, 116, 117, 119, 129, 142, 149, 152, 155, 158, 159, 171, 176, 177, 179, 182, 185, 186, 192, 193, 195, 197, 200, 205, 208, 217, 221, 244, 249, 255, 256, 259
promote, 244
promoter, viii, x, 43, 44, 45, 46, 47, 48, 49, 50, 52, 53, 55, 56, 57, 80, 81, 94, 97, 103, 106, 117, 150, 151, 152, 153, 156, 158, 159, 182, 193, 201, 233, 234, 235, 236, 240, 249, 254, 261
propagation, 144
prophase, 140
prophylactic, 44
prostaglandin, 247
prostaglandins, 28, 195, 218
prostate, 248, 249
prostate cancer, x, 39, 83, 100, 133, 134, 160, 179, 186, 191, 195, 214, 215, 216, 217, 218, 219, 220, 221, 222, 223, 224, 225, 226, 227, 228, 248, 249
prostate carcinoma, 217, 219, 220, 221, 223, 224, 225, 227
prostate specific antigen, 195, 215
prostatectomy, 194, 215, 218, 225, 226
prostrate cancer, ix, 89, 93
proteases, 93
protective mechanisms, 231
protein, xii, 245, 246, 250, 251, 253, 254, 255, 256, 257, 259, 260, 261, 262
protein family, 163
protein kinase C, 103, 110, 231, 240
protein kinases, 241
protein synthesis, xii, 253, 255
proteolysis, 260
proteomics, 52
proto-oncogene, 245
PTEN, v, ix, 89, 90, 91, 92, 93, 94, 95, 96, 97, 98, 99, 100, 101, 102, 103, 181, 191, 192, 193, 194, 195, 214, 215, 216, 217, 218, 219, 220, 222, 223, 224, 225, 226
ptosis, 163
public health, 183
pulmonary edema, 96
PUMA, 239
purification, 5
purines, 26
pyridoxine, vii, 25, 27, 30

Q

Quantitative Multiplex Methylation-Specific PCR, viii, 44, 50, 60, 63
quantum dot, 221
quinones, 247

R

Rab, v, viii, 71, 72, 73, 74, 75, 76, 77, 78, 79, 80, 81, 82, 83, 84, 85, 86, 87
race, 32, 38
radiation, xi, 27, 34, 37, 94, 135, 145, 189, 190, 192, 193, 194, 195, 196, 197, 198, 200, 201, 202, 203, 204, 205, 206, 207, 208, 209, 210, 211, 212, 213, 214, 215, 217, 218, 219, 221, 222, 223, 224, 225, 226, 227, 228, 244, 250
Radiation, xi, 41, 58, 189, 196, 215, 219, 220, 221, 224, 226
radiation damage, 222
radiation therapy, 190, 193, 197, 202, 207, 209, 211, 215, 217, 218, 219, 221, 222, 223, 224, 225, 227, 228, 244
radioactive isotopes, 190
radioresistance, xi, 189, 190, 191, 192, 196, 197, 200, 203, 208, 211, 212, 213, 214, 216, 221, 225, 226, 227
radiosensitization, 190, 191, 192, 193, 196, 200, 203, 205, 210, 214, 215, 217, 221, 223
radiotherapy, xi, 52, 189, 190, 193, 194, 195, 196, 198, 199, 200, 201, 202, 203, 205, 206, 207, 208, 210, 212, 214, 215, 216, 217, 218, 219, 220, 221, 222, 224, 225, 226, 227
rapamycin, 255
RARB, viii, 44, 49, 50, 51, 53, 54, 55, 56, 57
RAS, 245, 248, 262
RASSF1, viii, 44, 49, 50, 51, 53, 54, 55, 56, 57
rat, 254
RB1, ix, 89
reactions, 4, 27, 143, 244
reactive nitrogen, 244
reactive oxygen, 91, 95, 135, 210, 244, 248, 251
reactive oxygen species, 244, 248, 251
reactivity, 15, 19, 202
reagents, 38
reality, 163, 222
receptors, 75, 76, 77, 80, 82, 184, 190, 230, 245, 256
recognition, 48, 91, 107, 204
recombination, 5, 6, 7, 48, 139, 140, 145, 146, 245, 247, 248, 249, 250
recommendations, iv, 22, 99
recruiting, 87, 92, 143, 144, 158, 231
recurrence, xi, 51, 189, 190, 194, 199, 200, 207, 210, 214, 216, 223
recycling, 74, 78, 79, 80, 81, 82, 84
redistribution, 116
reduction, 244
regenerate, 36
regeneration, 41, 42, 128
regression, 158, 257
regulation, xii, 249, 253, 256, 259, 260
reintroduction, 179
relationship, 249
relaxation, 139
relevance, 115, 216, 220
remission, viii, 25, 32, 33, 34
remodelling, 47, 146, 147
renaissance, 124
renal cell carcinoma, x, 161, 162, 169
repair, ix, x, 12, 16, 21, 48, 49, 105, 108, 109, 117, 118, 130, 133, 135, 136, 138, 139, 140, 141, 143, 144, 145, 146, 147, 152, 158, 163, 200, 208, 210, 211, 212, 213, 225, 230, 231, 245, 247, 249, 250
replacement, vii, 25, 26, 27, 36
replication, ix, xii, 26, 32, 48, 105, 108, 109, 117, 130, 135, 141, 143, 144, 176, 230, 243, 244, 245, 249
repression, x, 46, 150, 151, 152, 155, 156, 157, 159, 160, 177, 179, 234, 240
repressor, 49, 117, 208, 232
reproduction, 140
resection, 51, 139
residues, 15, 93, 97, 110, 113, 114, 117, 118, 151, 152, 154, 231, 232, 238
resistance, viii, 25, 32, 33, 39, 40, 41, 103, 137, 191, 192, 193, 197, 200, 201, 202, 208, 210, 214, 215, 218, 221, 222, 226, 240, 247
resolution, 73, 96, 97, 134, 144, 156, 212, 224
respiration, 244
responsiveness, xi, 189, 190, 198
restriction enzyme, 48
resveratrol, viii, 25, 33, 183, 185, 187
retardation, 83
reticulum, 73
retinoblastoma, ix, 34, 35, 41, 89, 101, 131, 152, 158, 182, 203, 217, 225, 245
retinoic acid, 261
retinol, 111, 125
reverse transcriptase, ix, 133
rheumatoid arthritis, 98
ribose, 26, 27, 146
ribosomal RNA, 21
risk assessment, viii, 43
risk factors, 44, 57

RNA, 5, 21, 26, 32, 47, 101, 108, 115, 134, 184, 186, 195, 213, 215, 235, 254, 256, 262
ROS, 243, 244, 246, 247
Royal Society, 40

S

S6K, xii, 253
SAHA, x, 150, 153, 154, 155, 156, 159
saliva, 12, 20, 21, 23
Salmonella, 247
SCGB3A1, viii, 44, 49, 50, 51, 53, 54, 55, 56, 57
schema, 230
SCP, 202
screening, viii, 20, 43, 44, 45, 52, 55, 57, 58, 157
seborrheic dermatitis, 27
segregation, 115, 116, 128
selectivity, 153, 236
selenium, vii, 25, 29, 32, 38
self-renewal, 244
seminal vesicle, 195
senescence, 12, 35, 49, 83, 130, 136, 141, 142, 143, 147, 153, 160, 201, 221
sensing, 92, 99, 100
sensitivity, 23, 44, 50, 56, 81, 97, 118, 130, 131, 135, 137, 155, 195, 196, 201, 205, 213, 218
sensitization, 205, 215
sensors, xi, 229
sepsis, 102
sequencing, 4, 5, 19, 48, 134, 202, 228
serine, 2, 12, 101, 121, 127, 135, 164, 191, 220, 231, 235
serum, 4, 29, 31, 91, 197, 198, 211, 225
shape, 36, 93, 114
shelter, 141, 142, 143
shock, 94
shrinkage, 94
siblings, xii, 254, 257
side effects, vii, 25, 26, 30, 31, 52
signal transduction, xii, 87, 98, 106, 123, 190, 244, 245, 253
signaling, 255, 256, 257, 262
signaling pathway, ix, xi, 71, 77, 80, 84, 97, 98, 99, 103, 143, 162, 163, 164, 167, 183, 189, 190, 191, 193, 204, 220, 225, 231, 255, 256, 258
signaling pathways, 256
signalling, 49, 82, 84, 98, 102, 145, 220, 225, 240
signals, 28, 32, 56, 72, 96, 98, 154, 163, 176, 230, 232, 238, 254
Sinai, 39
Singapore, 71
siRNA, x, 137, 150, 195, 215
sites, 245
skin, xii, 2, 82, 91, 106, 240, 253, 254, 257, 258, 261
small intestine, 119, 121
smokers, 250
smoking, 22, 23, 246, 250
smooth muscle, 33
smooth muscle cells, 33
SOD, 244
sodium, 48
solid tumors, 73, 209, 245
somatic cell, 154
soybeans, 28
species, xii, 3, 12, 91, 95, 135, 179, 210, 243, 244, 247, 248, 251, 254
spindle, 108, 111, 113, 114, 115, 116, 117, 126, 128, 129, 172
squamous cell, 17, 73, 74, 169, 185, 223, 226, 249
squamous cell carcinoma, 17, 73, 74, 169, 185, 223, 226, 249
stability, 245, 249
stabilization, 108, 109, 111, 113, 141, 143, 204, 231
stages, xii, 243, 245, 246, 261
starch, 27
stasis, 187
statistics, 161, 169, 220
stem cells, xi, xii, 18, 35, 36, 41, 86, 109, 111, 121, 189, 190, 209, 210, 212, 213, 215, 216, 217, 219, 220, 221, 222, 227, 243, 244, 247, 248, 251
stimulus, 135, 198
stratification, 206, 214, 221
stress, xii, 243, 244, 245, 247, 248, 249
stretching, 115, 128
subgroups, 202, 211, 218
substitutes, 28
substitution, 9, 10, 12, 14
substitutions, 7, 15
substrates, 90, 131, 135, 152
subtraction, 162
suicide, 97
Sun, 21, 22, 38, 90, 94, 97, 100, 103, 131, 158, 183, 185, 186, 227, 260, 262
superoxide, 244
supply, 244
suppression, ix, xi, 35, 49, 81, 98, 103, 105, 107, 121, 124, 134, 143, 145, 147, 167, 168, 169, 175, 178, 179, 181, 206, 209, 225, 232, 233, 235, 239, 240, 247, 256
suppressor, xii, 243, 245, 259, 260, 261, 262
surveillance, 44, 136, 163, 245, 246
survival rate, 96, 195
survivors, 41
susceptibility, 23, 135, 136, 183, 186, 195, 233
suture, 84
sweat, 257

syndrome, 29, 33, 38, 73, 80, 82, 84, 85, 87, 91, 100, 101, 102, 103, 106, 115, 120, 136, 247
synergistic effect, 156, 194
synthesis, xii, 5, 15, 17, 22, 23, 26, 27, 31, 32, 38, 93, 109, 130, 131, 137, 233, 244, 245, 253, 255, 261
systems, 244

T

T cell, 102, 135, 254, 256, 259
T cells, 254, 259
T lymphocytes, 22
tamoxifen, 52, 53
targets, xii, 243, 245, 248, 254, 262
technical assistance, 19
telangiectasia, 135
telomere, ix, 35, 133, 141, 142, 143, 144, 147
telomere shortening, 35
temperature, 201
terminal patients, viii, 25, 26, 29, 32, 33, 34
testicular cancer, 26
testing, 32, 156
texture, 30
TF, 46, 178, 179, 218, 219, 222
TGA, 5, 6
TGF, 97, 99, 224, 256, 258
therapeutic agents, 119
therapeutic intervention, 191, 226
therapeutic targets, viii, 43, 81, 97
therapeutics, x, 133, 186, 235
therapy, xi, 25, 26, 27, 30, 33, 34, 36, 37, 52, 156, 157, 158, 160, 161, 175, 181, 182, 183, 185, 186, 189, 190, 193, 195, 197, 201, 202, 203, 204, 207, 208, 209, 210, 211, 214, 215, 216, 217, 218, 219, 221, 222, 223, 224, 225, 227, 228, 236, 244, 245, 248
thiamin, vii, 25, 26, 27, 29, 30
thiamin deficiency, 27
threonine, 28, 101, 191, 220, 231
thromboxanes, 28, 29
thymus, 91
thyroid, 74, 75, 83, 91, 100, 106
thyroid cancer, 100
tissue, vii, ix, x, 3, 25, 26, 27, 28, 35, 36, 40, 45, 48, 49, 50, 51, 52, 55, 56, 57, 73, 74, 75, 77, 79, 96, 101, 105, 106, 111, 119, 123, 125, 135, 149, 153, 154, 163, 176, 179, 194, 198, 199, 201, 202, 204, 206, 207, 211
tissue homeostasis, ix, 105, 106, 119
TNF, 94, 96
tobacco, vii, 1, 3, 12, 17, 19, 21, 23, 36, 250
tobacco smoke, 17
toluene, 251
toxic, xii, 243, 244
toxicity, 29, 31, 32, 193, 197, 246, 247
toxicology, 251
Toyota, 59, 68
TP53, v, vii, 1, 2, 4, 5, 6, 7, 8, 9, 11, 12, 13, 14, 15, 16, 17, 18, 19, 21, 22, 23, 49, 218, 225, 240, 245
TPA, xii, 233, 253, 254, 257
trace elements, 29
tracks, 26
trade-off, 41
training, 39
transcription, viii, x, 43, 46, 47, 49, 51, 81, 94, 96, 97, 107, 111, 116, 123, 129, 131, 135, 141, 144, 147, 149, 150, 151, 153, 155, 157, 158, 173, 176, 178, 179, 180, 181, 203, 204, 230, 231, 232, 233, 234, 235, 237, 240, 241, 245, 254, 256, 259, 262
transcription factor, 245, 254
transcription factors, 46, 81, 94, 107, 176, 178, 181, 245
transcriptional, 249, 259
transcripts, 186
transduction, xii, 87, 98, 106, 123, 135, 190, 236, 244, 245, 253, 261
transfection, xii, 194, 201, 253, 256, 257
transformation, xii, 5, 8, 49, 77, 79, 83, 122, 160, 165, 170, 178, 253, 254, 260, 261, 262
transforming growth factor, 100, 254, 260, 262
transgene, 109, 201, 217, 225
transgenic, xii, 253, 256, 257
transgenic mice, xii, 253, 256, 257
transitional cell carcinoma, 250
translation, xii, 97, 178, 253, 254, 255, 259, 260, 261, 262
translational, 261
translocation, 91, 107, 117, 163, 166, 167, 169, 235, 240, 245
translocations, 244, 246
transmembrane glycoprotein, 111
transmission, 106, 143
transplantation, 211, 247
transport, xi, 72, 73, 86, 108, 110, 113, 115, 129, 161, 166, 168, 171
transportation, 166
treatment methods, 203, 207, 214
trial, 28, 38, 39, 40, 186, 195, 196, 197, 199, 202, 205, 206, 209, 219, 220, 224
trichostatin A, 156
triggers, 32, 150, 235, 237, 251
trimolecular complex, 164
tryptophan, 28, 29
tumor cells, xii, 26, 31, 32, 33, 37, 39, 75, 78, 93, 106, 112, 119, 129, 162, 168, 170, 171, 196, 211, 253, 256, 259

tumor development, viii, ix, 43, 45, 105, 106, 111, 116, 185
tumor growth, vii, 25, 30, 32, 78, 162, 172, 184, 190, 193, 195, 196, 201, 204, 226, 227, 236
tumor invasion, 76, 120
tumor metastasis, 187
tumor necrosis factor, 38
tumor progression, 78, 80, 106, 120, 134, 152, 178, 191, 218, 219
tumor resistance, viii, 25, 193
tumorigenesis, viii, ix, x, 21, 43, 71, 73, 76, 77, 78, 80, 81, 105, 107, 109, 115, 119, 121, 122, 124, 128, 131, 133, 134, 135, 140, 141, 142, 143, 150, 152, 156, 168, 176, 203, 232, 260
tumors, vii, ix, xii, 20, 23, 25, 26, 27, 28, 29, 30, 31, 32, 33, 34, 36, 39, 50, 51, 55, 73, 76, 77, 78, 81, 89, 106, 109, 118, 129, 134, 135, 140, 150, 152, 158, 178, 179, 182, 183, 185, 190, 198, 200, 201, 202, 205, 206, 208, 209, 210, 211, 218, 221, 222, 223, 224, 230, 243, 244, 245, 246, 250, 257
turnover, 110, 115, 129, 164
tyrosine, ix, 29, 49, 76, 82, 89, 90, 98, 100, 195, 235, 245, 246

U

ubiquitin, xii, 253, 255
ubiquitin-proteasome system, xii, 125, 253, 255
ultraviolet, 257, 260
ultraviolet B, 257, 260
underlying mechanisms, 56, 81, 134
undernutrition, 33, 36
undifferentiated cells, 257
urinary bladder, 246, 250
urine, 28
urokinase, 178
UV, 2, 94, 135, 233, 235
UV irradiation, 2, 235
UV radiation, 94
UVB irradiation, xii, 253, 259

V

vacuum, viii, 43, 45, 52, 53
Valencia, 85
valine, 28
vascular endothelial growth factor (VEGF), 193
vector, 5, 193, 214
VEGF expression, 209
velocity, 197
venules, 95
vesicle, 73, 74, 86, 87
vesicular membrane traffic, viii, 71
vessels, 209
video, 40
viruses, 2, 16, 34, 111
visible, 245
visualization, viii, 25
vitamin B1, vii, 25, 27, 29, 30, 33, 40
vitamin B12, vii, 25, 27, 29, 30, 33, 40
vitamin B6, 33, 40
vitamin D, vii, 25, 32
vitamins, 26, 27, 28, 29, 31, 32

W

Wales, 189, 214western blot, 196, 213
Western countries, xi, 189
wild type, ix, 6, 78, 89, 96, 247
withdrawal, 209
Wnt signaling, ix, 48, 49, 80, 105, 107, 115, 118, 121, 167, 258

X

xenografts, 197, 204, 211, 215
X-irradiation, 240
xylenes, 251

Y

yeast, 5, 8, 19, 21, 22, 42, 110, 113, 126, 127, 152, 163

Z

zinc, 93, 180